Stretch Marks

Selected articles from The Mother magazine
2002 ~ 2009

Edited by
Veronika Sophia Robinson
and
Paul Robinson

Stretch Marks
Selected articles from The Mother magazine 2002 ~ 2009
Edited by Veronika Sophia Robinson and Paul Robinson
Cover illustration by Andri Thwaites
ISBN 978-0-9560344-3-4

Published by Starflower Press
www.starflowerpress.com
www.themothermagazine.co.uk

British Library Cataloguing in Publication Data.
A catalogue record for this book is available from the British Library.

Other books by Veronika Robinson, published by Starflower Press:
The Drinks Are On Me: everything your mother never told you about breastfeeding
The Birthkeepers: reclaiming an ancient tradition
Life without School: the quiet revolution (co-authored by Paul Robinson, Bethany A. Robinson, Eliza Serena Robinson)

Thank you to Bethany and Eliza Robinson, and Andri Thwaites, for various illustrations throughout Stretch Marks, and to the families who've shared their photos in The Mother magazine.

Thank you to Eliza for dreaming up the title of this book.

Dedication

*For all the families who've subscribed
to The Mother magazine since 2002,
as well as the writers, artists and photographers
who contributed their magic!*

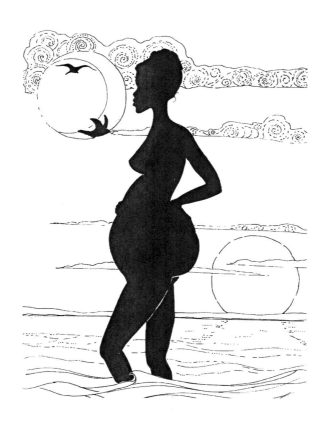

Contents

23 Fertility Awareness

29 Conscious Conception

51 Pregnancy

73 Birth

155 Breastfeeding

229 Health, well-being & natural immunity

259 Holistic Living

323 Sexuality

355 Fathers

373 Education and Learning

Introduction
by Veronika Robinson

The Mother magazine was conceived in Autumn, 2001, and the first issue birthed in February, 2002. This grassroots publication was born in my lounge room, by the fireside, and in amongst the laughter of our two young daughters as they played, did fine artwork and breastfed on cue.

It hasn't been easy publishing niche material and trying to be commercially viable. However, I've been blessed by so much support ~ financial and emotional ~ from families across the globe, and countless unseen angels. If the love we received through our mailbag could be measured in dollars and pounds, we'd be millionaires over and over again.

May you be inspired by the articles we've selected. Indeed, this is a selection, rather than a 'best of The Mother'. It had been my original plan to publish such a book, but that task proved impossible. To do so would have meant a book the size of the Oxford Dictionary. Rereading articles from back issues has been such a pleasure, and has inspired us as we've been reminded over and over again what a unique publication we're gifting to the world. Thank you to all the writers who've taken the time, energy and passion to offer us their work.

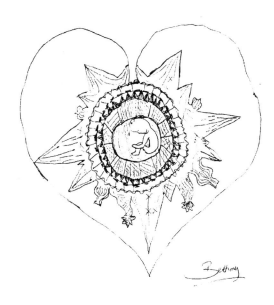

The Mother magazine's natural parenting glossary

It's understood that human babies are born about nine months 'early', which means they need the first nine months of life 'in-arms' to provide an optimal external gestation. The in-utero needs of warmth, movement, food and connection are now met by being carried all day, slept with at night, breastfed on cue (not demand), and by the mother living her life. Constant caregiving by the mother should ensure that all needs of the baby are met almost instantly. The fields of science, anthropology and medicine recognise that this traditional way of nurturing babies is best for short and long-term physical, emotional and psychological health and well-being. This is commonly known as attachment parenting, but is more suitably described as intact parenting.

Vaginal Birth After Caesarean (VBAC)
There was a time when women who underwent a caesarean were told 'Once a caesarean, always a caesarean'. This is completely false. Every birth is different, and no woman should ever believe that because of her past she can not birth vaginally. If you've experienced a caesarean, surround yourself with positive birth stories from VBAC women.

Natural Breech Birth
A small number of babies (about 3 ~ 4%) present for birth with their bottom down: this is called breech. Although caesarean is routinely accepted as 'normal' for such babies these days, there's no valid medical reason for a woman not to have a natural breech birth. Although the birth isn't as straightforward as a head-first baby, it isn't more difficult. Sadly, many midwives haven't carried on the age-old tradition of natural breech delivery, so people are losing their skills. Being on hands and knees is the best birthing position for a mother delivering a breech baby. There are 'treatments' to change the baby's position before birth, but it's important to remember that babies who present as breech do so because either they or their mother has a 'fear' of being head-first, and breech is a *symptom*, not a cause.

Freebirth/Unassisted Birth

The female body is designed to give birth quickly and easily, within about 20 minutes. We've been doing so for thousands of generations. The knowledge and instincts of our ancestresses have been eroded by a medical system which insists women need help to give birth. The interference of the medical establishment impedes a woman's mammalian ability to birth vaginally, with ease and pleasure. Women who choose to forgo medical supervision and interference are known as freebirthers, or unassisted birthers.

Lotus-birth

Lotus-birth is an honouring of the baby's first 'grandmother' ~ the placenta. This organ grew from the same cell as the baby, and supported it throughout pregnancy. By not cutting the cord at birth, the baby is able to separate from the placenta in a natural way. Modern births include the instant cutting of the cord, which is traumatic for a baby. Parents who choose Lotus-birth wrap the placenta in a nappy, and keep it tucked up beside the baby for a few days, until the cord dries and eventually snaps. Care of the placenta is easy: after the initial draining in a colander (and washing off of clots), it's sprinkled with salt, and lavender oil, on a daily basis. Lotus-birthed babies are believed to be more placid and content than they would otherwise have been.

Babymoon

Traditional cultures around the world which hold the mother and baby bond as sacred, engage in a Babymoon ~ a period of 40 days after the birth where the mother is nurtured, loved and protected in a circle of support from her community. Modern women are beginning to recognise the importance of this sacred space to be with their child away from the harshness of 21st century life.

Elimination Communication

Throughout human history, until very recently, mothers were in tune with their babies' elimination needs, and knew when they needed to urinate or defaecate, in just the same way as they'd know their own needs. Many modern mothers are discovering the joy of tuning-in to their babies this way, and right from birth the mother understands her baby's elimination instincts, and listens to the cues and patterns her baby communicates to her.

The Family Bed

Humans are the only mammals which separate from their young during sleep. At The Mother magazine we promote sleeping with our children. Counter to media scare tactics about Sudden Infant Death Syndrome and sharing sleep, this is a natural way of parenting which has spanned human evolution across the globe. Babies and children who sleep with their parents engage in important bonding, which provides warmth, security, protection, and the ability to breastfeed on-cue.

Full-term Breastfeeding

Although the World Health Organisation recommends breastfeeding exclusively for a <u>minimum</u> of six months, two thirds of British women have weaned by the time their baby is two weeks of age. All children are biologically encoded to expect to breastfeed (not exclusively) up to about seven years of age ~ the universal time of losing the 'milk teeth'. Commonly called extended breastfeeding, this misuse of language implies that the child is engaging in something beyond the 'right time', when in fact, weaning before the child is ready should be viewed as 'premature weaning'. Full-term breastfed children reach their optimal IQ, receive security and warmth, and social bonding. Studies show that such children are at far less risk of viral infections, childhood cancer, diabetes, and diseases of the heart.

Natural Immunity

The human body has developed an immune system based on the entire history of human evolution. A natural parent uses the ingredients of love, kindness, fresh water and air, adequate sleep, nutrient-rich fresh fruits and vegetables, blue-green algae, seeds and nuts to build up their child's immune system, and recognises that vaccination does not build an immune system.

Foreword

written by Veronika Sophia Robinson
(Editorial, from issue 37 of The Mother magazine)

My daughter, Eliza, and I were lazing in my bed one chilly and misty Autumn morning, when she apologised for causing the stretch marks on my belly.

"But I LOVE those stretch marks!" I protested, defensively and protectively. "They're a map of where I've been, and how I've grown." Each and every silvery-lilac ribbon corrugating my spongey belly is a picture-postcard of the journey in my mothering story: singing the hymns of the six babies conceived in the deep, dark depths of my womb ~ four rejected by my body, but not my heart ~ and two nurtured through to birth.

For a large part of my parenting, I've edited The Mother magazine. Stretch marks are par for the course when leading a niche, radical parenting publication through the cultural clouds of discrimination, prejudice, disempowerment and ignorance.

The Mother consistently asks parents-to-be authentic ~ to question our choices, not just one or two, like: is vaccination a way to build immunity, or does it cause and spread diseases, and destroy the ecology of the developing immune system?

Should boys play with violent toys, or does our spiritual evolution as a species ordain that we model peace, and show them (and their fathers) how to lay down their weapons of destruction? After all, just who are they imitating in their play, and why?

Is institutional learning best for today's children, or are alternative, human-scale schools more suited to their unfolding of mind, body and soul? What value do home education and unschooling have in the life of the modern family?

The Mother asks us to question everything, every day: formula drink for babies, is it a life-saving product or counterfeit poison? How long should a mother breastfeed? What about child-led weaning? We aren't scared to publish information showing that the peace, passion and purpose of a culture rests firmly on the breastfeeding foundations it has lain down for its children (minimum 2.5 years); or that introducing solids at six months is too early for the digestive system, short-circuits the absorption of iron, and the ability to build stores for life. This doesn't make us popular, but it does make our work authentic, and, ironically, given how long humanity has breastfed: pioneering.

Are plastic nappies ever acceptable when they not only use finite resources, but take hundreds of years to decompose? What about fabric nappies? Should they be mandatory for the sake of babies' bottoms and the ecology of Earth? The Mother wouldn't be a primal parenting magazine if it didn't encourage us to step outside the nappy bucket and ask "why not listen to the elimination needs of your baby, and do without nappies altogether?"

We also ask the perennial controversial questions like: is it ethical or peaceful to farm sentient creatures for human consumption, or should we adopt a cruelty-free lifestyle, and abstain? And if, as stated in a UN report, the single most effective act that any individual can do to lessen the effects of global warming is to become vegetarian, why are there still slaughterhouses on this planet? We ask about the ethics of using the by-products of creatures, as well as looking at the health of the human body, and issues such as eating foods in their natural state.

The Mother magazine is here to nudge us, a little bit more, every day. It's fair to say that very few people like to be nudged along. I understand that. It's far more peaceful to stay in our comfort zones. "Ignorance is bliss" is the chant of our culture, and shame on she who dares to rock the boat.

As the voices behind this publication, we're here to help families see another picture ~ that of intuition, and connection to our children ~ and ideally, to make informed choices for optimal parenting.

Every choice, decision, thought and action has an impact, not just on your family, but on the whole world. Such choices can be overwhelming, intimidating, and oh so stretching. We may not feel stretch marks as they're forming, but one thing's for sure: once we've stretched, there's no going back.

The growth which creates the stretch marks of a pioneering publication, like The Mother, is hard work, and that's without even factoring in the treacherous economic waters we're sailing in right now. Writing for the minority in our culture, with a publication that is definitely "not bubblegum for the brain", as one reader so succinctly described it, takes courage. In September, 2009, my courage and faith abandoned me as I sat despondent in the mire of ever-increasing lapsed subscriptions from this past year; and I decided to bring The Mother back into harbour, never to sail again.

I pulled my socks up, and with heavy heart shared this fait accompli with our family of subscribers who are on the e-group community. They wouldn't let me close the doors. They demanded The Mother stay at sea, and together they networked night and day to bring more readers on board. They showed me how many more sunrises we'd witness on the horizon each morning. And even if the weather was foul, they'd be there. Why? Because they had stretch marks, too! They'd grown enormously, and The Mother had been part of that growth ~ their spiritual placenta. "We'll help you", they cheered, praying, but also moving their feet by throwing out necessary lifeboats.

I don't believe there's a marketing company in the world that could promote this magazine with the pride, passion, soul and dedication that these families have shown.

I've learnt something that I've always known theoretically. The Mother network is our family. For most people, their family is held within the larger family of culture, and they take on all the beliefs associated with that. For those of us who hold The Mother as our culture ~ a small but not insignificant subculture within the counter-intuitive culture around us ~ we realise how precious and powerful our support of one another is, and why everyone in the family must nurture the other. It's too easy to feel alone and in exile when we watch mainstream parenting and live our lives from the fringes. For those who find their homeland in The Mother, we remind you of the stunning gifts you're giving to our culture by parenting with consciousness. You may not know other readers of The Mother, but I can assure you that this silent and invisible family that they form, is here, energetically, holding the space for your family's journey.

My family and I are a small but passionate and dedicated team at the hub of The Mother; our writers, photographers and artists are the spokes which spread the messages, and YOU, our precious reader, are the wheel which carries this magazine far and wide. You're our marketing department! Share your Mother today. Share what inspires you, makes you laugh, makes you cringe, makes you mad. Share, and watch the world change.

At this moment, The Mother is stronger than ever, but we don't wish to rest on our laurels, and so we ask that each reader considers how they can share their magazine.

We've been contacting our lapsed subscribers to hear why they've not renewed their subscriptions. As I suspected, in many cases they simply forgot, due to the business and busyness of mothering. This, I understand. I often put down something akin to a sub renewal/lapsed subscription form to deal with when I'm not making dinner, hanging out washing, hugging a child or taking a phone call. The piece of paper ends up under a child's drawing, other paperwork and bills, and somehow just disappears into the netherworld of paper, paper, paper. In some cases, though, I heard stories that put The Mother magazine's future back into harsh perspective ~ stories which stopped me in my tracks and lashed stinging tears across my eyes. Stories of tragedy and trauma...a sober reminder of life, and of other people's stretch marks.

I laugh now, to think of how often I rubbed coconut oil into my pregnant belly to ensure I wouldn't get stretch marks! My vanity and immaturity had no idea that at another time in my life I'd celebrate every lilac ribbon as if gaily dancing around a maypole; that one day I'd know the secret and beauty of life is held in growth. Clarissa Pinkola Estes, storyteller, says that a flower is blooming whether it's half, three quarters or in full bloom.

I pray that you, too, can see the beauty of your stretch marks.

Selected editorials

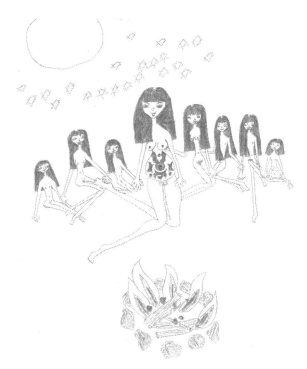

Tribal systers at the camp fire, by Bethany A. Robinson

ISSUE 1 ~ Spring, 2002

It's early February. Torrential rain lashes the window pane. The wind howls like a woman whose baby has been ripped from her very heart. I feel the pain of women whose babies have been ripped from them.

From the window, I can see for miles. I see our back garden, where last Summer's vegetable and herb patches lie barren. The bare plum trees sway in the wind like nurturing mothers who rock their babes. I'm a mother who sways when I wear my baby. Beyond this, the grassy fields stretch down to the creek. Then, on the other side the bosom-like hills rise up to become The Pennines. And like those swollen hills, my breasts, too, have been swollen...and filled with bounteous milk, they've risen to feed tiny mouths.

Long, stretched-out views nurture me. They always have. I hate being boxed in and not seeing my options and choices. It seems to me very symbolic of everything The Mother magazine represents: to stretch our vision, beliefs and world view beyond our current horizon; to know there's always more to learn. Always other options. Other choices. We don't have to be victims. We must not be content with mediocrity in our mothering. For this reason alone, I know that some readers will find the contents challenging. I know. I know! The Mother is here to challenge *all* of us; to remove us from the very inertia that holds humanity back from seeing its potential. For most of our readers, The Mother will be a breath of fresh air in a world filled with parenting magazines that tantalise readers with the wonders of modern-day obstetric drugs, and give 50 ways to make your baby independent before he's taken his first breath! We won't ever dilute our articles so that we can appeal to a mainstream readership. We'll never publish articles on why you should <u>abandon</u> your kids to "quality" day care. Kids need mothers! They need loving mothers. Strong mothers. Mothers who will let them know, by word and action, that nothing in the world is more important than being with them day and night. There's no substitute for a loving, full-time mother. The Mother magazine is here to speak for the children.

We don't accept adverts for disposable nappies, because we know it takes at least 500 years for each one to decompose. Never will we take adverts for plastic toys, when the best toys for our children are both ecologically sound and aesthetically pleasing. And we do want the best for our children.

We won't publish articles on why you should vaccinate when we know that vaccination doesn't support the immune system or prevent diseases. However, our purpose isn't to judge others. We trust that people will take responsibility for their own choices and the subsequent results.

I've come to realise that The Mother is not my magazine, but belongs to all of us.

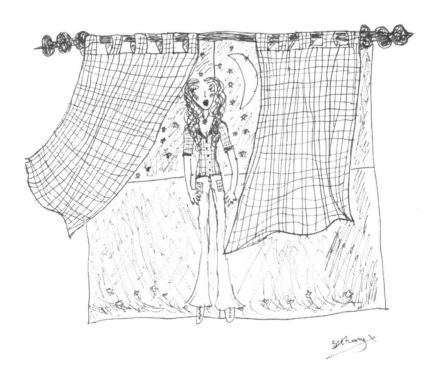

The Old Pepperina Tree
Issue 24 ~ Sept/Oct 2007

During the Summer, my daughter Eliza wanted to show me how good a climber she'd become, so I watched her go to the top of a cherry tree in our village.

I was struck by how confident and agile she is ~ rather like a monkey, but without the tail! 'When did she learn to climb like that?', I wondered. 'What was I doing that was so important as to miss this particular milestone?'

Most of the children in Britain don't get unsupervised, spontaneous play. My children consider the village to be their back garden, and go playing for hours. That's where they learnt to climb trees after they graduated from the plum tree in our garden.

Although I spent a lot of time up Enid Blyton's Magical Faraway Tree, my own magical tree was the imposing pepperina in our front garden. My childhood surroundings in Queensland, Australia, were a paradise for tree climbers ~ hundreds of acres, including mountains covered in eucalyptus, pines, wattles and pepperinas. There were the occasional wild apricot and lemon tree, too.

Despite being the middle of eight children, I spent the vast majority of my childhood playtime on my own, captivated by my imaginary friends and the world I invented for myself. The pepperina was a sanctuary: a place to escape, daydream, create, write poetry and love letters for undeserving schoolboys, and, last but not least, a place to spy on my siblings!

My bird's-eye view gave me a 360 degree lookout, and afforded me ample camouflage from the outside world. The tree's willow-like leaves disguised me time and time again.

If I was ever in trouble with my parents, which, given my mischievous nature, was rather a regular occurrence, I'd head straight for my other home.

It was, without doubt, one of my favourite places in childhood. I couldn't have claimed it as mine, however, unless I'd taken the risk to climb ~ to move away from the safe and familiar Earth beneath my feet.

I had to risk falling, being hurt, being told I was reckless, scraping my knee, getting covered in sticky sap, breaking an arm, meeting a tree snake or being bitten by a wasp. I don't remember actually ever giving much thought to these possibilities ~ my focus was always on navigating the hard-to-reach bottom branches so I could journey to the very top.

My beloved pepperina tree is a metaphor for my life as a parent. By choosing to climb up and away from the familiar parenting culture of our Western world, I discovered a new view. At the top of the holistic living tree, I found I could birth my baby in water, at home, by candlelight. My mother carried the candle up the tree for me, by birthing her last three children at home, unassisted.

By sharing the tree with my mum, I knew that breastfeeding was the only option for my children. I learned that I could breastfeed my daughters until they'd had their fill ~ which they took advantage of for seven years apiece! Society didn't like this one little bit. They called me sick, selfish, stupid. Ah well, never mind. From my tree-top lookout, I could see things that were impossible to witness from down on the ground. One day more people will be brave enough to climb the tree. And then they'll know...

My daughters didn't get sent off to nursery at three years of age 'like all the other children'. I ignored the voices manically calling to me from the bottom of the tree, and chose to let my girls 'wake up gently' to this world.

George Bernard Shaw said that trying to explain vaccination to a doctor was like discussing vegetarianism with a butcher. So I didn't invite the doctor anywhere near my children. At the top of our tree of life, we nurtured our girls through love, an optimal in-arms gestation, child-led weaning, pure water, slow parenting, plant-based wholefoods, cranial osteopathy, chiropractic care and quantity time.

Life at the top of the tree isn't to be confused with being on a pedestal, or up in an ivory tower. Far from it. Choosing this way of life comes with its own set of challenges. It is, indeed, the road less travelled, or the branches few choose to climb. A perfect life isn't guaranteed. And, it can be very, very lonely.

I doubt I'd have absorbed the enormity of what our culture does to us had I stayed on the ground, or even the bottom branch. There's simply no scope for perspective unless you can see the whole picture.

Climbing up, and away, and literally going out on a limb, is an absolute prerequisite to conscious parenting in this modern world. We may be more technologically advanced than at any time in our known history, but we couldn't be more backward or more blind, as a culture, if we tried! I've found the view from the top at times exciting, exhilarating, sometimes terrifying, and, at other times, downright depressing. At the top of the tree we see how brainwashed people are by the media, health 'care' systems, institutionalised education and government diktat.

The ascent can be challenging, precarious, and, for some, rather scary; but unless you do it, despite everyone at the base of the tree calling you back down, you'll never know how liberating the complete trust in yourself, and your family, can be. The most beautiful part is when you feel confident enough to reach to another, and give guidance along the branches.

I've often felt that parenting has stopped me taking risks, that I'm no longer the girl I used to be ~ the one who'd fly to a new country, on a one way ticket, with less than a tenner in her pocket, just 'knowing' everything would be ok.

My mum's advice throughout life has been "Just jump, the angels will catch you". And you know, I believed her! My mother was the perfect mother bird, guarding her nest at the top of the tree, knowing the right time to push her little chickadees out …"Fly", she'd say.

I often hear her voice in my head, and upon reflection, I realise I'm no less of a risk-taker now than I ever was. My day-to-day choices are seen as risks by modern culture, but to me, well, they're just part of everyday life, like breathing. Stepping away from mainstream thinking is as big a risk as we'll ever take. Personally, I think it's a far greater risk not to step away.

Tree climbing is an interesting experience upon which to draw strength, and belief in one's self. It's perfect that this happens in childhood. It's good and right that my girls have learnt to climb trees without me nearby wondering if they'll fall down!

I don't know if my magic pepperina tree is still standing, but I'd love to think another child spent time there, hearing the Divine Whisperer beckoning "Climb higher, my friend, climb higher"…

The Apron Strings
Issue 28 ~ May/June 2008

It's often said, by those in our culture who believe separation of mother and child should happen as early as possible, that it "can't be good for children to be at home all day tied to their mother's apron strings". Well, as someone who wears those apron strings, I'd like to share a view from the other side.

A couple of months back, I appeared on a US TV chat show, where the topic of discussion was stay-at-home mothers versus working mothers. I pointed out that every mother is a working mother. However, the audience was split. It seemed you could only be one or the other. How odd, I thought, when some of the most successful career women I know are those who are also full-time stay at home mothers. And what about all the mums who are able to take their children to work with them? Why does it have to be one or the other? Why do we have to have a war among the sisterhood? And why, in all these discussions on women's rights, do people fail to address the rights of the child?

The career mums in the studio audience were adamant that a mother would 'lose herself' if she didn't go back to work: something she'd always regret. They also chanted (as if under mass hypnotism) that "children NEED day care". Whoah!

In my twelve years of being a full-time stay at home mother, I couldn't disagree more with the statement that children need day care or that a woman will lose herself by staying at home with her children. I've changed enormously through being a mother. I've changed in ways that would simply have been impossible by being a career woman, no matter how spectacular or dazzling a career. And though I've had hellish days, I know for certain that going out to work wouldn't have made me a better mother or woman. The whole 'quality time' thing is, to my mind, a myth; something used when people wish to justify the adult part of the equation. Anyone can be nice if they're only with their child/ren for a limited time, but is that all we want our children to see of us? A mask? An act that we perform for a couple of hours? A perpetual parental-child courtship? Where's the integrity in that?

My children have seen all sides of me (some not so pleasant!), and yet they still fully embrace and love me. They're under no illusions about who I am as a person. But it works both ways.

Yesterday, my ten year old daughter, Eliza, and I were curled up on the sofa reading Indigo for Girls, a magazine she gets from Australia. Her favourite parts of the magazine are the reader profiles, where Indigo girls answer a series of questions. One such question is "Who inspires you?" I'm often intrigued, too, to see which well-known person's life has had an impact on these young girls' way of thinking.

In the kitchen last night, I said to Eliza that she could do the questionnaire herself, and then asked, as an example, "Who inspires you?" Without batting an eyelid or pausing for breath, she said, "You inspire me Mum because you still love me even when I'm being horrible." The truth is, I probably learnt that from my girls. They're incredibly forgiving of my weaker moments. They always have been, and perhaps it's what has helped me to grow the most: my evolution hastened because they've presented me with forgiveness in action.

Author, Eckhart Tolle, wrote in his book A New Earth ~ Awakening to your life's purpose, that to find out if you're enlightened, try spending a week with your parents! Well, that made me splutter my tea all over myself. OK, I can live with my Mum very easily, but I'd be challenged to spend a week with my Dad (much as I love him), so diametrically opposed are our views on just about every aspect of life.

It had me thinking though, how will our children feel about us when they're adults? Will they comfortably spend a week with us? Will they want to run for the hills?

As the one wearing the apron, I know that my mothering job is far from over; however, I also know that if I were to leave this Earthly life tomorrow, my girls have had such an incredibly secure foundation to their own lives precisely because they've been able to tug at my apron strings, pull on them, dance with them, trip me up with them, and leave their little finger stains upon them. They've been raised to know, without an ounce of doubt, that they're loved as much as is humanly possible. My actions have spoken far louder than my words.

I'm not a perfect mother. Far from it, much to my great disappointment. I have ideals as high as the heavens, and a parenting reality somewhere near mud level! So often I was busy looking for my gum boots (wellingtons) that I failed to notice that deep within the squelchy mud I was trying to avoid, my girls found pleasure in feeling it ooze between their naked toes. They built castles from the mud. I dare say they've tasted the mud, and they've used that mud to furnish the love in our home. The mud has been their growing soil, their nourishment, the fertility upon which their imaginations grew. It's the spring water in which they joyously bathe and drink ~ and all this because I chose to let them hang on to my apron strings.

At the swinging end of the apron strings, my girls have learnt about life, and not been hidden away, as common thought would have it. From the earliest ages, they knew about the menstrual cycle; how babies were created; birthed and fed; what it meant to live on a budget; how herbs are Nature's medicine cabinet; how to grow fruit, vegetables and herbs. They can make a great meal for a raw fooder, or vegan; they can cater for people on wheat-free diets.

The apron strings gave them a first-hand look at life when parents 'fail' and then have to brush off their knees and start again. My girls have witnessed me go through some painful losses and come through the other side. They've celebrated my joys and triumphs. Most importantly, they've witnessed that life is cyclical. They haven't been sheltered: they've been witnesses. They've learnt far more about life and from life, by dancing near my apron strings, than if they'd been separated from me several days a week.

As for losing who I am because of staying at home with my children, I've found the opposite to be true. Being present with kids 24/7 is the quickest way to discover who you are. It's the ultimate personal growth workshop. Children will bring up every last part of you that needs healing. This scares the life out of many people, and they'll use any excuse to remove themselves from their child's orbit.

To suggest a woman reduces her potential for self-expansion and identity because she chooses to stay at home and raise her child with motherly love is to be completely ignorant of what a mother and child need. It also fails to recognise that 'who we are' is never about what we do for a job, and indeed, can't be defined by a label. Our children know this; but most adults don't.

Bonding is in the realms of extrasensory perception. It isn't something which would make a lot of sense on a resumé. And like parenting, it's an unpaid job. What price can you put on being there for your child all day, every day? How do you measure love? How do you define the indefineable? You can't.

The apron strings of mothering are linked to our heart. They tell our stories, fill our children with tender moments, and act as the visible umbilical cord to our destiny link. Mothering my two feisty daughters has revealed the incredible potential in me as a human being. They daily challenge me to be more of who I am. There's no room for shrinking back, hiding away. My girls demand the best from me. I wouldn't have ever traded a single smile or cuddle, grazed knee or two-year-old meltdown from either of them for a day in the 'real world'. And I dare say they'd not have traded a day of apron strings for a motherless day care centre.

What happens in the home, at the end of a mother's apron strings, shapes our world. They say charity begins at home, and so too do joy, fun, laughter, companionship, humanity, compassion, kindness, humour, happiness, peace, satisfaction and love.

I may not have known how to wear the apron of motherhood, however, had I not had a childhood witnessing how beautifully my mother wore hers.

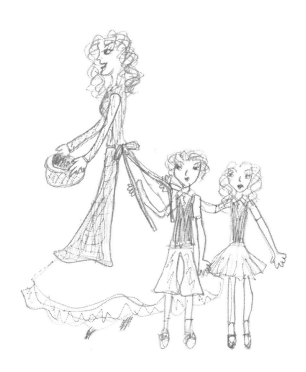

22

Fertility Awareness

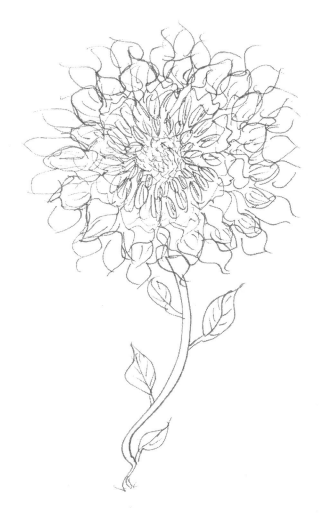

Ovulation Ceremony

This simple ritual involves aligning your cycle to the Moon. At days 14, 15 and 16 of your menstrual cycle, sleep with the light of the Moon shining on you. If the Moon is dark, use candlelight or a low lamp. Do this each month until you're cycling to the Moon.

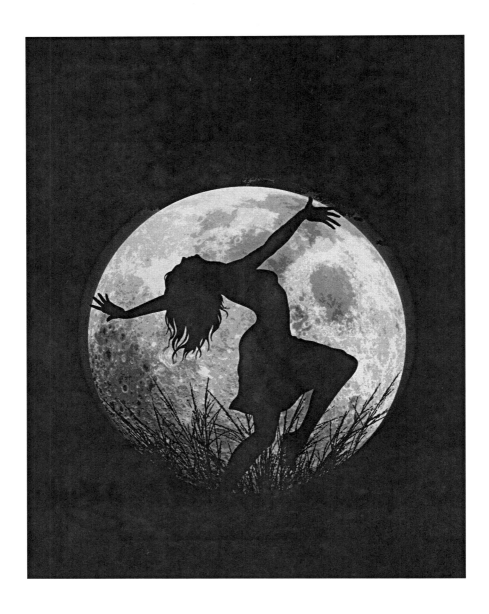

Fertility Awareness: a skill for the twenty-first century
By Liz Pilley

When I tell people we use the Fertility Awareness Method (FAM) for contraception, I see that look which tells me they think we've gone one weirdness too far. The glazed look, as they nod and smile, plainly says "you're mad". However, I have used it for over seven years now, both as a contraceptive method, and in order to conceive, and it has never let me down with either. It's a shame that fertility awareness has either had a bad press, or no press at all, as it's an easy, reliable, non-chemical and reversible way of planning your family. It needs no drugs or prescriptions, and it costs nothing. However, most people confuse it with the 'rhythm method', and tell the old joke: what do you call a couple who use the rhythm method of contraception? Parents!

Actually, the rhythm method and FAM are completely different, although they do share some techniques. The rhythm method relies on predicting a future menstrual cycle by average data from previous cycles. This is, of course, fraught with problems, as all sorts of things can affect the cycle, including stress, travel, insomnia, drugs, and the time of the year. FAM, in contrast, is a scientific method of tracking the course of each cycle as it happens, and learning to identify the signs of approaching ovulation. A pregnancy can only occur if there has been an egg released recently, as an egg only lives for 24 to 48 hours. Sperm can live for longer, but even allowing for that, there's only a fertility window of about six days in each cycle.

FAM isn't just a contraceptive ~ it's a method with which a woman can get to know her own body and its unique hormonal make-up. It gives you the tools to recognise your fertile and non-fertile times, and a set of rules so that you can use these observations to avoid a pregnancy, or to maximise your chances of creating one. You can decide what you do with the knowledge it gives you. If you're using it to avoid a pregnancy, you can choose to abstain from sex during fertile times, or to use a barrier method, such as a condom, at those times. If you're trying to conceive, it can pinpoint your fertile times, and tell you about the state of your reproductive health.

The damage that school biology lessons have caused is apparent in the everyday and erroneous assumption that every woman ovulates on day 14 of a 28 day cycle. This may be average (although in my experience, I doubt that), but many women have much longer or shorter, or completely irregular, cycles. This is where FAM is invaluable, both for calculating fertility, and helping to avoid or achieve a pregnancy, and for helping a woman to know where she is at any moment in her cycle. No more unexpected periods, no more worrying over late periods; it's truly empowering to finally understand your body and its individual idiosyncrasies.

Tuning-in to the ebb and flow of hormones throughout your cycle can give a real insight into Premenstrual Syndrome, especially symptoms such as cravings and headaches. It's fascinating to observe how your sex drive changes throughout the cycle, and interesting to see how travel, stress and different seasons, can affect your body.

I cannot understand why FAM is not taught in schools, as it gives you a different perspective on fertility, periods and hormones. Being able to monitor, on a day-to-day basis, the effect of various lifestyle choices on your menstrual cycle brings home to you what a delicately balanced system it is, and how easy it is to throw it out of kilter. It's not surprising that so many people have difficulty conceiving these days. I was astonished when I first saw how just a late or boozy night could delay ovulation, and how stress could stop it happening at all during that cycle. But is it as effective as a contraceptive? That's not as easy a question to answer as it should be. Contraceptive effectiveness is classified in two ways: method-effectiveness, and use-effectiveness. Most manufacturers quote method-effectiveness rates, which are misleading, as this is the effectiveness the method would enjoy _if_ it was used _perfectly_, which, in the real world, rarely, if ever, happens. So, the use-effectiveness rate includes reality: the missed pills, the condoms put on inside-out, the spermicide past its use-by date. FAM, therefore, has a use-effectiveness equivalent to condoms, and just below the 'combined' pill.

But, isn't it fiddly? I suppose that depends on your definition of fiddly. FAM relies on three indicators of hormone levels: cervical fluid, position of cervix, and Basal Body Temperature (BBT). The BBT has to be taken with a reliable thermometer at roughly the same time each morning before you get up. I've never found this a problem. I keep the thermometer under my pillow, and just get in the habit of taking my temperature when I wake up. You don't need to take it at exactly the same time each day, and missing the odd day doesn't matter. In fact, when you become experienced at FAM, you'll probably find, as I have, that you only need to take your temperature for the middle couple of weeks of any cycle anyway.

A lot of people are squeamish over the concept of cervical fluid. I never have been. It's just a fact of life that every woman must have noticed that some days in the month she has wetter discharge than other days. As soon as you start producing wetter fluid you're becoming more fertile. The day of wettest discharge is the day you're most fertile, and then the fluid dries up, and you're in your post-ovulatory phase. It takes a bit of experience to learn your particular pattern, but once you know it, the whole cycle seems obvious, and you wonder how you could have spent so much time in the dark.

Cervical position is the thing I've had the most trouble with, due to having a retroverted (backward-tilted) uterus. Basically, the higher up and softer the tip of the cervix feels, the more fertile you are. But the great thing about FAM is that the three fertility signs are there to cross-check against each other. If you have trouble with one sign, the other two are there to be interpreted.

This sounds complicated, and it is at first, but what in life isn't? Driving a car or making a cake sound horrifically complex when you try and explain them to someone who has never done either; and yet, if you take a lesson, you soon find it becomes second nature. If you want to be properly scrupulous when using FAM, there are a lot of rules to learn about when you may or may not be fertile. The best way to learn these is either from a natural fertility teacher, or from a decent book which you can refer to whenever you're in doubt. In my opinion, the best book is Toni Weschler's Taking Charge of Your Fertility, which gives detailed instruction on using the method both for pregnancy achievement and avoidance. It also includes sample charts, case histories, and an exhaustive list of special circumstances in which using FAM can be a challenge, such as while breastfeeding.

Whenever I talk to people about using FAM, someone inevitably says that they know someone using FAM who got pregnant. It's usually said as if this is a clincher that the whole method is useless. However, when I enquire further as to which rules they were using when this mishap occurred, it often turns out that they weren't properly charting or observing fertility signs at all, just vaguely avoiding the middle of their cycle. Of course, in that case, I never have to reply that I know someone who got pregnant when using a condom, and another who'd actually been sterilised. No method is perfect, and we're all going to know someone for whom a contraceptive method failed. The trick is to try not to be that person!

Another point often overlooked about FAM is its versatility. If it doesn't suit you as a contraceptive method, that's fine, but you may want to use it to help you get pregnant. With infertility figures rising, many couples find themselves unable to conceive when they plan to. For many people, the first port of call is the family doctor, for a referral to fertility or gynaecology specialists. But fertility tests are invasive and stressful, and should not be the first resort. Many doctors are unaware of how helpful charting using FAM can be in situations of less than optimal fertility. FAM can tell you the exact time of ovulation, to give fertilisation the best possible chance. It can also help pinpoint the exact nature of any problems: it can tell you if you're ovulating or not; if you're producing the right kind of cervical fluid to aid fertilisation; if you're having sex at the right time; and if your post-ovulatory luteal phase is long enough to allow implantation. It can arm you with a lot of useful information which could mean you don't need to see a doctor, or, if you do, rule out some problems from the outset.

In these days of quick fixes, the idea of learning a method, and applying rules, can seem like too much hard work. When I first started using FAM, I used squared graph paper to fill in my temperatures and make a nicely readable line graph. Soon after that, I found a chart in a book, which I photocopied and filled in with my own details. It had spaces for noting cervix position and type of fluid, too. But the thing which has transformed my use of FAM has been finding Ovusoft: a piece of computer software which allows me to fill in my fertility signs on my computer. It's taken the effort out of the thing. No longer do I have to remember the rules. I simply observe my fertility signs, input them, and the computer tells me if I'm likely to be fertile that day. When things can be this easy, there's really no reason not to give FAM a try.

Resources
Taking Charge of Your Fertility by Toni Weschler (Vermilion)
Cycle Savvy: The Smart Teen's Guide to the Mysteries of Her Body by Toni Weschler (Collins)
www.tcoyf.com ~ Weschler's support website, with forums and articles, plus Ovusoft
http://www.fpa.org.uk/information/leaflets/documents_and_pdfs/detail.cfm?contentid=159 – the Family
Planning Association guide to fertility awareness

Conscious Conception

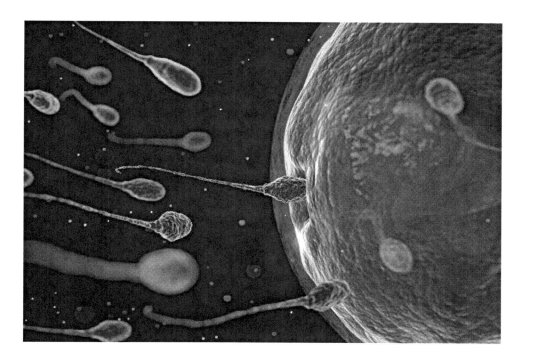

A Twinkle in your Parents' Eyes:
conscious conception and conscious pregnancy
By Bruce Lipton, PhD

This is an excerpt from *The Biology of Belief: Unleashing the Power of Consciousness, Matter and Miracles*, by Bruce Lipton, PhD, published by Mountain of Love Productions. Excerpted from Chapter 7, Conscious Parenting: parents as genetic engineers. This was printed as an article in The Mother, prior to the book's publication ~ with immense gratitude.

Research suggests that what is going on in the lives of the parents during the process of genomic imprinting has a profound influence on the mind and body of their child: a scary thought given how unprepared most people are to have a baby.

You all know the expression, "When you were only a twinkle in your parents' eyes" ~ a phrase that conjures up the happiness of loving parents who truly want to conceive a child. It turns out it's also a phrase that sums up the latest genetic research suggesting that parents should cultivate that twinkle in the months before they conceive a child; that growth-promoting awareness and intention can produce a smarter, healthier and happier baby.

Research reveals that parents act as genetic engineers for their children in the months before conception. In the final stages of egg and sperm maturation, a process called genomic imprinting adjusts the activity of specific groups of genes that will shape the character of the child yet to be conceived. [Surani 2001; Reik and Walter 2001] Research suggests that what is going on in the lives of the parents during the process of genomic imprinting has a profound influence on the mind and body of their child: a scary thought given how unprepared most people are to have a baby. Verny writes in Pre-Parenting: Nurturing Your Child from Conception: "It makes a difference whether we are conceived in love, haste or hate, and whether a mother wants to be pregnant...parents do better when they live in a calm and stable environment free of addictions and supported by family and friends." [Verny 2002] Interestingly, aboriginal cultures have recognised the influence of the conception environment for millennia. Prior to conceiving a child, couples ceremonially purify their minds and bodies. Once the child is conceived, an impressive body of research is documenting how important parents' attitudes are in the development of the foetus.

Again Verny writes: "In fact, the great weight of the scientific evidence that has emerged over the last decade demands that we re-evaluate the mental and emotional abilities of unborn children. Awake or asleep, the studies show, they [unborn children] are constantly tuned-in to their mother's every action, thought and feeling. From the moment of conception, the experience in the womb shapes the brain and lays the groundwork for personality, emotional temperament, and the power of higher thought."

Now is the time to stress that the New Biology is not a return to the old days of blaming mothers for every ailment that medicine didn't understand ~ from schizophrenia to autism. Mothers and fathers are in the conception and pregnancy business together, even though it's the mother who carries the child in her womb. What the father does, profoundly affects the mother: which in turn affects the developing child. For example, if the father leaves, and the mother starts questioning her own ability to survive, his leaving profoundly changes the interaction between the mother and the unborn baby. Similarly, societal factors, such as lack of employment, housing and healthcare, or endless wars that pull fathers into the military, can affect the parents, and thus the developing child.

The essence of conscious parenting is that both mothers and fathers have important responsibilities for fostering healthy, intelligent, productive and joy-filled children. We surely cannot blame ourselves, nor our parents for failures in our own or our children's lives. Science has kept our attention focused on the notion of genetic determinism, leaving us ignorant about the influence beliefs have on our lives, and more importantly, how our behaviours and attitudes program the lives of our children.

Most obstetricians are also still uneducated about the importance of parental attitudes in the development of the baby. According to the notion of genetic determinism that they were steeped in as medical students, foetal development is mechanically controlled by genes, with little additional contribution from the mother. Consequently, obstetricians/gynaecologists are only concerned with a few maternal prenatal issues: Is she eating well? Taking vitamins? Does she exercise regularly? Those questions focus on what they believe is the mother's principal role: the provision of nutrients to be used by the genetically-programmed foetus. But the developing child receives far more than nutrients from the mother's blood. Along with nutrients, the foetus absorbs excess glucose if the mother is diabetic, and excess cortisol and other fight or flight hormones if the mother is chronically stressed. Research now offers insights into how the system works. If a mother is under stress, she activates her HPA axis, which provides fight or flight responses in a threatening environment.

Stress hormones prepare the body to engage in a protection response. Once these maternal signals enter the foetal bloodstream, they affect the same target tissues and organs in the foetus as they did in the mother. In stressful environments, foetal blood preferentially flows to the muscles and hindbrain, providing nutritional requirements needed by the arms and legs, and by the region of the brain responsible for life-saving reflex behaviour. In supporting the function of the protection-related systems, blood flow is shunted from the viscera organs, and stress hormones suppress forebrain function. The development of foetal tissue and organs is proportional to both the amount of blood they receive and the function they provide. When passing through the placenta, the hormones of a mother experiencing chronic stress will profoundly alter the distribution of blood flow in her foetus and change the character of her developing child's physiology. [Lesage, et al, 2004; Christensen 2000; Arnsten 1998; Leutwyler 1998; Sapolsky 1997; Sandman, et al, 1994]

At the University of Melbourne, E. Marilyn Wintour's research on pregnant sheep, which are physiologically quite similar to humans, has found that prenatal exposure to cortisol eventually leads to high blood pressure. [Dodic, et al, 2002] Foetal cortisol levels play a very important regulatory role in the development of the kidneys' filtering units, the nephrons. A nephron's cells are intimately involved with regulating the body's salt balance, and consequently are important in controlling blood pressure. Excess cortisol absorbed from a stressed mother modifies foetal nephron formation. An additional effect of excess cortisol is that it simultaneously switches the mother's and the foetus' system from a growth state to a protection posture. As a result, the growth-inhibiting effect of excess cortisol in the womb causes the babies to be born smaller. Suboptimal conditions in the womb that lead to low birthweight babies have been linked to a number of adult ailments that Nathanielsz outlines in his book Life In The Womb, including diabetes, heart disease and obesity. For example, Dr. David Barker of England's University of Southampton has found that a male who weighs less than 5.5 pounds at birth has a 50% greater chance of dying of heart disease than one with a higher birth weight. Harvard researchers have found that women who weigh less than 5.5 pounds at birth have a 23 percent higher risk of cardiovascular disease than women born heavier. And David Leon of the London School of Hygiene and Tropical Medicine has found that diabetes is three times more common in 60-year-old men who were small and thin at birth.

The new focus on the influences of the prenatal environment extends to the study of IQ, which genetic determinists and racists once linked simply to genes. But in 1997, Bernie Devlin, a professor of psychiatry at the University of Pittsburgh School of Medicine, carefully analysed 212 earlier studies that compared the IQs of twins, siblings, and parents and their children. He concluded that genes account for only 48 percent of the factors that determine IQ. And when the synergistic effects of mingling the mother and father's genes are factored in, the true inherited component of intelligence plummets even further, to 34 percent. [Devlin, et al, 1997; McGue 1997] Devlin, on the other hand, found that conditions during prenatal development significantly impact IQ. He reveals that up to 51% of a child's potential intelligence is controlled by environmental factors. Previous studies had already found that drinking or smoking during pregnancy can cause decreased IQ in children, as can exposure to lead in the womb. The lesson for people who want to be parents is that you can radically shortchange the intelligence of your child simply by the way you approach pregnancy. These IQ changes are not accidents; they're directly linked to altered blood flow in a stressed brain. In my lectures on conscious parenting, I cite research, but I also show a video from an Italian conscious parenting organization, Associazione Nazionale Educazione Prenatale, which graphically illustrates the interdependent relationship between parents and their unborn child. In this video, a mother and father engage in a loud argument while the woman is undergoing a sonogram. You can vividly see the foetus jump when the argument starts. The startled foetus arches its body and jumps up as if it were on a trampoline when the argument is punctuated with the shattering of glass. The power of modern technology, in the form of a sonogram, helps lay to rest the myth that the unborn child is not a sophisticated enough organism to react to anything other than its nutritional environment.

Nature's Head Start Program

You may be wondering why evolution would provide such a system for foetal development that seems so fraught with peril, and is so dependent on the environment of the parents. Actually, it's an ingenious system that helps ensure the survival of your offspring. Eventually, the child is going to find itself in the same environment as its parents. Information acquired from the parents' perception of their environment transits the placenta and primes the prenate's physiology, preparing it to more effectively deal with future exigencies that will be encountered after birth. Nature is simply preparing that child to best survive in that environment. However, armed with the latest science, parents now have a choice. They can carefully reprogram their limiting beliefs about life before they bring a child into their world.

The importance of parental programming undermines the notion that our traits, both positive and negative, are fully determined by our genes. As we have seen, genes are shaped, guided and tailored by environmental learning experiences. We have all been led to believe that artistic, athletic and intellectual prowess are traits simply passed on by genes. But no matter how "good" one's genes may be, if an individual's nurture experiences are fraught with abuse, neglect or misperceptions, the realisation of the genes' potentials will be sabotaged. Liza Minelli acquired her genes from her superstar mother, Judy Garland, and her father filmmaker, Vincent Minelli. Liza's career, the heights of her stardom and the lows of her personal life, are scripts that were played out by her parents and downloaded into her subconscious mind. If Liza had the same genes, but was raised by a nurturing Pennsylvania Dutch farming family, that environment would have epigenetically triggered a different selection of genes. The genes that enabled her to pursue a successful entertainment career would have likely been masked or inhibited by the cultural demands of her agrarian community.

A wonderful example of the effectiveness of conscious parenting programming is superstar golfer Tiger Woods. Although his father was not an accomplished golfer, he made every effort to immerse Tiger in an environment that was rich with opportunities to develop and enhance the mindset, skills, attitudes and focus of a master golfer. No doubt, Tiger's success is also intimately connected with the Buddhist philosophy that his mother contributed. Indeed, genes are important ~ but their importance is only realised through the influence of conscious parenting, and the richness of opportunities provided by the environment.

Conscious Mothering and Fathering

I used to close my public lectures with the admonition that we are personally responsible for everything in our lives. Such a closure did not make me popular with the audience. That responsibility was too much for many people to accept. After one lecture, an older woman in the audience was so distressed by my conclusion, that she brought her husband backstage, and in tears vehemently contested my conclusion. She did not want any part of some of the tragedies she had experienced. This woman convinced me that my summary conclusion had to be modified. I realised that I didn't want to contribute to foisting blame and guilt on any individual. As a society, we are too apt to wallow in guilt or scapegoat others for our problems. As we gain insights over a lifetime, we become better equipped to take charge of our lives. After some deliberation, this woman from the audience happily accepted the following resolution: you are personally responsible for everything in your life, once you become aware that you are personally responsible for everything in your life. One cannot be "guilty" of being a poor parent unless one is already aware of the above-described information and disregards it. Once you become aware of this information, you can begin to apply it to reprogram your behaviour. And while we're on the subject of myths about parenting, it's absolutely not true that you are the same parent for all of your children. Your second child is not a clone of the first child. The same things are not happening in your world that happened when the first child was born. As I said above, I once thought that I was the same parent for my first child as I was for my very different second child. But when I analysed my parenting, I found that was not true. When my first child was born, I was at the beginning of my graduate school training, which was for me, a difficult transition fraught with a high workload accompanied by high insecurity. By the time my second daughter was born, I was a more confident, more accomplished research scientist ready to start my academic career. I had more time and more psychic energy to parent my second child and to better parent my first daughter, who was now a toddler.

Another myth I'd like to address is that infants need lots of stimulation in the form of black and white flash cards or other learning tools marketed to parents to increase the intelligence of their children. Michael Mendizza and Joseph Chilton Pearce's inspiring book Magical Parent-Magical Child makes it clear that play, not programming, is the key to optimising the learning and performance of infants and children. [Mendizza and Pearce 2001] Children need parents who can playfully foster the curiosity, creativity and wonder that accompanies their children into the world.

Obviously, what humans need is nurture in the form of love, and the ability to observe older humans going about their everyday lives. When babies in orphanages, for example, are kept in cribs and only provided with food, but not one-on-one smiles and hugs, they develop long-lasting developmental problems. One study of Romanian orphans by Mary Carlson, a neurobiologist at Harvard Medical School, concluded that the lack of touching and attention in Romanian orphanages, and poor-quality day-care centres, stunted the children's growth and adversely affected their behavior. Carlson, who studied 60 Romanian children from a few months to three years of age, measured their cortisol levels by analysing samples of saliva. The more stressed a child was, as determined by the higher than normal levels of cortisol in its blood, the poorer the outcome for the child. [Holden 1996]

Carlson and others have also done research on monkeys and rats demonstrating crucial links among touch, the secretion of the stress hormone cortisol, and social development. Studies by James W. Prescott, former director of the National Institutes of Health's section on Human Health and Child Development, revealed that newborn monkeys deprived of physical contact with their mothers or social contact with others, develop abnormal stress profiles and become violent sociopaths. [Prescott 1996 and 1990]

He followed up these studies with an assessment of human cultures based on how they raise their children. He found that if a society physically held and loved its children and did not repress sexuality, that culture was peaceful. Peaceful cultures feature parents who maintain extensive physical contact with their children, such as carrying their babies on their chests and backs throughout the day. In contrast, societies that deprive their infants, children and adolescents of extensive touch are inevitably violent in nature. One of the differences between populations is that many of the children not receiving touch suffer from somatosensory affective disorder. This disorder is characterised by an inability to physiologically suppress surging levels of stress hormones, a precursor to violent episodes.

These findings provide insight into the violence that pervades the United States. Rather than endorsing physical closeness, our current medical and psychological practices often discourage it. From the unnatural intervention of medical doctors in the natural process of birthing, for example, separating the neonate for extensive periods from the parents into distant nurseries, and to the advising of parents not to respond to their babies' cries for fear of spoiling them. Such practices, presumably based upon "science", undoubtedly contribute to the violence in our civilisation. The research regarding touch and its relationship to violence is described in full at the following website: www.violence.de

But what about the Romanian children who come out of deprived backgrounds and become what one researcher called "the resilient wonders". Why do some children thrive despite their backgrounds? Because they have "better" genes? By now you know that I don't believe that. More likely, the birth parents of these resilient wonders provided a more nurturing pre- and perinatal environment, as well as good nutrition at crucial points in the child's development.

The lesson for adoptive parents is that they should not pretend their children's lives began when they came into their new surroundings. Their children may have already been programmed by their birth parents with a belief that they are unwanted or unlovable. If more fortunate, they may have, at some crucial age in their development, received positive, life-affirming messages from their caretakers. If adoptive parents are not aware of pre- and perinatal programming, they may not deal realistically with post-adoption issues. They may not realise that their children did not come to them as a "blank slate" any more than newborns come into the world as blank slates, unaffected by their nine months in their mothers' wombs. Better to recognise that programming, and to work, if necessary, to change it.

For adoptive and non-adoptive parents alike, the message is clear: your children's genes reflect only their potential, not their destiny. It's up to you to provide the environment that allows them to develop to their highest potential.

Notice I do not say that it's up to parents to read lots of parenting books. I've met lots of people who are intellectually attracted to the ideas I present in this book. But intellectual interest is not enough. I tried that myself. I was intellectually aware of everything in this book, but before I made the effort to change, it made no impact on my life. If you simply read this book and think that your life and your children's lives will change, you're doing the equivalent of accepting the latest pharmaceutical pill thinking it will "fix" everything. No-one is fixed until they make the effort to change.

Here is my challenge to you: let go of unfounded fears, and take care not to implant unnecessary fears and limiting beliefs in your children's subconscious minds. Most of all, do not accept the fatalistic message of genetic determinism. You can help your children reach their potential, and you can change your personal life. You are not "stuck" with your genes.

Take heed of the growth and protection lessons from cells, and shift your lives into growth whenever possible. And remember that for human beings the most potent growth-promoter is not the fanciest school, the biggest toy or the highest-paying job. Long before cell biology and studies of children in orphanages, conscious parents, and seers like Rumi, knew that for human babies and adults the best growth promoter is Love.

A lifetime without Love is of no account
Love is the Water of Life
Drink it down with heart and soul!

"It makes a difference whether we are conceived in love, haste or hate, and whether a mother wants to be pregnant…parents do better when they live in a calm and stable environment free of addictions, and supported by family and friends."

…do not accept
the fatalistic message
of genetic determinism.

You can help your children
reach their potential,
and you can change
your personal life.

You are not "stuck"
with your genes.

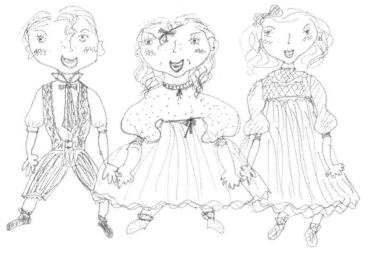

To consciously conceive
our children
is to embark on an awakening journey
of divine magnitude.
It moves us towards our spirituality
and onto a path
which enlivens
our magnificent potential.

Consciously Creating Tomorrow's Children
By Veronika Sophia Robinson

Why do we yearn to create a new child? Is it an expression of the love we feel for our partner, or is it because we want to re-parent ourselves? Is it a spiritual experience we're seeking, or is it as basic as some primal encoding which requires us to reproduce for the sake of continuing the human race?

To consciously conceive our children is to embark on an awakening journey of divine magnitude. It moves us towards our spirituality (regardless of our religious beliefs), and onto a path which enlivens our magnificent potential. It simply means conscious creation.

We live at a time where, collectively, we're in a hurry. We're even in a hurry to conceive our babies! Instant gratification has no part to play in conscious conception. Mother Nature has her own seasons and doesn't try to make things happen before their time. Likewise, a soul choosing to come Earthside has a lot of things to consider: such as country of birth; parents; siblings; environment; time in history.

Slow time

As a parent looking to consciously conceive, there are many steps we can take to align ourselves with our body and future baby. The most important is to learn to live in the present moment. Recognise and balance all of your six senses. Many of us focus on just one sense, e.g. vision. If you have a job which requires a lot of computer use, for example, sight will be the way in which you predominantly experience the world. It's inevitable that your other senses will be neglected, unless you make conscious choices in each moment to use and embrace them.

Sight

Make sure you exercise your eyes well by getting plenty of natural light, adequate sleep, and by using them equally for far and near vision. Ensure your diet contains vitamin A. Raw carrots are great! Learn to observe the beauty around you. Let this fill your consciousness.

The scenes of beauty which you choose to embrace before conception will become scenes within the being of your child.

Smell

Indulge in your sense of smell. Burn incense, or essential oils of your favourite scent. Smell the food you eat. Take the time to peel a mandarin, and absorb the wonderful citrus aroma. Try squeezing a eucalyptus leaf. Exquisite! Nature's perfumes are everywhere. Be conscious of them. Play with them. Smell is a sense we tend to ignore unless something incredibly vile assaults us. Write a list of your ten favourite smells, and actively seek them out on a regular basis. It's good for you! My own favourites from Nature are:

.fully Sun-ripened mango
.eucalyptus essential oil
.freesias
.pine needles
.freshly-mown grass
.jasmine
.rain
.my husband's skin
.my children's hair
.cinnamon bark

The pleasurable scents which nurture you before conception will become scents that live within the being of your child.

Sound

Which sounds warm you, soothe your soul? I love the sound of rain on a tin roof, my husband singing, and the dawn chorus of birdsong. Do you have music that calms you? What noises fill your day? Are they harmonious or jarring to your being?
The sounds which fall upon your ears before conception will become sounds that live within the being of your child.

Touch

To be touched is an important human need. Countless studies have shown how children in orphanages thrive when touched. Are you touched enough? What comforts your skin? Is it the hands of another human, or water, or clothing, or air?
The touch that sustains you before conception will come alive within the being of your child.

Taste

I wonder how many people really taste their food these days? Many people buy ready-made meals full of preservatives, as they're too busy to prepare their own food. Most people are in too much of a hurry to even eat their food as Nature intended. Are you someone who gulps each mouthful while watching the news and reading the letters in the post?

Think about the type of eating environment you want your child to grow up in. Do you care whether they grow up eating around a table and sharing family time? Does it matter to you whether your children eat breakfast cereal from a box, and heap even more sugar onto it while they watch breakfast television? Think about these things now before you conceive. These decisions form the basis of conscious conception.

The food you taste, and eating habits you form before conception, will become forces that dwell within the being of your child.

Intuition

Ah, the sixth sense. Often hinted at, but never really acknowledged. In many ways, I regard this as our most important sense, for it helps us to use and enjoy our other senses more fully. Intuition is about listening to the inner voice. Everyone has access to this sense. It's when we don't use it, don't acknowledge it, and don't trust it that we forget how to fully engage it. In many ways, it's like a muscle...it needs constant use to be strong.

Trust your intuition before conception, for it will grow to be your greatest spiritual resource as a parent.

Contentment

For as long as humans have existed, we've yearned for that grass just over yonder. It's as much a blessing as a curse. The downside is that we live always feeling like something is missing.

If you don't yet have your desired child, learn the art of contentment. Look at all you do have in your life. I know it's easy for me, a woman with two children, to say that, but the truth is that a life without children doesn't need to feel empty. It's a choice to see it through different eyes. There's an infinite number of ways to express our creativity while living on Mother Earth. Having children is just one way. If you feel such a strong maternal need then find ways to express it so you can still live in the present moment and ENJOY your life. Do volunteer work in a kindergarten, or children's hospice, for example. Go to Romania and work in an orphanage. Join Volunteer Services Overseas and teach in a small school. Babysit for friends.

A beautiful and dear friend in my life, now in her seventies, tried for ten years to conceive a child. She and her husband gave up and decided to adopt. The adopted baby arrived, and spent his childhood as a very ill boy. Regardless, his mother loved him with all her heart, and nursed him through his various illnesses. Six years after his adoption, this couple conceived a boy. Several years ago, their first son died. The grief this couple experienced could not have been any greater had he been born from her body.

Children don't always come to us from our own body. Children are conceived in our heart.

Appreciation
Hand in hand with contentment is appreciation. The more we appreciate our life, the more life brings us. Want more love in your life? Give more love. Want more energy in your life? Give energy to something. Appreciation provides a direct link with our soul.

It's been said that the religions of the world are divided into two types of people. Those who pray "Help me! Help me! Help me!" And those who pray, "Thank you! Thank you! Thank you!" Learn the art of saying thank you in advance. That's the secret of life.

Questions about parenting
If you already have a child or children, and you want to conceive, spend some time thinking about current world population statistics. How do you feel about bringing another child into a world already overloaded? Those of us in abundant countries are fooled into thinking there's plenty for all. The truth is we're disastrously overstretched. Mother Earth is being drained, raped and mutilated in ways that are heart-wrenching. There's no right number of children for any family to have. And I certainly think China's 'one child only' rule is

going to backfire badly: a generation of children without siblings? I shudder to think. Those of us who have a desire for larger families really do need to question this outside of our own needs. We must think of our global family. I urge anyone in this situation to read The Last Hours of Ancient Sunlight by Thomm Hartman. What do you currently do to walk lightly on the planet? Are you actively taking part in recycling schemes, buying locally, etc. What else can you do? Are you willing to do this? Do you live simply so that others can simply live? Our lifestyle choices in First World countries do affect those in less fortunate countries.

Your children in a high-tech world

My husband recently did a stint as Santa Claus where he'd see about 20 children an hour, over a period of five weeks. The majority of these children wanted Playstation 2 (whatever that is), a computer or a mobile phone for Christmas. The average age of these children was five. This is the world you're bringing your children into. These are the peers of your future children. How do you feel about this?

What steps in your personal lifestyle can you take now, before conception, to counteract this high-tech age where children imitate parents, and don't have a natural childhood? What example in your own life are you offering? What holistic practices can be implemented now? Arm yourself with studies so that your child doesn't become another brain tumour statistic because his/her little brain was fried by the ever-essential mobile phone. How will you say no to the pressures of modern living? Learn to say yes now to a healthy, conscious and holistic lifestyle.

Imagination

Our greatest tool for consciously creating tomorrow's children is not to be found outside ourselves. Yes, there are many remedies, allies and therapies which can greatly aid and enhance our path towards conscious conception; however, it's our very own imagination which will play the pivotal role of bringing our children forth. You're limited only by your own consciousness. Thoughts held in mind, produce after their own kind. This ancient metaphysical teaching has inspired many people. In terms of your own fertility and childbearing, what it means is to avoid thoughts and feelings of barrenness and infertility. Replace this 'empty' feeling that screams of 'failure'. Replace all feelings of incompleteness by using your wonderful imagination to CREATE life as you wish it to be. It's been said that the best way to predict the future is to create the future! To consciously create our future we must imagine it already exists. Marry your thoughts and feelings and they will produce. i.e., they'll create. Imagine the life with children that you want, and feel it exist within the depths of your being, so that you're imagining in the present, rather than the future.

*Imagine yourself welcoming a soul into your world.

*Imagine yourself making love with your partner ~ with love, beauty, reverence, honesty and joy.

*Imagine the combined love and welcome, emanating from <u>both</u> of you, acting as a beacon in the etheric world.

*Imagine your brilliant and beautiful auric lights joined as one ~ and the child of your dreams seeing the rainbow of your invitation. Imagine this soul-baby being drawn towards you and your life-creating partner.

*Imagine creating a safe and sacred space within your womb ~ a bed on which new life can grow.

*Imagine the incredible thrill of discovering you're pregnant!

*Imagine the pure joy of sharing this news with family and friends.

*Imagine your baby growing inside you, strong, healthy, and happy.

*Imagine the awesome magic of your babe's birthing day. Hold your baby. Make eye contact.

*Imagine each age and stage of your child's life.

Go to sleep every night imagining life with your children. Wake up each day, smile, and be filled with gratitude. Appreciation is the highest form of love.

Allies to conscious conception
Preconception cleanse:
Begin a preconception cleanse at least six months (ideally two years) before you plan to conceive. This cleanse includes:

Physical
Take stock of your eating habits. Eat plenty of fresh, organic fruit and vegetables, especially leafy greens. Avoid processed foods. Be sure to take Omega 3, 6 & 9 oils in your diet on a daily basis. You can get this vegan mixture from your local health store. Both men and women should include rich, natural sources of zinc, B vitamins and folic acid in their daily diet.

Ensure you're drinking plenty of pure water.

Sleep in a well ventilated room.

Exercise daily: a brisk twenty minute walk.

Breathe fresh air.

Keep houseplants.

Clean your environment. Avoid using chemicals and poisons within your car, home and place of work. If you use a computer, get a radiation screen fitted.

Limit your use of computers, television and mobile phones. Avoid microwaved food.

Detox from synthetically-produced hormonal contraception.

Avoid light pollution when sleeping (e.g. street lights, clock radio lights, etc.). Allow your body to fall into sync with the moonlight so that your hormones and glands can function naturally.

Emotional

Having children is the ultimate personal growth course. Children have an incredible ability to bring up our core issues for healing. It's in everyone's best interests to heal deeper issues before giving birth, or at the very least to be aware of what drives them. Look at your relationship with your life partner. Have you talked about what it will be like having children? This might seem rather basic, but it's amazing how many people never talk about which parenting style they'll follow when they have children! Develop complete honesty and openness in your relationship, based on respect and care. Allow yourselves to feel safe and to trust one another. In the more difficult moments of your parenting journey you'll need each other more than ever. It's far better to be united as friends, than enemies, in those darker hours. Talk about such things as religion/spirituality, vaccination, schooling, in-laws, etc., before you have children.

Mental

Are you prone to depression or anxiety? Can you treat these from Nature's Medicine Cabinet? Consider getting professional help from an understanding and holistic therapist.

Spiritual

What do you believe? What will you teach your children? This isn't about religion, so much as the fundamental beliefs we hold about life. What is your guiding force? What morals and ethics do you hold strongly? What will your children inherit from your belief system? How much value do you place on honesty, trust, love, happiness, empathy, integrity and peace?

Remedies and Therapies

Our path to conception can be shared and aided by many therapies and remedies. To name but a few:
Cranio Sacral Therapy
Shiatsu
Emotional Freedom Technique
Chiropractic
Remedial Massage
Homeopathy
Herbs
Acupuncture
Osteopathy
Reflexology
Aromatherapy
Reiki
Bowen Technique
Counselling
Flower and crystal essences (e.g. She Oak flower essence for difficulty conceiving)

Enjoy your journey. Bless each step. Give thanks.

Soul Welcoming Ceremony

Some parents choose to have a conception or Soul Welcoming Ceremony. It can be as simple or elaborate as you feel comfortable with. Below are some ideas for you to work with. Make them your own.

Conception Mandala

This is a wonderful way for parents-to-be to join their energies. Find a secluded place in Nature. A stone circle can feel energetically vibrant. Collect stones, or shells if on a beach, leaves, twigs, berries, pine cones, etc. Together, make a spiral, working from the inside out. IMAGINE the slow movement outwards mimicking a foetus wrapped up in your womb. This very symbolic act is a way to embrace slowness, and to feel yourself as part of creation.

Conception Meditation

You can meditate alone, though for the purpose of conception it's far more powerful to meditate together. Some couples choose to do this just prior to lovemaking. It's entirely up to you as individuals how you do this. Some people light a candle first to represent Divine Light. The main focus is of reverence and welcome. It's about creating a space in your heart and mind, and asking ~ inviting ~ the child of your dreams to walk with you on Earth. Be attentive to any hunches or inspiration that you may get during this time, or shortly afterwards.

Conception Altar

As with meditation, the way in which you approach this will reflect your own personality. An altar is a dedicated space, whether it's on an altar table, windowsill or bookshelf. It may be in your garden on an old log. Place things which represent new life. It may be eggs or berries or even a baby's bootie. Perhaps you could place a picture of a beautiful child. The altar is a place to pause, to slow down, and to be aware of the incredibly powerful act of conception.

Conception Vows

This is a very moving experience which needs to be done with integrity, honesty and absolute intimacy between the couple. At this time, you share vows about how you'll create a child; how you'll parent this child; and how you'll continue to love and nurture each other. Example: "I take you, my life partner, to share my body, my heart, my life, and to create new life with me. I promise to parent fully and faithfully with you. I will honour you each day for who you are as a person, and as a parent. I will honour your presence within our child."

You can add to the sanctity of any sacred ceremony by including music, readings, vows and symbolic acts, such as candle lighting or planting a seed.

Pregnancy

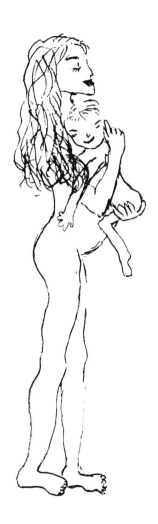

Isolation, rejection and communion in the womb
By Thomas Verny, MD, DPsych, FRCPC

Most people, whether they're lay people, scientists or academics, cling to a whole slew of erroneous beliefs about prenatal life. Two of the most prevalent ones are: firstly, that the uterus is a place of perfect peace, harmony and joy; and second, that our mental faculties start to develop only after birth, i.e., that babies prior to birth are mindless creatures. Why this stubborn resistance when evidence to the contrary is so overwhelming? I think it's due to the presence of a collective unconscious defence against the threat of re-stimulating and re-awakening deeply repressed feelings of intrauterine rejection, isolation and separation.

Even a person who, as a pre-nate, had miraculously escaped exposure to any toxic maternal or paternal feelings, would find re-experiencing this state of prenatal bliss, compared to his present existence, painful. In other words, no matter whether you had a good or a bad prenatal life, you don't want to be reminded of it. On the other hand, those who've faced and overcome their fears, are willing to look at the facts. One of these facts is that unborn children respond to, and are affected by, maternal emotions. Here I'll attempt to examine those maternal feelings and attitudes that promote the formation of a strong ego and a healthy mind-body continuum, and those that create feelings of dejection and despair in the unborn. I'll examine the effect of parental messages on the unborn and newborn, and not the mechanisms of parental-foetal communication, a subject I have dealt with previously.[14,15] The focus is on negative parental foetal communication, though the effect of positive prenatal parenting will also be briefly studied.

Pollutants of the amniotic Universe

There are many ways in which future parents and pregnant parents expose themselves, and in turn, their unborn children, to a variety of noxious and potentially harmful influences. Briefly stated, these toxins fall into two categories: external toxins and internal toxins.

External toxins

These are produced by agents outside the bodies of the parents, and may be listed as:

[] environmental toxins and radiation
[] psycho-active drugs, hallucinogenic substances, tobacco and alcohol
[] obstetric tests, such as amniocentesis, chorionic villi sampling, ultrasound and many others

The question arises: how much conscious control do parents have in this area? It is my belief that they have a lot, either by choosing to be addicted, or by choosing to ignore information about the detrimental effects on the baby of such things as radiation and amniocentesis on the baby.

This article deals with the second category, that is, the internal toxins.

Internal toxins

By internal toxins I refer to a variety of neurotransmitters, stress, and sex hormones, as well as thoughts, feelings, and behaviours produced by the pregnant mother and her partner. I will focus on the quality of parental messages and their effect on the unborn and newborn, and not on the mechanisms of parental-foetal communication[1].

I should point out that I consider human beings as mind-body entities, so that every thought and feeling is both a mental and a physical phenomenon. Every hormone or chemical in our bodies is produced either in response to some mental representation or feeling state, or, once produced, induces an effect on the psyche. Consequently, a pregnant mother who bombards her baby with stress hormones, is sending a certain message to her baby, as is the mother who has a persistent preoccupation with aborting her baby, or who wishes that her baby were a male child. With this in mind, let us turn our attention to some extreme forms of parental-foetal toxic communication.

Consider, for a moment, the Greek myth of Oedipus. Oedipus was the son of Laius and Jocasta, King and Queen of Thebes, respectively. After Laius married Jocasta, he was informed by the oracle that he would perish by the hands of his son. To prevent the fulfillment of the oracle, he decided never to approach Jocasta sexually. His solemn resolution was violated in a fit of intoxication induced by the Queen. The Queen became pregnant, as was her desire. Laius, still hoping to avert the evil, ordered his wife to destroy the child at birth, if it was a boy. Upon birth, the mother gave her newborn to a domestic, with the instruction to expose him to the elements. The servant suspended the baby boy by the heels from a tree on Mount Cithaeron. There, a shepherd found him and took him to Polybus, King of Corinth, who was childless, and raised him as his own, calling him Oedipus.

Freud's interpretation of this story concentrates on Oedipus' unconscious wishes to be intimate with his mother and to kill his father. Yet, in the actual myth, young Oedipus, on being told by the oracle of his fate, tried strenuously to avoid it, by leaving Corinth. Freud makes no mention of this, or of Laius' fear of having a son. But most importantly, he does not make it plain that Oedipus' real parents attempted to kill him.[12]

If Freud had allowed himself to pay more attention to the events leading to Oedipus' birth, then perhaps he would have defined the Oedipus complex more correctly as belonging to a person who, exposed to rejection and abandonment by both parents pre and post-natally, exhibited severe sexual abnormalities and murderous rage as an adult.

When you consider the fact that Jocasta must have been ridden with anxiety and guilt during the time she carried Oedipus, I think it stands to reason that he would have been severely traumatised in the womb. If we were to represent on a graph the intrauterine experiences as going from the truly blissful to the most toxic, then surely, at the negative end of this spectrum, from a psychological point of view, are babies whose mothers wish to abort them. What happens to babies who survive such wishes by their mother?[3] Research from Finland, Sweden and Czechoslovakia is instructive in this respect.

Blomberg[1] observed that all the differences in his study (which is the Swedish study) were uniformly to the disadvantage of the unwanted children. In the Finnish study, which is still continuing, the incidence of infant mortality, cerebral palsy and mental retardation was significantly higher among the unwanted children than the controls.[7]

The Prague cohort follows the development of 2290 children born in 1961-1963 to women twice denied abortion for the same pregnancy, and pair-matched controls, from age nine through ages 21 to 23. An excellent and thorough discussion of this research may be found in the book Born Unwanted - Developmental Effects of Denied Abortion, by David, Dybrich, Matejcek and Schüller.[4] All the differences noted were consistently in disfavour of the unwanted children.

Over the years, these differences widened, and many that had not been statistically significant at age nine became so at age 16 or 21. The findings of the Prague study, and also of the Scandinavian research, support the hypothesis that children rejected prenatally, will, more likely than controls, show developmental, psychological and social handicaps.

In a paper published last year, Ann Coker[3], an epidemiologist from the University of South Carolina, found that infants born of unwanted pregnancies are more than twice as likely to die within a month of being born than wanted children. The group studied was of married, largely middle income women who were all receiving prenatal care. Low birth weight or congenital anomalies were not found to be factors in this study.

A study at Wayne State University[6] of close to 15,000 singleton live births showed that mothers with broken marriages have a higher incidence of low birth weight infants than comparable groups of married or single mothers. This was attributed to poor foetal growth, because preterm birth was not increased. Apart from a conscious wish for an abortion, prenatal rejection can also occur unconsciously for a variety of reasons, and find expression in a number of ways.

One such condition is the denial of pregnancy by an otherwise healthy and "normal" woman. Brezinka[2] from the University of Innsbruck, reports on 27 women who professed they did not know they were pregnant until term, or until contractions set in. In this group, there were four foetal deaths, three premature babies, one case of intrauterine growth retardation, and one case of possible intended infanticide. Obviously, these outcomes are grossly abnormal.

The following case study illustrates some of the salient features of a denied pregnancy[16].

This pregnant woman was raised by a mother who didn't want to be a mother. The subject stated that her mother was always youth-conscious, and she never told people she had a daughter. When her daughter became pregnant, the mother refused to talk about it because she didn't want to be a grandmother. All of the subject's life, her mother said to her "I doubt if you'll ever get pregnant." (The subject rarely had a menstrual period, and even her doctor was convinced she wouldn't be able to get pregnant, yet she did.)

Three days after her expected due date, the baby had not arrived. The subject informed this researcher that she wanted the baby to be late by four weeks so she could receive more money for her maternity leave. Fifteen days after the expected due date, the doctor tried to induce labour, giving her pitocin for six hours. Nothing happened.

Twelve days later in the hospital, pitocin was given intravenously for 14 hours. She began dilating, but had no feelings of contractions. She dilated to one centimetre. The next day she was given more pitocin, dilated to two centimetres, but still she felt no sense of contractions. At this point, the nurse broke her water and inserted an internal foetal monitor. The foetal heart rate was falling and there was meconium in the amniotic fluid. She felt three very painful contractions. Because of the meconium, and the signs of foetal distress, the doctor ordered a caesarean delivery. The subject had the option of being awake, or totally anaesthetised. She chose to be anaesthetised.

The baby was born in severe foetal distress. Meconium was released and entered the baby's lungs, and her blood vessels became very constricted, causing a cardiac arrest. The baby was rushed to another hospital, which had a Neonatal Intensive Care Unit. The mother saw her new daughter on the fifth day, but was not able to hold her. The following day the baby had a cardiac arrest. The next morning she died. The mother held her baby for the first time after the baby had died. The main theme of this woman's belief system was that she would never have children. This would also entail not experiencing pregnancy, labour or delivery. The subject did not ever touch, hold or nurse her daughter when she was alive. The baby's existence was never validated, just as the subject's mother had never validated her existence[16.]

My next example is taken from research on observations of prenatal life with ultrasound, as reported by Dr. Alessandra Piontelli[8,] from Italy.

Mrs. B., a woman in her mid-thirties, was very anxious when she came for the first observation. This was her third pregnancy, and the second one had ended in stillbirth, due to abruptio placentae. She was accompanied by her husband, and all her attention was directed towards the placenta: its insertion, its shape, etc., and she kept repeating the same questions about it throughout the observation. Her husband, a man also in his mid-thirties, sat by her side, and, though rather silently, appeared to foster her fears. No reassurance seemed enough to placate her obsessive questioning and her anxiety that something could happen at any time. The anxiety, and the endless repetitive questioning, remained constant features throughout the pregnancy.

On the second observation, Mrs. B. came accompanied by her seven year-old daughter, and both now seemed obsessed also by another question: sex. Though one could already tell rather clearly that it was a boy, the question was repeated over and over again: what was its sex? Was it a boy or a girl? Was that the penis?, etc. Very little attention and space were given otherwise to the child.

During ultrasound observation, Gianni, the name given to the baby, later, remained immobile, crouched in a corner of the womb, with his hands and his arms so tightly folded and crossed as to almost cover his face. His immobility seemed born out of tension, if not terror. With his arms raised above his head sheltering his eyes and face, he looked very much like a figure out of a painting by Munch.

When the term approached, he had not yet turned, and was still tightly crouched in a corner of the womb, in the transverse position. Since the child gave no sign of wanting to turn, and Mrs. B.'s blood pressure continued to rise, a caesarean section was decided upon. The obstetrician later told me that the child was so crumpled in a corner of the womb, that she had considerable difficulty pulling him out. She said, "He would never have been born." Once she had pulled him out, the obstetrician was also struck by his immobility, and by his fixed and sad look. "He looked old . . . 100 years old . . . it was somehow frightening to see the immobility of his face . . . "

During the next two months Gianni continued to be practically immobile. Whenever I saw him, his arms were kept at his sides, his head was bent backwards, his eyes were closed, and he seemed immersed in a deep sleep. When his mother put him to her breast, he sucked slowly, frowning, with his eyes tightly closed and his arms at his sides, but he also clung to the breast for hours on end.

When Gianni was six months old, his mother decided to go back to work. After that, she said: "I feel as if I am breathing again . . . he seems better too . . . " and funnily enough, while she was saying this, Gianni let out two heavy sighs which sounded like relief. Though his gaze continued to be rather fixed and vacant, Gianni sometimes looked at me and smiled. He also accompanied his mother's endless inquiries about gynaecology and sex with long constant sounds, which reminded me in their tone of the endless talking of his mother. His main contact with her was still the breast, and Mrs. B. continued breastfeeding him until he was ten months old. At the age of one year, Gianni looked rather backward in his development. Though he could certainly sit and apparently crawl, he preferred to sit in a corner, always holding the same toy, and almost never moving about. So far I have heard from him only sounds, and no words.

I think this case study clearly shows how the unborn child is assailed by his mother's anxiety, and how from the beginning, he tries to escape from it by moving into the furthest reaches of her womb. Of course, there is no escaping her obsessive ruminations, he is a helpless victim. He was not cared for lovingly, either before or after birth. His chances of developing into a normal adult are slim.

THE EFFECT OF POSITIVE PRENATAL COMMUNICATION ON THE UNBORN CHILD

There is a growing literature on affectionate communication, both verbally and non-verbally, with the unborn child, and its long-term beneficial effects on post-natal bonding and personality. Renee Van deCarr1[3] (1992), Donald Shetler[10] (1989), Thomas Verny[14] (1991) and William Sullenbach[11](1994) are just a few of the many scientists who have studied the impact of a systematic program of prenatal communication between parents and their unborn, usually along a multiplicity of modalities such as speech, touch, music and others.

In many studies of psychotherapy, in which regression is tolerated or encouraged, we find verbatim reports of good and bad womb experiences. Perhaps because most of the subjects are psychotherapy clients, the recovered memories are predominantly negative. However, there are still plenty of happy, blissful moments that are re-experienced vividly, especially in LSD Therapy ~ as described by Grof[17,] Kafkalides[5] and in the recent work of Piontelli, with which I would like to close my article.

Mrs. D., a woman in her late twenties, was expecting twins. In her first ultrasonographic session her little boy (Luke) seemed much more active than her daughter (Alicia). Luke kept turning and kicking and changing position and stretching his legs against the uterine wall. As his mother remarked, "Oh my God! ...look at him . . . he is so small, and he's already fed up with being in there. He conveyed the same impression to me. From time to time he would interrupt his motor activities and turn his attention towards his sister. He reached out with his hands, and through the dividing membrane he touched her face gently, and when she responded by turning her face towards him, he engaged with her for a while in a gentle, stroking, cheek-to-cheek motion. From then on they were nicknamed by us 'the kind twins'. His sister, Alicia, initiated contact less frequently than he. Most of the time she seemed asleep, or else moved her head and her hands slowly, almost imperceptibly, but each time responded to her brother's gentle stimulation.

Mr. D. was also present from the second observation. Rather shy and reserved, he was very gentle and loving.

After the delivery I went to visit her in hospital. Mrs. D. was very pleased to see me, and told me about the delivery, saying, "He came out first . . . then she came out too . . . their difference of weight is very noticeable . . . he is all skinny and bony and looks like a small bird . . . and their character, you know . . . just like we had seen inside . . . He's very lively and alert. You remember how he used to move and play all the time? She's completely different. She's very calm."

At one year of age they could walk, and were beginning to talk, and took a great delight in playing with each other. Their favourite game had become hiding behind a curtain, and using it a bit like a dividing membrane. Luke would put forward his hand through the curtain and Alicia would reach out with her head, and their mutual stroking began, accompanied by gurgles and smiles.

This case, though very much condensed from the original, clearly demonstrates the effects of positive parenting and a good mother-father relationship on the unborn child. Furthermore, it shows persuasively that prenates are not, as commonly believed, in a so-called state of primary narcissism, or, that they are autistic, i.e. non-interactive socially. The twins in Piontelli's study are very much interested in reaching out to each other. In fact, there is a stunning contrast between poor Gianni hiding in isolation in a corner of his mother's womb, and continuing to be reclusive after birth, and the "kind twins" playing with each other prior to and after birth.

SUMMARY

Every unborn child is bombarded in the womb by toxins that may be physical, chemical, hormonal or psychological in nature. At the same time, the unborn child is also the recipient of positive, nurturing and loving communications from its immediate environment, the mother, and the larger world outside the mother, such as father and siblings. The organic and emotional development of every child will be determined in a large measure by the balance between these opposing forces. I've attempted to examine maternal and paternal messages that were largely of a negative nature. The effect of positive prenatal parenting was briefly examined. Looking at this material, we are reminded of the overriding importance of conscious parenting.

Conscious parenting, in its most ideal sense, involves the following three principles:

[] Personal growth work by each future parent, to process any psychological complexes that may interfere with them becoming loving and caring parents.

[] An examination by each partner of their relationship to each other, and a willingness to engage in open and honest communication.

[] An appreciation of the essential humanity of the unborn child, and his or her need for love and affection, both pre and post-natally.

The future of mankind may well depend on how successful we are at conveying to the world this simple but powerful message: as you do unto your own unborn children, so will they do unto the world. Or, to put it in less biblical and more modern terms, there can be no world ecology without womb ecology.

REFERENCES

1. *Blomberg, S. (1980). Influence of maternal distress during pregnancy on post-natal development. Acta Psychiatrica Scandinavica, 62, 405-417.*
2. *Brezinka, C, O. Huter, W. Biebl, and J. Kinzl (1994). Denial of Pregnancy: obstetrical aspects, J. Psychosom. Obstet. Gynecol. 15, pp1-8.*
3. *Bustan, Muhammad N and Ann L. Coker (1994). Maternal Attitude toward Pregnancy and the Risk of Neonatal Death, Am J Publ Health, Vol. 4, No. 3 pp411-414.*
4. *David, Henry P., Zilenek Dybrich, Zilenek Matejcek & Vratislav Schüller (1988). Born Unwanted - Developmental Effects of Denied Abortion. Springer Publ. Co. New York.*
5. *Janus, Ludwig, (1991). Die frühe Ich-Entwicklung im Spiegel der LSD-Psychotherapie von Athannassios Kafkakalides, Z.f.Individualpsychol., 16. Jg., Ernst Reinhardt Verlag München Basel, S, 111-124.*
6. *McIntosh, Lisa J, Nabil E. Roumayah and Sidney F. Bottoms, (1995). Perinatal Outcome of Broken Marriage in the Inner City, Obstetrics & Gynecology, vol. 85, No. 2, pp233-236.*
7. *Myhrman, A (1986). Longitudinal studies on unwanted children. Scandinavian Journal*

of Social Medicine, 14, 57-59.

8. Piontelli, Alessandra (1987). Infant Observation from Before Birth. J. Psycho-Anal. (1987) 68, 453.

9. Piontelli, Alessandra (1989). A Study on Twins Before and After Birth. Int. J. Psycho-Anal (1989) 16, 413.

10. Shetler, Donald J (1989). The Inquiry into Prenatal Musical Experience: A Report of the Eastman Project 1980-1987, PPPJ, 3(3), pp 171-189.

11. Sullenbach, William B. (1994). Claira: A Case Study in Prenatal Learning. PPPJ, 9(1) pp33-56.

12. Taylor, David C. (1988). Oedipus's Parents were Child Abusers. Br. J. of Psychiatry, 153, 561-563.

13. Van deCarr, Renee, and M. Lehrer (1992). The prenatal classroom: A parents' guide for teaching your baby in the womb. Atlanta, GA, Humanics Learning.

14. Verny, Thomas and P. Weintraub (1991). Nurturing the Unborn Child:A Nine Month Program for soothing, stimulating and communicating with your Baby. Delacorte Press, New York.

15. Verny, Thomas R and John Kelly, (1981). The Secret Life of the Unborn Child, Summit Books, New York.

16. Wulfert, Kimberley Ann (1986). The Relationship Between A Primigravida's Belief System Regarding Childbirth and the Course and Outcome of Labour and Delivery. PhD Thesis, William Lyon Univ. 1986.

17. Grof, Stanislav (1976). The Realms of the Human Unconscious, E.P. Dutton & Co., New York.

Miscarriage
By Sara Simon

I miscarried my second pregnancy at the end of the first trimester whilst travelling in New Zealand, and it helped me greatly to keep a pen and paper by the bed. I scribbled pages and pages in the dark, sometimes with tears falling onto my words. Almost four years on, I've decided to share some of what I wrote in the hope that it might give some perspective to other mothers who lose a baby before they've even met. I no longer grieve, but I think about her often.

I hoped I'd never be in a position to write about this from experience, but now am strangely glad I can. I have experienced another facet of life. I understand something that so many women go through, but never tell. It's so often forgotten, pushed into the past, 'dealt with'. I've witnessed a complete cycle of life at once: birth and death ~ or death and birth?

Sometimes I can detach myself and tell myself that it's natural; that my body is doing the right thing; that this baby was never meant to be born. Other times I feel too unbearably sad about the death. I can feel so empty; like I will be sucked into the void inside me. I don't know how to deal with that. Of course both are right ~ feelings are never wrong. They are a natural part of the process, starting with conflicting ideas that gradually merge to make some kind of sense.

I've been given a leaflet called Understanding Miscarriage. It's very informative and helpful, but I can't take it all in, partly because I don't want to be told how I'm feeling, or how I will feel after this. Just as I will let my body deal with it naturally ~ it knows what to do ~ I want to trust that my mind and spirit can, too. I don't want anyone else messing with me.

As I lie awake feeling the cramps fill my belly, I'm actually welcoming them. This pregnancy has ended, so there's nothing I should cling to. The best stuff is in memory, anyway. I need to feel closure on these past days of bleeding, yet resting in the desperate hope that somehow I could keep it all in. The pain is not so upsetting any more ~ I welcome the passing into the next phase of my life. Everything IS as it's supposed to be. However you look at it: non-viable sperm/egg; problem with mum; spirit passed because it had already completed its mission on Earth ~ this experience will teach me something. I'm still entitled to grieve, and I will, for a long time. The dream has ended, the hope dashed, the excitement obliterated, the bond severed, a life ended. My husband says he feels some detachment, and is mostly sad for my loss. He's constantly there for me, without question. I didn't even look pregnant. I am so thankful that I have a son, already. I know I can carry a baby to term, and birth.

I told the world about my pregnancy ~ and miscarried at 12 weeks, after a week of bleeding. I don't regret telling them ~ I just have to be prepared for unwanted intrusion. I want to stay in my bubble for now. Well-meaning relatives don't need to ask how I'm coping; to look at me sympathetically, but not know what to say. I will find my own way of moving through the pain, and no outsider would have a clue about where I'm really at. I may seem to be working through it okay with those closest to me ~ partly to spare their helplessness ~ but I burst into tears when they go. My Mum is distraught. Part of me wishes I could just go to her and be mothered, but the other part is glad I'm so far away from everyone right now.

There's a tendency for people to expect a positive answer when asking how you are doing. We're expected to keep difficult emotions to ourselves. But this means that most of us don't know how to deal with the loss of a loved one. I couldn't even bear to be at my own cat's funeral, never mind a human being. How messed up is that?

I wish I had the strength to stop people who are just not helping ~ like the male medical student at the hospital who was clearly bluffing his way through. I had to report him for the sake of the next woman going through something like this. Sometimes you just need another woman! We need to educate the system about our emotional needs. We shouldn't have to say 'yes' when asked if we're okay, just to avoid unwanted awkwardness. Often, we just want a woman to bring a box of tissues and give us a hug while we cry. Sometimes we want to be left alone. Sometimes we just want to be listened to. All these things can be difficult to find when we're going through something so personal and devastating, and are afraid to say 'hold me'. We cry behind closed doors, and some of us have even forgotten how to. We're numb. After years of bottling up my feelings, it's a relief to feel that I deserve to feel this grief without judgement. I so need to cry.

In a perverse way, it is good. It's potentially a healing experience that's been presented to me. Do I feel I deserve it? Actually, yes ~ because I think that ultimately I will grow and be a better, more whole person for it. I can own this. I don't have to compare it with how others are feeling, like when a relative or friend dies. I'm learning more about myself.

I try to remember that we attach human and societal values to all our experiences. Other animals generally don't feel the same attachment to outcomes as we do. There are ways to keep things in perspective. I haven't lost my parents yet, but it's inevitable. This has made it real ~ I need to cherish the time they have left.

It felt so good to come home and breastfeed my son.

The hospital sonographer told me there was no baby in there, yet her little body filled the palm of my hand. What do they know? We buried her in a beautiful windswept place overlooking the sea, and decorated her grave with shells, flowers and a candle. We all said a few words, and I explained to Niall (age 2½) why Mummy cried a lot: I was sad that I would never meet Eve, but that I'd loved having her in my tummy. I wanted him to experience her death in a healthy way, and to have a way of remembering her.

I'm sure it was a girl. I felt a strong feminine presence in the night before the bleeding started, and the name 'Eve' was there over and over. This has helped my healing so much. My confidence in spirituality had been floundering for some time, and this experience has brought it back into focus.

I look at the sea, a river, the clouds, the changing seasons... the circle of life goes on. I think I've found my way back to the path, so to speak.

In the middle of the night when my mind is racing, it helps a lot to release my feelings onto paper. One day I'll type this up, if I can read it by the light of day.

Eve

My belly is empty now
But my heart will never be.
I thank you for being with me for those ten short weeks.
Your brother talked to and hugged you every day.
You warmed my belly and gave me joy in anticipation.

Then there was blood and pain
and finally the bittersweet taste of release.

They ask how I am coping...
How can I be bitter when in your short time here
you brought me so much?
You taught me how to cry again.
You were a gift and will be with me forever.
I love you.

The tears fall and I sob because I can.
There is nobody here to say
I should be brave for my son.
There are no people who think I'm 'losing it'
when I can smile with tears rolling down my face.

It is MY grief, MY loss, my honour.
I CAN FEEL. It is not good or bad, it is both pain and even joy,
it is mine and it is real.
Such love.

I think I 'knew' when your name came to me.
I feared the loss would kill me inside when I had to birth your tiny body,
but didn't know you would breathe such life into me as you passed.
Thank you.

Ultrasound: reasons for caution
By Dr. Sarah Buckley

Ultrasonography is a very recent technology, and was originally developed in World War II to detect enemy submarines. Its use in medicine was pioneered by Dr Ian Donald in Glasgow, who first used ultrasound to look at abdominal tumours, and later, babies in-utero, in the mid 1950s. (Oakley, 1986)

Ultrasound in pregnancy spread quickly, and developments in this technology have lead to the use of "real-time" (i.e. moving) images, as well as doppler ultrasound, which is used in specialised scans, foetal monitors and hand-held foetal stethoscopes ("sonicaids").

Even more recently, ultrasonographers have been using vaginal ultrasound, where the transducer (the equipment that sends out the ultrasound wave) is placed high in the vagina, much closer to the developing baby; and three dimensional ultrasound, which promises to show expectant parents their baby's face in-utero, but isn't used for routine scans .

Medical ultrasound uses equipment which sends waves with a frequency of 10 to 20 million cycles per second ~ well above audible sound, which is 10 to 20 thousand cycles per second ~ deep into the body. A picture of the underlying tissues is built up from the pattern of "echo" waves which return.

Ultrasound in pregnancy has become almost universal in Westernised health care systems.

Here in Australia, 99% of pregnant women have at least one scan, for which our federal government, via Medicare, pays part of the fee. In 1997-8, Medicare paid out $AU39 million for obstetric scans, compared to $54 million for all other obstetric Medicare costs. In the US, it's estimated that 90% of pregnant women are scanned, despite an official statement from ACOG that recommends against routine ultrasound. With each scan costing around $300, this represents a cost of approximately $1.2 billion by the 4 million women pregnant each year in America.

Ultrasound may be offered to a pregnant woman in two situations: either to investigate a possible problem at any stage of pregnancy, or as a routine scan at around 18 weeks. If there's bleeding in early pregnancy, for example, ultrasound may predict whether miscarriage is inevitable.

Later in pregnancy, ultrasound can be used when a baby isn't growing, or when a breech or twins are suspected. In these cases, the information gained from ultrasound can be very useful in decision-making, and generally most professionals in the area would support the use of ultrasound in this context.

However, the use of routine prenatal ultrasound (RPU) is more controversial, as this involves scanning all pregnant women in the hope of improving the outcome for some mothers and babies. When RPU is used, there are four main areas of information that can be gained.

First, a due date may be estimated. Dating is most accurate at the early stages of pregnancy, when babies vary the least in size. At 18 to 20 weeks, expected date of delivery (EDD) is accurate to within a week either side. Some studies have suggested that an early examination, or a woman's dates, can be as accurate as RPU. (Olsen and Clausen, 1997; Kieler et al, 1993)

Second, ultrasound is used to discover unsuspected physical abnormalities. While many women are reassured by a normal scan, in fact RPU detects only between 17% and 85% of the 1 in 50 babies that have major abnormalities at birth. (Ewigman 1993, Luck 1992)

A recent study from Brisbane, Australia, showed that ultrasound at a major women's hospital missed around 40% of abnormalities, with many of these being difficult or impossible to detect. (Chan et al, 1997)

Major causes of intellectual disability such as cerebral palsy and Down's syndrome, are unlikely to be picked up on a routine scan, as are heart and kidney abnormalities.

When an abnormality is detected, there's a small chance that the finding is a "false positive" diagnosis, where the ultrasound is wrong, and the baby is, in fact, normal.

A UK survey showed that 1 in 200 babies aborted for major abnormalities were, in fact, normal. (Brand 1994)

There are also many cases of error with more minor abnormalities, which can cause anxiety and repeated scans, as well as conditions which have been seen to spontaneously resolve. (e.g. see Saari-Kemppainen 1990)

As well as false positives, there are also uncertain cases, where the ultrasound image cannot be easily interpreted, and the outcome for the baby is not known. In one study involving women at high risk, almost 10% of scans were uncertain. (Sparling et al, 1988)

This can create immense anxiety for the woman and her family, and the worry may not be allayed by the birth of a normal baby.

In the same study, mothers with "questionable" diagnoses still had this anxiety three months after the birth of their baby.

In some cases of uncertainty, the doubt can be resolved by further tests, such as amniocentesis. In this situation, there may be up to two weeks wait for results, during which time a mother has to decide if she would terminate the pregnancy if an abnormality is found. Even mothers who receive reassuring news have felt that this process has interfered with their relationship with their baby. (see Brookes, 1995)

The third area in which ultrasound can give information is location of the placenta. A placenta which is very low-lying at birth (placenta praevia) puts mother and baby at risk of severe bleeding, and usually necessitates a caesarean section.

However, 19 out of 20 women who have placenta praevia detected on RPU will be needlessly worried: the placenta will effectively move up, and not cause problems at the birth. (MIDIRS, 1995) Furthermore, detection of placenta praevia by RPU has not been found to be safer than detection in labour. (Saari-Kemppainen, 1990)

Lastly, ultrasound can detect the presence of more than one baby at an early stage of pregnancy.

Again, there are no documented health advantages for mother or babies, and, without RPU, almost all multiple pregnancies are discovered before birth. (MIDIRS, 1996)

Supporters of RPU argue that availability of this information should lead to better outcomes for mother and baby.

While this would seem logical, researchers have not found evidence of significant benefit from RPU, and the issue of the safety of ultrasound has not yet been resolved.

From a research perspective, the most significant benefit of RPU is a small reduction in perinatal mortality ~ the number of babies dying around the time of birth. However, this is a statistical, rather than a genuine reduction.

When a baby is found to have a fatal abnormality on RPU, and the pregnancy is terminated, perinatal mortality is improved because deaths below five to six months gestation are not counted in perinatal mortality statistics.

Supporters of RPU presume that early diagnosis and termination is beneficial to the affected woman and her family. However, the discovery of a major abnormality on RPU can lead to very difficult decision-making. Some women who agree to have an ultrasound are unaware that they may get information about their baby that they do not want, as they would not contemplate a termination.

Other women can feel pressured to have a termination, or at the least feel some emotional distancing from their "abnormal" baby. (Brookes, 1995)

Furthermore, there's no evidence that women who have chosen termination are, in the long-term, psychologically better off than women whose affected baby has died at birth. In fact, there are suggestions that the reverse may be true, in some cases. (Watkins, 1989)

In choosing a possible stillbirth over a termination, women at least get social acknowledgement and support, and are able to grieve openly.

Where termination has been chosen, women are unlikely to share their story with others, and can experience considerable guilt and pain from the knowledge that they themselves chose the loss. (MIDIRS, 1996)

When minor abnormalities are found, women can feel that some of the pleasure has been taken away from their pregnancy. Occasionally, minor abnormalities found on RPU have been seen to spontaneously resolve. Another quoted benefit of RPU is a reduced risk of being induced for being "overdue", due to more certainty with RPU dating.

Around one in five women have their dates changed by scan, and usually the date is put later. (MIDIRS, 1996) There is, as yet, no clear evidence that this leads to less women being induced, and the chance of induction is more determined by hospital or doctor policy than by availability of RPU. (MIDIRS, 1996)

Many supporters of RPU claim that it's a pleasurable experience, and contributes to "bonding" between mother (and father if he is present) and baby.

While it's true that it can be exciting to get a first glimpse of one's baby in-utero, there is no evidence that it helps attachment or encourages healthier behaviour towards the baby. (MIDIRS, 1996)

Ultrasound waves are known to affect tissues in at least two ways.

First, the sonar beam causes heating of the highlighted area by about one degree celsius. This is presumed to be non-significant, based on whole-body heating in pregnancy, which seems to be safe up to 2.5 degrees celsius. (Am Inst of Ultrasound Medicine Bioeffects Report, 1988)

The second recognised effect is cavitation, where the small pockets of gas which exist within mammalian tissue vibrate, and then collapse.

In this situation "…temperatures of many thousands of degrees celsius in the gas create a wide range of chemical products, some of which are potentially toxic." (Am Inst of Ultrasound Medicine Bioeffects Report, 1988) The significance of cavitation effects in human tissue is unknown.

A number of studies have suggested that these effects are of real concern in living tissues. The first study suggesting problems was a study on cells grown in the lab. Cell abnormalities caused by exposure to ultrasound were seen to persist for several generations. (Liebeskind, 1979)

Another study showed that, in newborn rats (which are at a similar stage of brain development to humans at 4 to 5 months in-utero), ultrasound can damage the myelin that covers nerves, (Ellisman, 1987) indicating that the nervous system may be particularly susceptible to damage from this technology.

A 1999 animal study by Brennan and colleagues, reported in New Scientist (June 12, 1999), showed that exposing mice to dosages typical of obstetric ultrasound caused a 22% reduction in the rate of cell division, and a doubling of the rate of cell death in the cells of the small intestine.

Studies on humans exposed to ultrasound have shown that possible adverse effects include premature ovulation (Testart, 1982); preterm labour or miscarriage (Lorenz, 1990; Saari-Kemppainen; 1990); low birth weight (Newnham, 1993); poorer condition at birth (Thacker 1985; Newnham, 1991); dyslexia (Stark et al, 1984); delayed speech development (Campbell, 1993); and less right-handedness (Salvesen et al, 1993: Kieler et al 1998).

Non right-handedness is, in other circumstances, seen as a marker of damage to the developing brain. One Australian study showed that babies exposed to five or more ultrasounds were 30% more likely to develop intrauterine growth retardation (IUGR) ~ a condition that ultrasound is often used to detect. (Newnham, 1993)

Two long-term randomised controlled trials, comparing exposed and unexposed children's development at 8 to 9 years old, found no measurable effect from ultrasound. (Salvesen et al, 1992; Kieler et al, 1998) However, as the authors note, intensities used today are many times higher than in 1979 to 1981. Further, in one of these trials

(Salvensen, 1993), scanning time was only three minutes.

More studies are obviously needed in this area, particularly in the area of Doppler ultrasound, where exposure levels are much higher, and in vaginal ultrasound, where there is less tissue shielding the baby from the transducer.

A further problem with studying ultrasound's effect is the huge range of output, or dose, possible from a single machine. Modern machines can give comparable ultrasound pictures using a lower, or a 5,000 times higher dose (Meire, 1987), and there are no standards to ensure that the lowest dose is used. Because of the complexity of machines, it's difficult to even quantify the dose given in each examination. (Taylor, 1990)

In the US, as in Australia, training is voluntary (even for obstetricians), and the skill and experience of operators varies widely.

In all the research done on ultrasound, there's been very little interest in women's opinions of RPU, and the consequences of universal scanning for a woman's experience of pregnancy.

In The Tentative Pregnancy, Barbara Katz Rothman's thoughtful book on prenatal diagnosis, the author suggests that the large numbers of screening tests currently being offered to check for abnormalities makes every pregnancy 'tentative' until reassuring results come back.

Ultrasound is not compulsory, and I suggest that each woman consider the risks, benefits and implications of scanning for her own particular situation.

If you decide to have a scan, be clear about the information that you do and do not want to be told. Have your scan done by an operator with a high level of skill and experience (usually this means performing at least 750 scans per year), and say that you want the shortest scan possible.

If an abnormality is found, ask for counselling, and a second opinion, as soon as practical.

And remember that it's your baby, and your choice.

Birth

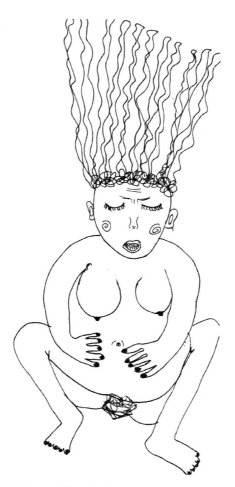

Squat and birth, by Eliza Robinson

Shamanic Midwifery:
hands that heal birth
By Jeannine Parvati Baker

I first heard my call to assist women becoming mothers, to realise birth as a spiritual, as well as a natural, rite-of-passage, by birthing my own babies consciously.

My initiation in giving natural birth was in January of 1970. It was the first time an obstetrician had seen a woman squat on the delivery table to give birth. Postpartum, when I wouldn't be separated from my newborn, Loi Caitlin (as they had no rooming-in arrangement), they put me back in the labour room with my baby.

A labouring mother in the next bed was screaming, "Ah Dios, Dios!" How she suffered: my heart went out to her, and I soothed her from my bed, my first experience as a spiritual midwife.

About this time in my life, I began to teach childbirth education and prenatal yoga classes. My goal was to help more babies be born consciously ~ thus, creating a sustainable future for my own child ~ and future grandchildren.

I had a significant dream during these years. In my dream, two brilliant white doves flew to me.

I watched them land on my hands, and when they walked from my hands, now tingling with energy, up my arms, to my heart, I was filled with radiant light. I understood at that time that my hands and heart were agents of the healing light.

It was a while later that I met this archetype in the Greek myth of the two midwives who flew to the birth of the twins, Artemis and Apollo, in the form of doves.

By then, I was well known as the "baby lady" of my community, and preparing for my next challenge in reclaiming birth.

My second and third births were twins, and when I was in the hospital, they x-rayed me and announced that my pelvis may be too small, and I would need a caesarean section.

I checked myself out of the hospital, and went home to give ecstatic birth to my footling breech baby, Oceana Violet, and her head-first twin, Cheyenne Coral.

From that point on, 1974, I have only birthed and midwifed at home. I clearly saw what a distraction hospitals can be when giving birth.

After my third birth, I understood that I needn't hire anyone to be paranoid for me when labouring to bring forth my young.

In 1975, I became a spiritual midwife whose main tools are my faith in the naturalness of birth, my healing hands, and word medicine. My community made me a midwife, by asking me to attend births.

Rather than getting trained by an institution, and learning a medical set of rituals to take women through birth, I apprenticed directly to birth itself. My promise as spiritual midwife is to honour the journey, be attentive to what presents itself, and remind a mother by my presence that she already knows how to give birth.

I trust that if a woman consciously conceives her baby without the help of experts, she is able to give birth unassisted by the medical experts. My "back-up" is whatever God-Us is "on call" that night ~ in over a generation of attending births, every woman I have midwifed has given spontaneous birth.

Once, I was called to a birth and forgot to bring my birthing kit. Then I realised that I am my midwifery kit ~ I had my ears through which I could hear the baby's heart, I had my hands through which I could feel the baby, and I had my heart ~ which loves the baby Earthside.

After that experience in 1980, I founded HYGIEIA COLLEGE, a mystery school in womancraft and lay midwifery. I teach the "inward skills" ~ how to cultivate intuition, and know our embodied perception is the medicine bundle or midwifery kit, par excellence.

At this writing, mid '90s, there are over 600 students currently enrolled in Hygieia College, studying an essential midwifery which locates the power to give birth in the God-Us ~ a divine life-force which brings our babies to the light.

It's an international mystery school which, I am proud to say, graduates midwives who practise differently than I. Each midwife serves her own community, and is responsive to what is best-for-life in the moment. Rather than a method, or a training course, Hygieia College is a journey to the sources of healing, and an un-training of erroneous beliefs and actions which interfere with spontaneous childbirth. I see this un-training process akin to removing the mind-swaddling of the prevailing technocratic culture. From attending birth mindfully, I recognised that there's a lot of work to be done to heal fertility, specifically the abortion epidemic, and on the other extreme, infertility. Women who've had abortions, as well as those who've had difficulty conceiving, are more likely to have difficulties surrendering to the power of the birth-force.

In 1986, my partner, Frederick Baker, and I, published the tome Conscious Conception: Elemental Journey through the Labyrinth of Sexuality. In this book we articulate the practice of fertility awareness as an opportunity for self-realisation, in the specific focus of fertility.

My work in spiritual midwifery includes conscious conception, and I often connect with a family before they conceive their baby, in the capacity of midwife.

What I notice is that a baby who's consciously conceived, who's desired by both mother and father, already has the foundation for health, wholeness and holiness in place.

A baby who's not wanted, on the other hand, is spiritually handicapped in that their Source, the Earthly mother and father, are disconnected. Children who are not wanted are more likely to be abused, and "act out" for negative attention ~ for it's better to be wanted by the police, than not at all.

According to research reports, babies who are born in violence (standard obstetrical management of birth in hospital) are more likely to be involved in violent crimes as youths and adults. (See the Jonn Vascocellos congressional report from California.)

My work in conscious conception, toward making every baby a wanted baby (rather than a mistake in a contraceptive method), contributes to a more peaceful society.

My firstborn son, and fourth baby, Gannon Hamilton, was our first freebirth. We didn't pay anyone to be responsible for our baby's birth, and in 1980, my partner ~ the baby's father ~ and I experienced a most powerful spiritual initiation. There were no other adults present to distract us from the immense sexual bonding of the original lovers greeting their newborn together.

The Holy Trinity has new meaning for us since Gannon's birth ~ Mother/Father/Baby. And we honoured the Son as he is ~ already enlightened, whole, perfect. Needless to say, no circumcision.

When I conceived and birthed my fifth baby, Quinn Ambriel, in 1985-86, I prepared for these experiences as a vision quest. I was given a vision which has sustained me spiritually ever since. When I ecstatically gave birth underwater to my fifth baby, Quinn, I saw every mother on this Earth giving birth with her lover between her legs ~ in a unique, and creative expression of love. No masked man, no paid paranoid in attendance ~ only the original lovers who first invited the new one to join them in holy family. I see this as central to what will bring peace and an authentic self-sufficiency to the world.

Once parents birth their own babies, in a balanced partnership, they know they can also take care of this baby. The trust that is established in a freebirth, a delivery free of MANipulation and medical control, lasts a lifetime. The fear-based imprint of hospital birth is "the institution will take care of me."

The consequence is socialised welfare ~ the institution of government taking care of our own responsibilities.

Again, the experience of being my own midwife has made me freer ever since, and the sequel of homebirth naturally follows: natural healing at home (no paediatricians), homeschool (no teachers), and the living experience of spirit (no churches).

We do not rely on institutions to mediate or make life safe for us. Birth is as safe as life gets.

As a spiritual midwife, my primary responsibility is to empower the mother to give birth spontaneously. The tendency is to enrol in the cult of experts who say, "I know more about your body than you do."

My responsibility as a healer is to return any projections of power upon me to the family I'm serving. The truth is that I am not medically nor surgically skilled ~ I cannot deliver a mother's baby for her. Rather, I remind the mother that she's the only one able to give birth (her other option is to be delivered) ~ and I support her every way I can. In this way, I am able to respond to my original calling: to be the guardian at the gate.

To aspiring healers who are called to attend childbirth, I advise the following: first, midwife, heal thyself. Next, do no harm.

Remember your own birth, and forgive any trespasses upon your soul. And always, listen to the still, small voice within ~ and the voices of countless mothers before who gave birth with dignity, and as a natural expression of sexuality.

Last, realise that mothers who give freebirth can connect with the Source of all creation and be the God-Us in action.

It's an honour to see the original face of any new one. Each baby born holds the light very purely, and as a spiritual midwife, I greet the new one with celebration and gratitude for the ordinary miracle of birth.

Humility, patience, trust, integrity ~ these qualities are essential to a spiritual midwifery practice. I was called as a young woman, myself, yet traditionally it is the grandmothers who are asked by Spirit to be midwives.

Now that I'm a grandmother, I see the wisdom in first being seasoned by life before answering the call.

Therefore, I encourage young midwives to be who we really are ~ if we have children, to give a living model to the families we serve by being real mothers, and taking care of our own children.

Hygieia College was founded, in part, to meet the needs of mothers desiring to increase the upward mobility of their minds as mothers. Our college holds all gatherings and workshops with children not only invited, but honoured.

At the edge of the millennium, more midwives are being ordained by the God-Us to heal birth without being indoctrinated nor controlled by medical licensure. In that legal definition of a licence, is permission to do what society considers "dangerous or immoral" We are choosing to be midwives based on authentic need. Homebirth is not dangerous or immoral ~ actually, the converse is true ~ hospital birth is dangerous and immoral. The US is 20th in the World Health Organization's statistics on perinatal mortality and morbidity.

In other words, there are 20 other countries in the world where it's safer to give birth than in an American hospital. The other countries with better statistics almost exclusively use midwives rather than doctors.

But what about the "consumer" or "patient" ~ do they not need protection?

Let me clarify that I'm not suggesting a "buyer beware" attitude toward midwifery. If a midwife is capable, she will stay in practice. If a midwife is not serving her community, she will eventually not be asked to attend any more.

We do not need the State in our bedroom; for indeed, birth is a woman's expression of sexuality ~ and in my practice, not under legal or medical jurisdiction.

Traditionally, midwives are the wise women, the herbalists and psychologists of their communities. They knew who was sleeping in whose lodge ~ and being attentive to the sexual dynamics of their communities, could facilitate the sexual energy of birth.

A major eradication of wise women took place in the Dark Ages, and most midwives were destroyed as "witches". It has taken a long time for a renaissance in birth to occur. Midwives today must be courageous to practice in our constrictive and litigious climate.

Sometimes the most courageous amongst us are targets of litigation.

Midwives need the support of the entire healing community to face the challenges ahead.

In 1986, I gave birth underwater to my last baby, Halley Sophia. As in our last three births, we hired no expert to attend "just in case". All my work is devoted to making every mother a midwife ~ so I practise what I preach.

I live in a state where parents have the right to choose where and with whom they give birth, so we broke no law.

Yet, in my neighbourhood there was an unease, which, in my pregnant, intuitive condition, I sensed.

I went to my neighbour's church on a fast and testimony meeting day, and addressed the congregation all at once. I said, "I have prayed about this birth, and have been told that being home is our sacred place. However, I have one fear, and that is, if something goes wrong in this birth, I'm concerned what you would think. So, I now ask that you pray for a perfect delivery at home."

After the meeting, the very ones who'd been in the most fear about our upcoming unattended birth, now were enrolled as allies, for they soothed me with stories of their own relations' various births at home, and promised to pray for us. With all these prayers, during Halley's ecstatic birth, I had a vision where I had eyes all over my body and could "see" multi-dimensionally.

I realised that I was like the White Hole in astrophysics ~ that source point where something new comes into material existence, the opposite of a Black Hole. My uterus is the Universe ~ I am the stargate.

As mother, I am the means by which life creatively expresses itself, and giving freebirth is akin to the origin of stars. In other words, I know how God-Us must've felt giving birth to the Universe.

How can my personal experiences in birth serve the world now? One idea of how evolution works is the morphogenetic field theory of Rupert Sheldrake. It has been popularised by Ken Keyes in his book, The Hundredth Monkey.

What this idea states is that there are leaps of evolution, for an entire species, which occur simultaneously amongst all members regardless of geographic location.

In regards to childbirth, I observe the phenomenon of morphic resonance in this way ~ more and more families are choosing to freebirth, all over the world. When a critical mass is reached of ecstatic rather than suffering birth, there just may be a leap of faith.

All mothers may remember that
we're co-creators of life
and have totally within each of us
the capacity to show the world what our
love looks like
in the
form of a baby.

Whenever I give a talk or workshop, I imagine that the one mother who is the "critical mass" for freebirth may be attending, and inspired by my word medicine to reclaim birth.

Indeed, each mother I speak with, in my mind, is the hundredth monkey, a change agent for evolution, as well as the God-Us incarnate. For as the canon of Hygieia College states, Healing One Mother is Healing the Earth. Blessed Be the Babies!!

A baby who is not wanted...
is spiritually handicapped in that their Source,
the Earthly mother and father,
are disconnected.
Children who are not wanted
are more likely to be abused,
and "act out" for negative attention
~ for it is better to be wanted by the police, than not at all.

Orgasmic childbirth:
an interview with Laura Shanley, author of Unassisted Childbirth.

Veronika: Some people wonder how you can possibly use a pleasurable sexual experience like orgasm to describe what most people know (from experience) to be an excruciatingly painful event in a woman's life. When did you first come across the idea, indeed the experience, of women who've had pleasurable births? What does an orgasmic birth really mean?

Laura: I first learned about orgasmic childbirth when I was a sophomore in college. My roommate and I were discussing the concept of painless birth when she said, "My Mom actually had an orgasm when she was giving birth to me."

In the years since then, I've come across this phenomenon again and again in books, newsletters, and magazines. I think it's much more common than people realise, although it certainly isn't the norm. Some people have speculated that the orgasm is triggered by the baby moving over the G spot, the clitoris, or another sexually sensitive area. It's also possible that the intensity of the contractions can bring on orgasm. It's a known fact that intense menstrual cramps can cause a woman to have an orgasm, so it doesn't surprise me that childbirth can, as well.

However, when I talk about orgasmic childbirth, I'm not only referring to the small number of women who spontaneously experience orgasms in labour. Many women bring themselves to orgasm in labour. It's almost impossible to experience pain and pleasure at the same time. So sexual stimulation can be a wonderful way to alleviate labour pain. It also increases blood flow to the uterus and vagina, which makes for an easier birth. And last but not least, it produces a wonderful feeling of relaxation. Ann Douglas and John R. Sussman, M.D., authors of the book The Unofficial Guide to Having a Baby, claim that a single orgasm is thought to be 22 times more relaxing than the average tranquiliser. When you add to this the fact that the average vagina widens 2" during sexual arousal, it only makes sense to fantasise, masturbate or make love in labour ~ that is, if a woman feels motivated to do it.

Even if a woman doesn't have an orgasm in labour, she can still benefit from having sex with her partner. It's a little known fact that there's a hormone in semen called relaxin which softens the cervix and lengthens the pelvic ligaments. During conception, it softens the cervix to allow the sperm to easily pass into the womb, and during labour it can soften the cervix to allow the baby to easily pass into the world.

Veronika: How can a woman create for herself a pleasurable childbirth (with or without orgasm)?

Laura: Birth, like all bodily functions, is designed to be pleasurable. Most women, however, are unable to experience it this way primarily due to fear. Grantly Dick-Read, author of Childbirth Without Fear, explained it in this way: when a woman is in a state of fear, messages are sent to the body telling it there is a danger out there that must be fought or run away from. Blood and oxygen are instantly sent into the arms and legs, enabling the frightened woman to fight the danger or run away. In order for this to happen, however, blood and oxygen must be drained from other organs which the body considers non-essential for fight or flight. This is why we turn white when we're afraid. The body assumes that our leg muscles need blood and oxygen more than our face does.

Unfortunately, when it comes to fight or flight, the uterus is considered a non-essential organ. According to Dick-Read, the uterus of a frightened woman in labour is literally white. Because it is deprived of "fuel" ~ blood and oxygen ~ it cannot function correctly, nor can waste products be properly carried away. Hence, the labouring woman experiences not only pain, but a multitude of problems. The solution, he believed, was twofold: "Not only do women need to stop being afraid, but doctors need to stop interfering in the process."

Labouring women do not need to be poked, prodded, and drugged. Instead, they need to be calmly encouraged, or simply left alone so their bodies may work unhindered. When we allow our bodies to work the way they were designed, birth becomes a pleasurable experience.

Veronika: Have you heard of women who've had an orgasmic childbirth in a hospital setting in the presence of staff, or is it, to your knowledge, a gift bestowed upon those who birth at home?

Laura: I know of several women who've had orgasmic births in hospitals, but overall, I would say it's more likely to happen at home because of the privacy factor.

Veronika: Women who've experienced a traumatic birth often need to talk or write about it in order to heal themselves....and to move on in their life. Unfortunately, what most often happens is the message that "Childbirth is Traumatic/Painful" is continued. Indeed, the woman is not healed. How can we change this pattern? That is, nurture and honour a woman's painful experience, and help her to move forward, to empower herself and to choose another way if she desires?

Laura: In order for a woman to heal from a bad birth experience, she needs to take responsibility for it. Certainly, doctors, nurses, and even midwives can traumatise a woman in birth. But the bottom line is, no-one forced the woman to put herself in their hands. By continuing to blame the medical establishment for our trauma, we're actually perpetuating it. We need to forgive them for their ignorance, and more importantly, we need to forgive ourselves. All of us have been raised in a culture that fears birth. It's understandable that we would have problems. Birth attendants who insist on subjecting women to dangerous and unnecessary interventions generally feel they're helping women. Many of us know they're not.

Veronika: Childbirth is a sexual experience ~ a continuum of our sexual nature as women. And sex itself is undoubtedly one of life's more pleasurable experiences. Yet for many people the reverse is also true. It isn't just women who've suffered sexually. So have men. I believe women are more likely to verbalise their past experiences. How does the average man deal with this jungle of unexplored terrain prior to his partner's birth? And does he need to in order for a woman to give birth easily?

Laura: As strange as it may sound, I believe men actually have more sexual trauma to deal with, because of circumcision. And to make things worse, because the trauma isn't consciously remembered, many men refuse to acknowledge it. I've often heard men say, "I was circumcised and I turned out fine." But the fact is, the emotional scars remain. Still, those who are willing can heal from the trauma ~

whether it occurred during circumcision or later in life ~ using the principles of forgiveness mentioned above.

If a man doesn't choose to face his sexual traumas, however, I believe his partner can still have a good birth. But she will have to look more within herself for support, rather than relying on her partner.

Veronika: In my own experience, I've seen many women who've wanted a waterbirth, for example, and their mother or partner has been hesitant (usually because they don't understand the breathing mechanism of a baby). Time and time again I've seen these same women forfeiting their ideal birth (subconsciously) because of the transferred fears of someone else.

Laura: The difference between an intervention-free birth and a medical birth is almost always fear. This is where we need to heal. I agree. It's sad to see a woman give up her dreams out of a misplaced respect for her partner's wishes. But often, he's merely reflecting her own unfaced fears of birth. If a woman truly believes in her own abilities, she will go through with her desired birth in spite of her partner's objections.

Veronika: It seems to me that women who are comfortable with their menstrual cycle, and indeed celebrate their Moontime and body, approach childbirth similarly.

Laura: Yes, and by that same token, women who are comfortable with their bodily functions (elimination) and their sexuality, do better in birth than those who aren't. Unfortunately, many women are taught to believe that their bodily functions are shameful, and that sex is dirty. This belief can manifest itself in numerous ways, not the least of which is a difficult childbirth.

Thankfully, we can change what we believe about our bodies, and rid ourselves of fear, shame, and guilt. In my own life, I've accomplished this through the use of visualisations and affirmations.

Veronika: I've noticed that when a woman has had a difficult time birthing, family and friends who report it seem to 'enjoy' perpetuating the 'Childbirth is Painful/Dangerous' tag.

Laura: For some people, pain is a badge of courage, something to be proud of: "Oh, look what I (or my friend or relative) endured for the sake of a child!" For others, it's a way of purging themselves of guilt. But suffering in birth doesn't help anyone.

As far as family and friends perpetuating the idea that childbirth is dangerous, this allows them to continue justifying their devotion to doctors and other authority figures. In doing so, they avoid facing their own fears of accepting responsibility for their health and their lives.

Veronika: Your book Unassisted Childbirth has been a God-send for so many women, myself included. When I read it, I kept thinking, "Yes. Yes. Yes!" And yet my own mother had three unassisted home births herself. It wasn't a new idea to me, but seeing the message in black and white ~ in public ~ gave it a new slant. Do you think the average woman who chooses an unassisted birth does so because of a previous traumatic birth or simply because it feels right from the word go?

Laura: Unfortunately, many women come to unassisted childbirth (UC) only after enduring a traumatic, medically-managed birth. Others, however, come to it after successfully giving birth with doctors or midwives. Rather than crediting their attendants with the successful outcome, these women credit themselves, and see no reason why they can't do it unassisted next time. And still others choose UC for their first birth simply because, as you said, it feels right.

Veronika: Why did you write Unassisted Childbirth? What have you learnt since having your children and publishing your book? Is there anything you would do differently?

Laura: My births were such incredible, life-changing experiences, I couldn't help sharing my feelings with other people. Long before I wrote the book, I had begun telling people about them. Then during my pregnancy with my third child, in 1982, I felt compelled to write an article.

Much to my dismay, however, no-one wanted to publish it. It was finally published by a magazine called Reality Change in 1991. The following year, I received a catalogue from Bergin & Garvey (somehow I had gotten on their mailing list) with books by Michel Odent and Nancy Wainer Cohen. From the description of the books, it felt to me that these authors were one step away from advocating unassisted childbirth. I sent Bergin & Garvey my one published article, along with a book proposal, and lo and behold, they accepted it!

As far as what I've learned since its publication, I've learned that I'm not alone. Women all over the world (whether or not they're aware of my book) are discovering the truth about birth, and the joy of believing in their own abilities. I've also learned that giving birth to a child is a lot easier than raising one! That, for me, has been a greater challenge.

Laura: Would I do anything differently? As far as the births, no. All of them were wonderful. As far as the rest of my life, yes, but I'll save that for my next book.

Veronika: The birth presentation of some of your babies could have left a doctor or midwife in a panic. Yet you managed just fine. Why? Can you describe each of your births?

Laura: My first three babies were born in the "wrong" position: face first, breech, and posterior. However, other than my breech birth, I wasn't aware (at that time) that babies weren't "supposed" to be born this way. My ignorance, in this case, was probably beneficial. I didn't panic, and therefore didn't trigger the fight/flight response. Consequently my babies were born easily.

I went into labour with my first child, John, on his "due date". It was about three in the afternoon, and at first I thought it was gas pains. About midnight, I lost my mucus plug and knew it was the real thing.

We called up several of our friends who had wanted to be at the birth, along with a filmmaker who was making a film about us. I took a shower, and basically just relaxed. The contractions weren't painless, but they weren't anything I couldn't handle. It was very clear to me that I shouldn't interfere in any way, nor should I let anyone touch me "down there". With this birth, I had no desire for sex. About 1.30, I was sitting on the toilet, when my water bag broke. Seconds later, my body began pushing. After two or three involuntary pushes, I felt the baby's face at my perineum, and decided I'd better get over to the bed. I was on my hands and knees and was about to turn over (since I thought women were supposed to give birth on their backs), when I heard a voice inside my head say, "Don't turn over." I didn't, and a second later, John came flying out. My husband, David, caught him in mid-air. I believe I may have torn slightly, although believe it or not, I never checked. In any case, I healed fine. About 45 minutes later, I delivered the placenta into the toilet.

When I became pregnant with my second child, I decided I would give birth on my hands and knees, since that had worked so well with John. But in a dream, I was told otherwise.

In the dream, I was watching a woman giving birth standing up. She was straddling a little plastic baby bathtub, and catching the baby herself. As I watched her, I heard another woman very gently say to me, "Tell her to remember not to do too much." I understood what the woman was saying, and the peaceful feeling of the dream stayed with me for the remainder of my pregnancy. I want to say, at this point, that I don't follow every dream I have, but this dream was different. It seemed to be coming from the deepest part of my being.

And so, I decided to follow it faithfully ~ I would catch my baby myself as I stood over my little bathtub, and I would move out of the way, and essentially do nothing to interfere with the process.

On the morning of August 17, 1980, I began to feel contractions. David and I made love, and I remember feeling an orgasm, followed immediately by a contraction. The rhythmic contracting of my uterus during the orgasm felt almost identical to that of the contraction. They seemed to have the same pattern (although, I must admit that the orgasm felt better!).

A few minutes later, I was walking across the room, when my water bag broke. I took out my little bathtub, and stood over it as I had been shown in the dream. At that point, I couldn't feel the contractions, but I knew I was having them because when I put my hand inside my vagina, I could feel my pelvic muscles rhythmically contracting around it.

A few minutes later, a foot appeared between my legs. I wasn't expecting a breech birth, although a friend of mine told me during my pregnancy that he had dreamt he saw the baby inside me standing right-side-up.

David and I said belief suggestions that everything would be all right, and then we patiently waited for Willie to be born. Little by little his foot got lower, and soon his other foot popped out. When I felt the time was right, I gave one push, and gently pulled him out by the feet. David and John had been in the other room, but walked in just as Willie emerged.

David yelled excitedly, "You did it!", and Willie immediately began to nurse.

(Incidentally, twelve years later I read that Michel Odent says that for a breech delivery a woman should always be in a "standing squat" or "upright" position, and an attendant should do absolutely nothing to interfere if at all possible. This had been the message of the dream.)

Soon after the birth, I dreamt that Willie was speaking to me. He told me that part of the reason his birth had been so fast and easy (he was born two hours after the first contraction) was that he hadn't been afraid either. Babies are always picking up on our beliefs, both before and after birth, so <u>a fearless mother means a fearless baby.</u>

When I became pregnant again a year and a half later, I thought I might like to give birth alone. As it turned out, David was at the campus library on the morning of November 17, 1982, and the boys were sleeping when I felt my first real contractions.

I took a shower, and allowed myself to relax as much as possible. The water was soothing, and soon I felt that the birth was imminent. I took out my little baby bathtub, and straddled it. I didn't push, as I'd already learned from my other births that birth works best when it's "allowed" to happen, rather than "made" to happen.

Slowly, the baby's head appeared, with the water bag still intact. It broke as the rest of her body gently slid into my hands. She looked straight up at me with a gaze that defied her age. Instantly, we knew each other. The thought went through my mind that she was the most beautiful gift I'd ever received.

Never have I felt the bond between mother and child as intensely as I did in that moment.

I wrapped her up in a big towel, and set her down in her baby seat. The placenta slid into the baby bathtub, and I tied and cut her cord.

For the next hour, I laid on the couch with her peacefully sleeping by my side. Soft bells and the sound of ocean waves filled my head.

This, I thought, must be what Grantly Dick-Read meant when he said childbirth gives a woman a feeling of exhaltation.

Michelle's birth, four years later, was about as easy as they get.

On a Sunday morning, at about 7 am, I began feeling contractions. David got up and went out on the couch to read the paper. I didn't tell him I was in labour. As with Joy's birth, I wanted solitude. As I lay in bed, I said belief suggestions that I was totally co-operating with my body. "I'm not fighting this in any way."

I felt myself slip into a state of complete relaxation. There was not a tense muscle in my entire body. At 8.15, I got up and walked across the hall to the bathroom. "You taking a bath?" David asked. "Yes," I answered, still not informing him that I was in labour. I turned on the bath water, sat down on the toilet, and noticed the water bag between my legs.

It popped, and seconds later a head appeared. I gave a little push and Michelle slid into my hands. The cord was wrapped loosely around her neck, and I unwound it. She gave a little cry and immediately began nursing.

"David," I called out, "will you come here a minute?" David had heard the cry, but thought there was a cat in the bathroom. He came down the hall, looked in the bathroom, and saw me sitting there nursing a newborn. Needless to say, he was surprised!

A few minutes later, he washed a pair of scissors and cut the cord. This time we didn't bother to tie it, and it healed just fine. Shortly thereafter, the placenta slipped into the toilet.

That afternoon, Joy, Michelle and I went to a baby shower some friends of mine had unknowingly scheduled for that afternoon. I had thought my due date was towards the middle of the month, so I hadn't objected when they wanted to have the shower on the 5th. Everyone was amazed to see Michelle on the outside of my body!

Veronika: What are your children's feelings about their births? Are they inclined toward unassisted childbirth for their own children?

Laura: All of my children are proud of the way they were born, although Michelle is sometimes embarrassed to tell people she was born on the toilet! I tell her to just say it was a waterbirth ~ which it sort of was. None of them are planning on having children anytime soon, but they've all expressed a desire to have unassisted births.

Veronika: When is the presence of a midwife/mother/partner a hindrance or a help?

Laura: Anyone who is fearful at a birth is a hindrance, whether they're a friend, relative, partner, or paid attendant. Anyone who instructs a woman as to how to give birth (when or when not to push, what position to be in, etc.) is a hindrance. Instructions, by the way, are different from suggestions when asked for. Anyone who insists on checking for dilation, or timing contractions, in spite of the mother's wishes, is a hindrance. When a birth attendant refuses to acknowledge this, and instead tries to tell a woman how to give birth, she's robbing her of one of the greatest gifts of motherhood.

Of course, many people would say that a midwife or doctor can save the life of a mother or baby by intervening in a difficult delivery. However, because I believe we create our own reality according to our desires, beliefs, intentions, and expectations, difficult deliveries can only occur when a mother has refused to deal with her limiting beliefs (primarily those relating to fear, shame, and guilt) either during the pregnancy or before. If a woman truly believes in her own abilities, she can give birth with little or no help. If she doesn't, then outside help may become a necessity. But it all gets back to belief. Complications don't "just happen" unless we believe they do.

Veronika: What is the greatest gift we can give to ourself and our baby in birth?

Laura: Fearlessness, because when we're not afraid, we can experience ecstasy both in birth and in life.

Vaginal Birth with Herpes
by Stephanie Shiffler

I'll tell you how the birth went. Your CD (*Peaceful Pregnancy* by Veronika and Paul Robinson) was really relaxing during my pregnancy. It helped me to remember the natural process when everyone else was treating pregnancy and birth like an illness.

The birth went wonderfully. I had a friend come down from the States who is a birth assistant and doula, and she helped my husband and I through the birth.

We were in our apartment listening to piano music, and breathing. They were massaging me, washing my feet in warm water (there's no hot water in the Caribbean!), talking to me and encouraging me.

My blood pressure was high for the last week, and the doctor wanted to give me a c-section, but I convinced her to let me rest and wait for my friend Crystalline to come and help me.

The baby was due on November 25th, and finally on the day of the full Moon, we worked on getting my contractions going with nipple stimulation, a labour support tincture, homeopathic remedy, and massage.

The nipple stimulation really worked. Anyway, we were checking my blood pressure constantly with a cuff, and finally it was a little too high, so I said I wanted to go to the hospital (hospital birth planned)... the taxi ride was interesting... and when I got there I was eight centimetres dilated! Success!

The doctor basically left my friend and husband and I alone to work through the contractions in the labour room ~ the nurses were sleeping, and I was walking down the hall to the bathroom, moving around. The hospital was very old fashioned ~ with an old labouring bed and everything, but I was so happy to just be in control that I wasn't worried about the lack of anything.

About five hours later, Rio was born.

We named him Rio because the rio Magdalena (Magdalena River) could be seen shining silver gray in the full moonlight from our apartment window while I was labouring.

We stopped the doctor in time from giving me a routine (!) episiotomy. I didn't even tear, and was able to leave the hospital eight hours later feeling great! In fact, I think that I feel worse now (muscle aches, back pain, lack of sleep, etc., from carrying baby around) than after the birth!

Rio was purple coming out, and had the cord wrapped twice around his neck. The doctors were so pleased with him: said he was healthy and perfect, and they were pleased with themselves because they said that they usually wouldn't take that risk; they'd do a c-section.

My doctor said that never in fifteen years of birthing babies has she ever NOT cut a woman. She has ALWAYS done episiotomies because she thought they were necessary all the time!

My goodness!

I felt that the birth was a terrific success because I really communicated, and pushed my doctor for what I wanted; and thanks to my friend, Crystalline, and my husband, Jose Rafael, who advocated so much for me when I was busy with other things (like pushing!), the birth went just as I'd wanted.

No oxygen, no pitocin, no enema, no shaving, no episiotomy, no painkillers. The doctors couldn't believe that either ~ a birth without an epidural!

I felt sort of alien, the doctor kept telling the nurses "This birth is different, just do what I tell you", because they were so unaccustomed to straying from protocol.

It just goes to show that if you really push for what you want, it pays off.

I appreciate all the women who wrote to me about birth, and herpes, too. Because of the support that I got, I felt empowered to take control of my own birth.

The birth was natural and my baby is fine. Thanks for keeping in touch. It's made me feel more connected to a larger community than this place in another country that doesn't share my beliefs about hardly anything!

Herpes ~ what is it?
By Veronika Robinson

Genital herpes is a viral infection. About 25% of sexually active adults have the virus and have had 'outbreaks'. A significantly higher proportion of the population carry the antibody.

The virus appears during an outbreak as small fluid-filled blisters. They tend to be red and painful, lasting for a few days. During this time they are contagious.

Once the blisters have erupted they dry to form scabs. The first outbreak is the worst. At this time, the whole body comes down with a flu-like fever. Glands swell, muscles ache, severe neuralgia in the thighs or associated nerve pathway is experienced, with fever and a general run-down feeling. The pain and blisters can last for up to 21 days.

The blisters can appear on the vagina, bottom and anus. Before they appear, there'll be a nerve 'warning' as either tingling or pain (neuralgia) around the nerves which are affected.

Learning to recognise this sign is vital for those mothers wishing to give birth vaginally without the usual medical hijacking. In some babies who've been born during an initial herpes outbreak, there have been incidences of blindness and severe illness. This is far less likely during a repeat outbreak. The first outbreak is always the worst.

With each outbreak the body builds up resistance.

If you have genital herpes, don't be bullied into a routine caesarean. Empower yourself with the holistic and medical facts.

Flower Essence of Crab Apple
Useful for people who feel disgust or shame, particularly sexually. Helps with clearing on all levels.

Natural Immunity
Though it's believed by the medical community that once you've had herpes you'll always have the virus, it's important to remember that the body wants to heal itself.

If you're having recurrent outbreaks, take that as a sign to make radical lifestyle changes. If you allow herpes to make you feel like a victim, it will happily oblige. There's no need to feel sexual guilt. Anyone with lowered immunity (physical, emotional, mental, spiritual) is susceptible to infection. Outbreaks are the result of a run-down body due to a stressful and unhealthy lifestyle. Slowly incorporate healthy habits and healing rituals into your daily living.

Are you getting fresh air in your home or work environment? Do you allow air to circulate into the room you sleep in?

What exercise do you do on a regular basis? Our bodies are meant to move! Try bellydancing or salsa, go for long walks, swim, try yoga, tai chi, cycling, mountain climbing...the list is endless. Do it solo or join a team or class. Do it fast, do it slow, just do it.

Keep a food diary. Lyseine is an amino acid which can greatly inhibit outbreaks. Try fresh vegetables, sprouts, legumes, brewer's yeast and soya beans.

Argenine (amino acid) can predispose a person to recurrent attacks if other areas of their lifestyle are unhealthy. Avoid chocolate, coffee, popcorn, sugar, tea, peanuts.

The Mother's Magic Medicine Bag!

To relieve the discomfort of blisters and to aid healing, mix the powder of L-Lysiene (available from good health stores) with a few drops of pure 100% tea tree oil, and mix to a paste. This works both with genital herpes and cold sores on lips. This easy to prepare application will greatly reduce and often eliminate the blisters forming if done at the first sign of tingling. It can be helpful to take the tablets up to 1000 mg, 2 to 3 times daily during an outbreak.

Build immunity by increasing foods rich in zinc (pumpkin seeds), vitamin A (carrots), vitamin C (citrus, peppers berries) and E (avocados).

Learn yoga or meditation; deep connected breathing; bring peace and calm into your life and your relationships.

Can you see a pattern between incidences (triggers) and outbreaks?

Avoid electric blankets, saunas, and heat in the genital area. Sea salt added to your bath can be soothing. During an initial outbreak it will greatly help to urinate in a low bath or tub of warm water (to dilute the urine as it passes over the blisters).

Essential Oils

You can use these oils safely on herpes blisters: lavender; tea tree; clove; thyme. Mix 20 drops of oil with 30ml of water. Apply several times a day. St John's wort oil can help ease the pain. To care for the healing scabs apply oil, ointment or tea of comfrey; also, oil of Vitamin E.

Stimulating the lymphatic system through exercise is vital for healing herpes. Rebounding on a mini-trampoline is excellent for this.

Herbs for Internal Use ~ Echinacea,; garlic; dandelion root; calendula.

Studies have shown that propolis (tree resin) is helpful in minimising the virus, as does olive leaf extract.

Honouring placenta and cord
By Keeley Farrington

Keeley is a full time mother of three wyld and wonderful witchlings, living near Guildford in Surrey. She's the founder of The Red Thread Mothers' Circle, a holistic mothering support group. When family life allows, she's also a doula and celebrant.

While you have breath, give thanks. The art of ritual celebration in our culture has been steadily eroded over time, and to some, almost lost altogether. As a society, it seems that the majority of people drift through life on autopilot, barely conscious of, let alone connected to, the abundance all around. We coast through weddings, birthdays and funerals, more concerned with convention and polite tradition than actually bringing meaning to these events. Sugar-laden birthday cakes and plastic horse shoes are taking the place of true depth and symbolism in our transitions. Life flows effortlessly and gives endlessly if we're ready to receive ~ from the moment of our birth, through each age and stage, until the end of our time here on Earth. Each life is a treasure hunt, strewn with precious gem-like moments and unique events. Increasing numbers of us are choosing to wake up to the beauty of each moment, and to live life alive and consciously. In doing this, we not only notice, but actively honour and give thanks for, the treasured moments of our lives: both day by day and at important times.

There are some events that unite us all in our human adventure, and birth is one of them. Through all of human history, birth and death have been recognised and celebrated as the fundamental rites of passage for humankind. These are the times when the veil between worlds is thin, and we can gain some sense of our multidimensional selves and our true potential. It's no wonder that many rituals can be found from all parts of the world that express and try to capture some of the awe that we feel when in the presence of the great magic and mystery of birth.

I've been looking at rituals and lore surrounding the placenta and umbilical cord, and what I've found is an incredibly rich seam. In Western culture, sadly, the placenta has long been considered as little more than medical waste, regarded as a tiresome extra bit of effort after the hard work of childbirth. It's examined, and then discarded with the other rubbish for incineration, and known as the 'afterbirth'.

However, in other traditions the world over, the placenta is held in great esteem. It's regarded by some as the new baby's younger or older brother, and is accorded respect as such. The Ibo of Nigeria and Ghana believe it to be the dead twin of the live child, and it's buried with solemn ceremony. Malaysians consider it to be the older brother, and if the baby smiles in his sleep he's said to be playing with the spirit of his older brother.

In many places, the connection between child and placenta is believed to reach far beyond the womb time, and the placenta is regarded as a focus for sympathetic magic. For example, in Siberia, if the child becomes sick, the placenta is thought to be uncomfortable, its grave site is treated, and it may be dug up and reburied. Filipino women, and other cultures, bury the placenta with books to ensure a smart child, or with a token of their tribe, perhaps as a type of cultural insurance for the future. Among the Hmong of South East Asia, the soul is thought to retrace its steps after death, back to the burial place of its placenta, before departing this life.

The Maoris of New Zealand bury the placenta in their native soil. They name it whenua, which is the same as the Maori word for land. Native Americans customarily bury it within the boundaries of their reservation, as a tie for the child to the ancestral home and heritage.

Indeed the placenta is the first homeland of the child, where it dwells for their first nine months. It's the physical link between you and your baby, growing with her/him from the very first stages of pregnancy. Throughout gestation, it's their constant companion, soft pillow to snuggle, and first playmate!

The ritual that fully honours the role of the placenta is Lotus-birth. This is when baby and placenta aren't separated at birth, but cared for and kept together until natural separation of the umbilical cord occurs. This is a much more gentle entry into the world, and allows for a very real 'in-between' time, a pause, as baby and family rest after birth, but before fully stepping into the world. Lotus born babies are said to be very peaceful souls.

If Lotus-birth is not for you, then spending some time with the placenta after birth may be enough. Look at it and really take it in, in all its glorious textures and details. I found it an amazing organ, with such a strong presence, even though its birth signifies the end of its purpose. Silently thank it for its important role, and give thanks to whomever you choose to that it's done its job so beautifully.

Many people bury the placenta as a symbolic gesture, signifying the new arrival Earthside, and welcoming the child to their Earthly home. A tree or shrub can be planted over the site, so that the placenta can then go on to feed the tree as your child grows. If you don't have a favourite place where you're able to plant, you can use a large pot in which to bury the placenta and plant a tree. Don't forget, though, to make your pot large enough, as a placenta is very rich, and can sometimes 'burn' a root system if buried too closely. The burial can be with as much ceremony as you please. It can take place soon after the birth, later, as part of a welcoming ceremony for the child, or even at their first birthday celebration.

Another idea is to make a print of your placenta after the birth. To do this, you'll need some heavy-duty watercolour paper fixed to a hard surface or a board, where it can stay until the prints are dry. You can keep the placenta for a few days in a sealed container, at room temperature (so long as your waters were clear), as you're unlikely to feel like jumping up and doing it right away after the birth! If you put it in the fridge, it will change the texture and shape. There's plenty of blood and fluid within the tissues to make a print, but if you want to use paints, it would be wise to wash the placenta first. Don't forget that when you print in blood, the colours will change and go brown over the next few days. The two sides of the placenta have completely different textures and patterns, so go ahead, explore and be creative! If you've done any birth art during your pregnancy, what a wonderful addition to your collection a print of your baby's placenta would be.

One traditional ritual act that we all recognise in Western culture is the cutting of the umbilical cord, which over time has come to be a powerful symbol of our first physical transition here on Earth. Taking a little time to focus, and maybe pray, at the moment of cord cutting, can reclaim the ritual significance of this moment ~ which is so often lost in the flurry of post birth activity, especially if you birth in hospital. It will be useful to think about this beforehand, and request that midwives leave the cord uncut until you're ready and you feel the time is right, at least until after it's stopped pulsating. The umbilical cord is usually long enough to allow you to hold your baby skin to skin and have your first cuddle, whilst still attached. So as long as you state your wishes clearly beforehand, and there are no medical complications, then giving yourselves this time shouldn't be a problem. When you feel ready, you or your partner could ask to cut the cord along with a spoken blessing for your baby's first rite of passage: from the warm womb, into the warm loving arms of your family.

In many cultures, the umbilical cord is buried with ceremony and planted with a tree or shrub to protect it. Often the cord is buried with tokens to symbolise the dreams that the parents hold for their new baby. In Turkey, as in many other places, it's traditionally thought that how you treat the cord affects the life of the child; for example, they bury it in the grounds of a mosque for the child to be devout, or in the grounds of a school to ensure a love of learning.

The umbilical cord can also be dried and kept. You should gently squeeze the blood out of the length of cord, and then you can twist it into your chosen shape, before air drying on a piece of gauze. The drying should take a week or two. It could be dried into a heart, a circle, or spiral ~ all sacred shapes, symbolising the family and the cycles of life. In some cultures, an amulet made with a piece of the umbilical cord is believed to confer protection and good health, and is worn from childhood throughout life. You could sew a pouch for your child, and keep the dried cord in it for them as both a powerful charm and a reminder of their journey from the stars.

My feeling is that any act to which we can commit our full presence and focused intention can be considered a ritual. It can be small or large; silent, or given your fullest voice; a captured, spontaneous moment or a well planned event; in short, what makes a ritual is your intent ~ be it to honour an event, a person or a moment in your life. At birth, we're fully open on many levels: physically, emotionally, spiritually and energetically, moreso than at any other time in life. Marking events, observing quiet moments of reflection, and expressing gratitude can help as part of the closing down and rebalancing process that must happen after birth for the health and strength of mother and baby. Observing rituals, and the keeping of tokens from our transitions ~ such as the umbilical cord, can help us to feel a strong sense of closure: enabling us to move forward in our lives with no unfinished business.

Honouring the placenta and cord also offers us the opportunity to fully connect with our bodies in a visceral way not generally encouraged in our body-phobic culture of sterile birth. It enables us to reconnect and ground in the very physical reality of birth and human experience ~ which can be intensely moving and satisfying. If your birth was all that you'd hoped it would be, of course you'll want to preserve something of this magical time for yourself and your child. However, if your birth was less than perfect, or felt in any way traumatic, then any of these suggestions can be hugely cathartic and a big step in accepting and healing. If this applies to you, I urge you to make sure that you and your baby are well supported emotionally and spiritually through any rituals or ceremonies that you hold, as through the healing process as a whole. The intensity of the energy around this time can be overwhelming, especially where there has been wounding. Be gentle with yourself, take things slowly, and be ready for what healing these practices may bring. *"Kindle kindness, especially towards yourself, embracing the sweet silence of your own soul. Fear nothing. Accept what you are, and ~ while you have breath ~ give thanks."* ~ Anon.

As conscious participants in our life's journey, we can choose to fully live each moment, and breathe each breath in gratitude and acknowledgement of all that we are and all that we have. I believe there's no more perfect time to celebrate this life than at the dawning of a new one.

It could be dried into a
heart, a circle, or spiral
~ all sacred shapes,
symbolising the family and the cycles of life.

BIRTH TRAUMA:
Why children need chiropractic care
by Dr. Rozeela Nand

Conscious parents often do all they can to give their baby the best possible chance of a healthy life. That includes a toxin-free pregnancy, childbirth without violence, avoidance of drugs and medical procedures (except in emergencies), and breastfeeding. You have your baby's eyes, heart and ears checked, so why not their spine?

Your baby's spine houses her nervous system (brain, spinal cord, nerves), which regulates every cell in the body. Through chemical and electrical messages, it instructs the lungs to expand and contract with each breath; begins the peristalsis of your baby's digestive system, etc. If there is any disturbance to this intricate highway of communication, your baby's health diminishes. This neurological disturbance is called a subluxation, and it may result in the failure of one or more parts of the body, as well as health in general. Subluxations can also foster the onset of sickness and disease as the body weakens. The doctor of chiropractic specialises in the detection and correction of subluxations. Instead of treating the symptoms of the disease, the chiropractor corrects the subluxation, so that normal body functions may take place. By having subluxations corrected throughout childhood, your child will have a better opportunity to be as healthy as possible.

For over a hundred years, doctors of chiropractic have often observed dramatic responses from infants after a chiropractic spinal adjustment, with conditions as varied as Erb's palsy; unbalanced facial and skull symmetry; foot inversion; colic; torticollis (twisted neck); nervousness; and ear, nose and throat infections.

Eighty percent of the time the first subluxation occurs at birth.

Imagine a ripe peach being squeezed, stretched, pushed, and pulled with 90-140 pounds of pressure through a 10cm tube. Then imagine the force of vacuum pressure or cold metal tongs pulling the peach out the rest of the way. Now replace that ripe peach with an infant's skull. Birth is, potentially, the first trauma our children endure. Whether it's a natural vaginal delivery, or a caesarean, or reinforced with ventouse, birth can leave irrecoverable damage to the spine and nervous system if left unchecked. It can be argued that babies have been born since the beginning of time and haven't received chiropractic care, yet have still led fairly healthy lives. However, the majority of births these days are seen as a medical emergency, and not as the natural cycle of life Mother Nature intended. Far fewer women are having homebirths in a squatting, gravity-dependent position. Most women give birth, or have their baby delivered, in hospital. The routine use of epidurals, mothers birthing in a supine position, the use of vacuum extraction and forceps, all attribute to the shocking rate of infant problems after birth.

As the late Larry Webster, D.C., of the International Chiropractic Pediatric Association, said: "With the birth process becoming more and more an intervening procedure ... the chiropractic adjustment becomes even more important to the child's future."

Greater complications during delivery result in greater neurological insult to the newborn, due to injury to the head and neck. Because of this, babies should have their spines checked as soon as possible after birth. In accommodation, the foetus's cranial bones overlap to decrease the circumference as it journeys through the birth canal. This can leave the baby with an odd-shaped head, and upper cervical problems. In some cases the cranium will regain its natural shape as the baby suckles, cries and yawns. However, this unmoulding process is often incomplete, especially if the birth has been difficult. As a result, the baby may have to live with some very uncomfortable stresses, and neurological problems. There is a sweet window of opportunity to assist with the proper moulding of the baby's head and cranial sutures before permanent damage occurs. Optimal success has been reported in the first three months of the baby's life. After the suture starts to close, it's harder to adjust and align the cranial bones. It's crucial that the cranium be able to expand evenly to allow for the growth of the brain.

Bruce Kaufman, MD, a pediatric neurosurgeon, says that "more than fifty percent of brain growth occurs in the first year of life, so when one or more sutures prematurely close, the brain cannot expand in that area, and therefore must expand in another direction." Such growth can result in pressure on the brain and disfigurement of the skull.

From a random group of 1,250 babies examined five days after birth, 211 suffered from vomiting, hyperactivity and sleeplessness. Spinal abnormalities were found in 95% of this group.

Spinal adjustment frequently results in immediate quieting,

cessation of crying, muscular relaxation and sleepiness. The authors of the study noted that an unhealthy spine causes many clinical features, from central motor impairment to lower resistance to infections, especially ear, nose and throat infections. In another study, of 1093 newborns, 298 had upper neck stress and early signs of scoliosis.

How do I know if my child is subluxated?

Unfortunately, 90% of subluxated babies are often asymptomatic, so the only way to really know what's happening with your baby's spine and nervous system is to get them checked by a chiropractor.

Some may have immediate symptoms, such as respiratory depression, colic, inability to breastfeed, lowered immune system, etc. Subluxations may also interfere with internal organ function, resulting in the inability to produce chemicals responsible for raising and lowering body temperature as needed. Research has also indicated that the body's immune response in the production of anti-viral and anti-bacterial agents to fight infection is greatly compromised due to vertebral subluxations.

How can chiropractic help?

A chiropractor will gently examine the baby's head for overlapping cranial sutures, unevenness (one side of the head not matching the other), and missing, or unusually large or small, soft spots. The techniques used are to encourage the body to correct itself. Touch manual therapy is used to encourage the body's self-correcting mechanisms. Generally, using about five grams of pressure, or about the weight of a small coin, the practitioner evaluates the body's craniosacral system, which plays a vital role in maintaining the environment in which the central nervous system functions. It consists of the membranes and fluid that surround and protect the brain and spinal cord, as well as the attached bones, including the skull, face, and jaw ~ which make up the cranium, and the tailbone area, or sacrum.

What problems can chiropractic help with in babies?

The following is not a comprehensive list. It's an example of the sorts of conditions chiropractors see regularly and have success with. Remember, chiropractic doesn't aim to treat symptoms, but actually addresses the underlying problem, which, in more cases than not, is a neurological disturbance. Once your baby's body is in equilibrium and homeostasis, there isn't much she can't fight off naturally.

.*Boosting immune system*
.*Crying*
.*Colic, sickness, and wind*
.*Feeding difficulties*
.*Sleep disturbances*
.*Recurrent infections*
.*Ear infections*
.*Asthma*
.*Brachial plexus problems (Erb's palsy)*
.*Breastfeeding problems*
.*Sinus and adenoidal problems*
.*Behaviour problems*
.*Learning difficulties*
.*Cerebral palsy*

Chiropractic paediatric specialist Larry Webster says there are six times in a baby's first year of life when spinal examinations are especially important:
.*After birthing*
.*When the baby starts to hold her head up*
.*When the baby sits up*
.*When the baby starts to crawl*
.*When the baby starts to stand*
.*When the baby starts to walk*

Build your own waterbirthing pool
by Alex Kramer

Alex lives off the grid in rural Ireland with his partner and their two children.

When Siobhán was pregnant with Joe, we decided that we'd like to have a birth pool for our planned homebirth. I initially looked into hiring one, and found that the prices for two to four weeks ranged from about £120 - £200, which seemed a lot for something you don't even get to keep.

I priced up some bits and pieces, and figured that I could build one of my own for half that cost. I found a site in Western Australia that had some good tips for construction, and away we went. We still have this pool, and it has been in service for the birth of Rhiannon and the births of two of our friends' babies, too.

<u>What you'll need:</u>
[] One piece of 8ft x 4ft plywood
(3/4 inch)
[] 16 square metal hinges with three holes on each side.
[] 100 rounded cross-head bolts with wing-nuts
[] 2 pieces of heavy-duty builders' plastic (at least 4^2 metres each)
[] Some old blankets and cushions
[] A long length of rope

<u>Method</u>
Take the piece of ply, and cut it in half lengthways so that you now have two pieces measuring 2ft x 8ft. Now cut each length into 2ft pieces so that you end up with eight pieces measuring 2ft x 2ft.

Take one piece of ply, and position a hinge about 2 inches from the top of one side, with the central part of the hinge standing clear of the wood. Now take a pen and mark on the wood where each hinge hole is. Do the same thing with a hinge 2 inches from the bottom of the piece of wood. Drill holes where the pen marks are (wide enough for the diameter of bolt you have).

Push the bolts through the wood and then through the hinge holes, securing the hinge then with the wing-nuts. The hinge will be on the outside of the birth pool. On a level floor, stand the next piece of wood next to the first piece with a small gap (for the central part of the hinge) between them. Mark on the second piece of wood where the holes from the unsecured parts of the hinges lie, and drill holes here, too. Push the bolts through, and secure the hinge.

Now you have two pieces of ply that are hinged in the middle and should stand up on their own if the hinge is bent in the middle. You can now take the third piece of ply and stand it next to the second; place hinges across the two of them, top and bottom, at the same level as the other hinges, and mark the holes. Drill the holes, and fit the hinges.

Continue doing this with all the pieces of wood until you've gone all the way round and made an upright octagonal hinged ring.

Important: Now take a thick permanent marker, and go round the inside of the ring, and mark the pieces 1-8, with an arrow showing which way is up, and an arrow showing which way you're going round with the numbers (clockwise or anti-clockwise). If you don't do this, matching the pieces with hinges when assembling will be difficult.

Take the first piece of plastic, lay it over the assembled pool, and push it down so that it goes right down to the floor and into all the corners. Then get the blankets, and lay them over the edges of the pool, to soften them a bit.

Take the cushions, and place them on the floor of the pool. These make it more comfortable to kneel and sit.

Take the second piece of plastic, and lay it over the pool, pushing it right down, as with the previous piece.

Now tie the rope around the top of the pool (over the plastic) a few times, and tighten. This keeps the plastic out of the way, and prevents it slipping into the pool.

Now fill the pool, and use a thermometer to keep it just above body temperature (People vary with this. It shouldn't really be more than body temperature, but I figure that it's best a little too warm to begin with, and it will probably have cooled by the time things start hotting up with the mother). To fill it, I used a hose connected to the shower.

To empty, I used one of those pumps that you can connect to an electric drill. These aren't ideal, though, as they burn out if for some reason the water stops going into it, and I think it's a bit hazardous having a power tool so close to a lot of water, especially if it's being drained after the dizzying process of receiving a baby. A much better option is to get a submersible pump. If there's a drain at a lower location than the pool, then one can also use the siphoning method (get the water flowing though a hose [e.g. by sucking it through], and it will then continue on its own).

Before planning on having a pool, you have to consider whether you have a strong enough floor to hold one! Anywhere on the ground floor is fine, but an upstairs floor might not be strong enough for a pool full of water. It's possible to make the pool smaller by taking out some panels. For the birth of Rhiannon, we only used five panels (making a pentagonal shape), because we didn't have much space on the floor of the mobile home. Actually, this was more than enough room for Siobhán to move around, and was easier to fill and empty.

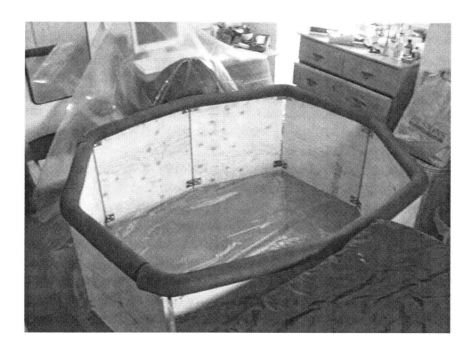

A brief history of vitamin K
by Lynda Cook Sawyer

Vitamin K is an essential clotting factor used by our blood to form a clot and slow bleeding from a large wound. It's a by-product of normal bacterial colonisation of the stomach. Since babies are born from a sterile environment, their stomachs (the entire gastrointestinal system, actually) are sterile also. They begin to ingest bacteria ~ normal flora from the environment ~ as they pass through the vagina into the world, and then again, as they nuzzle around the breast, eventually latching on. As they nurse, they transfer more normal skin bacteria into their sterile systems.

In this manner, the newborn is gently colonised with the mother's home/regional "normal" bacteria, while at the same time receiving her antibodies to neutralise an overgrowth creating an infection.

It takes about 6 - 8 days in a healthy term infant for the vitamin K to be manufactured in the gut, and then, to reach main bloodstream levels in an amount considered "effective" to stem a blood loss. (Thus, in Judaism, God's command to wait until the 8th day for circumcision? Hmmmmm....) When attempting to save very premature babies, it was found that if they were medicated with vitamin K at birth, the frequent leaking of blood into their brains following a vaginal birth was decreased markedly. It became routine for premmies ~ 36 weeks gestation, and earlier.

When haemophilia became a well-researched diagnosis, family histories that included a haemophiliac family member had their newborns given vitamin K at birth. It became routine for all newborns with positive family histories for "bleeding disorders".

When circumcisions became a common medical procedure, it was convenient for the physician to "do it while he was in the hospital already making rounds". Of course, a healthy newborn bleeding to death from an elective circumcision done at 24 - 48 hours of life would not be a profitable venture for the MD ~ so, a vitamin K injection became routine for all male infants whose parents wanted their newborn circumcised. And, well my goodness, now we're medicating 75% of all newborns with an injected vitamin K compound...the healthy, term baby girls are being neglected...better just give it to them, too.

And so it goes: 20 years of this practice has now made it: A REQUIREMENT OF THE MOST GRAVE IMPORTANCE.

Ephrem's Birth
Welcoming our first child in the clear water of the ocean
by Clara Scropetta

I tried several times to put this story on paper, but I was always disappointed. I was missing something, although apparently I didn't forget any detail. Then I read again the wise words of Jeannine Parvati Baker, talking about shamanic and spiritual experience (Rituals for birth, The Mother magazine, Spring 2002). I went back also to the powerful book of Vicki Noble "Shakti woman", and I understood.

My birth report was a profanation of a sacred moment. It was necessary for me to talk about it in a different way, touching the essence of this experience, that had absolutely nothing to do with measurements of any kind (like time, dilatation, contractions) and other practical events. All that is outside, instead of inside. I had to find different words, another language, another perspective to share what happened to me in that special moment of my life. I had to dive again into that fantastic altered state of mind to be sincere, accurate and incisive. I had to forget quite all I read about birth, and especially all the pictures I saw. I had to distance myself from the appearance, and bond again with the real essence.

So, here is the story of Ephrem's birth on the 20th of October 2000. It was just the beginning of the warm season in Mauritius. Close to the full Moon I was feeling really complete, yet I knew, from within, these were our last days. I enjoyed walking every day to the little beach we chose for giving birth, and unconsciously preparing my nest: the last plants and seeds in the garden, some cleaning of the house, some letters and e-mails to friends.

I was feeling beautiful. I wasn't scared, I wasn't anxious. I wasn't counting, but simply living the moment. It was like I was vibrating together with this life inside me ~ we were pulsing together. I was quiet.

One early morning, under the light of a waning Moon, I discovered something jelly, pink and wonderful-smelling between my legs.

I went back to bed and the embracing arms of my partner Yann-Vaï, knowing that I was going to give birth.

For several hours I ate tropical fruits, listened to the music we loved, and enjoyed loving attention from Yann-Vaï. I gave the last massage to Ephrem through my womb under the scent of incenses and oils.

We were starting to dance together with the gentle first movements of my body, and me diving into these still unknown sensations. Like the rest of this pregnancy, I was quiet and sure. The message from Ephrem was still clear. Everything was perfect and was proceeding as it was supposed to. It was important for me to just let go, let go, accept. Suddenly, I felt it was time, and we left for the beach with all that we thought we'd need (Laugh! Now I would pack half or even less!) with a kind of "quiet excitement". Immediately there my 'dance' started to get a different taste. I had made a bed of leaves under a magnificent tree. It was ready, and the tree itself was decorated for the occasion with corals and shells we had collected there. Jasmine and rose incenses started to burn. I no longer talked, but was simply present just for the birth.

Yann-Vaï kept on preparing the beach. He made a big fire for heating the water which we would later want for bathing Ephrem. He came with me every time I wished to enter the sea and follow the waves. He paid attention if somebody was coming, and asked a few (astonished) people if they would go away.

It was a cloudy, windy, fresh day. This beach was not so much visited except by some fisherman, but they knew about our plan, and respected our wish for intimacy. He truly protected me and took care of me.

I was becoming attuned with other realities and cycles. My body was following the suggestions that were coming from all elements. I remember well how I felt to be a kind of channel between sky and Earth: a strong ray of light and warmth was filling me, until I was simply one with All.

I felt the ground under my feet, soft coral sand and the wise life of that big tree offering support to me when I needed it. I felt the water of the ocean, full of resonance and messages, mixing with the water of the lagoon. I felt the wind.

Sea water and wind gave me movement, the ground and tree stability. The sky and Earth opening, and roots.

I enjoyed the birth dance. I trusted my body was looking for what it needed: a change of position, some seawater or some tree root, a drop of ylang-ylang, or a drop of rescue remedy.

I was moving and acting in a kind of dream, following a primal instinct. A lot of infinite circles designed from my pelvis. I was transforming myself into a tiger: I discovered my voice, the animal one. It was the voice of a tiger.

I was somewhere else, closer to the stars and the spirits. I remember my surprise seeing the Sun going down. I lost connection with time. It seemed to me such a short afternoon!

UN SOFFIO DI VENTO, UN BATTITO D'ALI DI FARFALLA!

Suddenly, I stood up and told Yann-Vaï: "I must go in the water."

I walked the few metres separating me from the shore. I touched and held with my hand the head of Ephrem coming out.

Under the glimmering light of the Moon, in the silence of the evening, the wind stayed still. Like a queen I entered the sea; on my knees I welcomed Ephrem, he was floating towards me like an angel. His fantastic open eyes looked deeply into my soul. His face was full of wisdom.

It was eternity. I stood up and walked back to our bed of leaves, with this new being close to my heart, still connected to my womb through the cord.

That's the story of Ephrem being born, and it's also the story of Clara. Still a young girl, despite her age of thirty-four. After nine intense and beautiful Moons of preparation, she opened herself to experience the connection between sky and Earth. She accepted the mystery and the perfection of life. She understood her position in the Universe, finally received her missing initiation to womanhood. And she became a mother.

Let's honour the silence and the mystery. Let's give thanks to the wonder of life.

Our theoretical background was just the book of Leboyer "Si l'enfantemente m'etait contè" (Birth without Violence). We knew nothing about Michel Odent or other spiritual midwives; we didn't even know there was a name for what we were doing: unattended childbirth. We knew nobody who'd done it. We were pioneers.

The place we chose to give birth was fantastic, yet now I would look for a more intimate corner, just the next tree would have been enough. We preferred the big tree because of its beauty, but overlooked the fact that it was in the middle, open towards the east. The shore offered very little sense of protection to me.

We cut the cord (after it stopped pulsing, but still felt it was too early). Yann-Vaï offered him the first bath in warm seawater (without removing the casex). We went back home to find a letter from Israel with the meaning of the name Ephrem: between the sea and the Earth ~ fertility! I give thanks to the power of Nature and the energy of life that supported me and offered me such a magical experience.

Afterword

From very early in the pregnancy I received and accepted the message that everything was all right and it would be possible to give birth unassisted. Me and my partner Yann-Vaï made the decision to go to Mauritius even before that, with the purpose of taking advantage of the warm, clean ocean. We had in mind a waterbirth because of the incredible attraction towards this element. Life is a marvellous source of suggestions. I had the privilege of visiting Flores, the most western Azorean island. In that paradise I met an Italian-French couple who had just had a baby at home. At that time, I was not so much interested in all these topics, I didn't even really talk with this woman about her experience, but it was the first time I'd heard about giving birth outside the hospital, and I wasn't going to forget it. At that time I was looking for novels, films, conversations, "culture", so they lent me several books. Among them was one of a Portuguese writer telling the dramatic story of all the poor Azorean women who had to give birth at home with no appropriate assistance, many of them damned to death after a lot of suffering, etc.

I can't explain in a logical way, but since that time I kept a kind of "seed" inside me, like a subliminal imprint: clearly there was something to investigate. Not very long after, I was in Berlin visiting an exposition called "Meergeboren", seaborn; I wasn't giving too much attention to all there was about birth. The exposition was generally about our relation with the sea, indeed there was something about Chris Grisgom giving birth in the sea. I remember very well lying on a water mattress, listening to the whales' songs, and feeling how right it was to accept that the origin of life is in the ocean. It was like nurturing that seed I already had in me. It was amazing: the mix of these beautiful islands full of waterfalls; volcanic lakes; powerful waves of the open ocean; with the concept of homebirth and the understanding of the origin of life.

Of course, the angels brought Yann-Vaï to me, as a lover and father, a young man of 24 that knew the work of Leboyer and also the story of the Russian waterbabies ~ what a coincidence!

A Beautiful Breech Birth
by Eve Kieran

It's one year since my second child was born. On the eve of her birthday I remember the events leading up to her meeting with the outside world, and am amazed that, with so much doubt around me, I was able to be calm and to trust that it was going to be OK.

Meditation with the baby in-utero, and regular Shiatsu treatments, had developed an awareness that served us so well in the last couple of weeks of pregnancy.

At 12 days over my due date (which, it turned out, was wrong), I was starting to receive advice from my midwife that induction was necessary. I knew that we were going to go as long as we safely could before we agreed to that, so I kept them at bay ~ by not showing up at the hospital or answering the phone. I needed my space. At my Shiatsu treatment that day, Therese Hawkins, not only my practitioner, but my sage and source of great strength and confidence, said she thought the baby would come in five days.

On day 14, I went to have the baby monitored at the hospital, and it was only then that we discovered she was breech. I was strongly advised to have a caesarean, or at least attempt to have the baby turned manually. The message from all sides was that the health professionals were not happy with breech births. However, nobody panicked, and I did not suffer any pressure from the community midwives at Helston in Cornwall, who had been in touch with me throughout the pregnancy, or even from the obstetrician, Rob Holmes, at Treliske hospital in Truro, over the following days. They were very respectful of my wishes, which came as a huge relief, as I've experienced the opposite in the past, and have heard stories from other mothers about the pressure that they can suffer at such a vulnerable time. I also really appreciated the way that Paul, my partner, stood between me and the people at the hospital, allowing me to feel absolutely protected and safe to make my own decisions. He literally would stand up to greet whoever came to talk to us, placing himself between me and them, and had no fear of interrupting them if he felt what they were saying was going to cause unnecessary upset. I loved him so much for doing that.

Over the next few days I spent as much time as possible with a tree that I love ~ a huge old oak by the creek, which had become an essential source of support. I sat with the tree, and became aware of its roots entangled with my own, anchoring me with a force that was almost physical, into the Earth. I felt steady and calm, and the thought came to me ~ this tree endures all without worry or complaint, life just passes on. So I'll be like the tree. I had a lot of options to think very deeply about ~ I certainly wasn't dismissing any of the suggested interventions out of hand, I just wanted to make the right decision.

On day 17 overdue, my labour began in the evening. Therese was right! It wasn't just <u>my</u> awareness of the baby that mattered, but hers too. We had given up hopes of another homebirth when we found out the baby was breech ~ we live an hour from the hospital, and felt it was too big a risk to take. So off we went, feeling excited but calm. As we settled in to our room, my contractions continued every few minutes but didn't get stronger. My body knew the space was not yet ready. Our promisingly old and experienced midwife and obstetrician had a lot to say about what might go wrong, and said I would be monitored throughout the labour. I said I would not be monitored at all. So they asked me to sign a disclaimer. When all the talking was over and we were left alone, Paul made me a cup of raspberry leaf tea, and I took an Arnica 30. I quite swiftly moved into second stage, and within 15 minutes the baby's body was out, then her head was eased out by the obstetrician's hand. No drugs, no forceps, no injections ~ we did it!!! I was quite sure that my body had waited for all the talking and the interveners to go away, and then had pushed the baby out as fast as possible before they could get back in and start interfering.

I'm not suggesting that this is how anyone else should approach a breech birth. I'm just glad to share a good news story that may offer support and encouragement in deciding which path to take, and in being strong with the health professionals, who, by their own admittance, give advice that is affected by fears of their own liability. We need and value their advice and expertise, but if anyone puts us under pressure to choose a certain path for our baby's birth (even our partners and families), the intuitive voice inside must remain the loudest, and will always tell us what we need to know. We just need to practise listening; and I'm sure that my meditation and Shiatsu helped me do that. Thank you Therese. Thank you tree.

Tarka's Birth
by Gina Sewell

(Tarka means *little water wanderer*, and is also the name given to male otters [by our ancestors], who once lived upon the land.)

The sky is filled with a million stars. The sea washes gently over the rocks, and the Moon spills a golden path over the water. I stand at the window with this tiny new soul in my arms, and feel overwhelmed with love for him.

When my daughter Mia was born, just over two years ago, I was left feeling as though something horrific had happened. I remember the terror of being left in a small, early-labour room, overwhelmed by the intensity of each contraction, clinging to my partner, Ash, and begging him to somehow make it all stop. I remember the fear and worry in his eyes, and I remember the helplessness. Reduced to tears by an overbearing, bullying, cold midwife, I begged for an epidural. Numb and frightened, I lay in a white, clinical, delivery room, clinging to Ash's hand, desperate to block out the sound of a woman in the opposite labour room, screaming and crying her way through her baby's birth. I felt the urge to push even through the anaesthetic, but it seemed I had given up the right to birth my baby myself. My legs were placed in stirrups. I was surrounded by midwives, and an obstetrician forced my head onto my chest, and told me when and how to push. They performed an episiotomy, and a few minutes later, Mia was pulled from inside me, and placed onto my chest.

For a few moments, there was bliss, just me and this beautiful little being gazing at one another. I remember whispering 'Look at her, look at her.' Then, it was over. She was whipped away from me, and I heard her screaming for me as she was weighed and dressed, and, God knows what, when she should have been wrapped in the warmth of my arms, nestled against my skin, finding her way to my breast.

My initial feelings after her birth were of relief. It was over, we had a beautiful daughter, and I would never have to go through that private hell again. But, I felt so damaged. I held my beautiful daughter and cried and whispered I'm sorry into her crinkly, dark hair. I thought I'd never recover from what had taken place in those 12 hours. But then I gave birth to Tarka on the 22nd August, 2006. Oh, how much those words mean to me now.

For, I really did give birth to Tarka. When I discovered that Tarka was growing quietly inside me, I knew that I needed to heal the pain of Mia's birth. I began to seek out inspirational stories of birth. I read books by Ina May Gaskin and Sheila Kitzinger, and devoured The Mother magazine!

Ten days after Tarka's 'due' date, the birth began. At lunchtime I was having mild contractions. I bounced on the birth ball and sought inspiration by re-reading birth stories in The Mother magazine! I was frightened, but Ash was so strong and supportive. He knew we could do it, and his confidence supported me so deeply.

Suddenly things speeded up. I stood up to go to the loo, and massive tightening doubled me over. Then my waters gently broke. We left the house, and drove to the birth centre. As we travelled, I watched the clouds move softly over the grey sky. The air was warm and the Sun slanted hazily through the trees. I closed my eyes and searched within myself for the strength to stay with the sensations that were embracing my body.

When we arrived, I was examined and found to be five centimetres dilated. The sensations came thick and fast, and I found I needed to use some gas and air. Ash held me by rubbing my back in deep, comforting circles as we waited for the birth pool to fill.

Oh the bliss of shedding my clothes and stepping into the warmth of the water! I felt my whole body give a shuddering sigh, and relax. I knelt down and held Ash's hands. After only two or three minutes of stepping into the warmth of the water, I knew the time had come. 'The baby is coming' I said, frightening the life out of the student midwife, who scurried off to get help.

Ash was so calm, so centred and strong, that I knew I could give birth to this baby, and I felt waves of almost euphoric excitement. I wasn't numb this time, and yes, it was painful, but oh how I love the healing power of that pain now. I was so entirely present. As each tightening faded away I wanted to shout 'I'm ok, I'm ok, I can do this!'

I was overwhelmed by the intensity of sensations that washed over me. I was somewhere outside of time and place. Even now, I feel that although I was there in that small room, nestled in the birthing pool, I could feel the pull of the Moon, the ocean; see the stars and feel the timelessness of the Sun, the wind and rain. I opened my eyes. I looked down and saw Tarka's head as he birthed into the water, and I'm so glad I did. For me, it was a moment of pure bliss, and it healed so much that was hurt: to see our baby suspended momentarily in the gentle water at the moment of birth, his hair like wisps of seaweed against my thighs; and then I breathed him out into the safe haven of the warm water and up, up into my arms. He fed at my breast, and gazed into my eyes. I held him all night. The Moon travelled across the sky, alight with a thousand stars. I held him, and the night passed gently around us. The Sun rose, bringing light to a new day and a new beginning.

I know now that giving birth to a new life is about so much more than just the moment itself. The power of finding your strength as a woman through birth resonates for the rest of your life. It shapes you as a person, and as a parent. I believe that because I was so fully present at Tarka's birth, I now have an innate confidence in my ability to be a mother, in my ability to take responsibility for my children's well-being. We choose to co-sleep, breastfeed, wear a sling, not vaccinate, and home educate, because we have the confidence to say this is what we believe is right for our children.

Our daughter Mia is a vibrant little soul and my deepest wish is that her life will be enriched by what I hope will now be her instinctive knowledge of birth as a conscious, joyful experience, filled with love, awe and thankfulness.

So, thank you Tarka, our little water wanderer! Your beautiful waterbirth has changed everything, and my heart overflows with love for you.

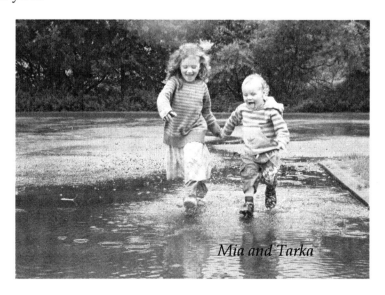

Mia and Tarka

Lotus-birth
by Gina Cox Roberts

I'm not sure when or how I first came to hear of Lotus-birthing ~ leaving the umbilical cord uncut so that the child and placenta remain attached, until the cord drops away naturally. It would have been at some time during my years of avid reading about all things birth-related, which eventually led to me becoming a doula. I do know that my feelings about it had remained consistent for some time: I considered it a perfectly valid choice, but one that, when I did eventually have a child, wasn't going to be for me. I could see the physiological benefits of not cutting the cord until it had stopped pulsating, and possibly even until the placenta had been delivered, but after that, I couldn't see how leaving it attached would be beneficial. If anything, I imagined the extra work involved in keeping the placenta clean, and doing whatever else needed to be done to prevent it from becoming a smelly, rotting mess, would be an extra burden in those joyous first few days. I simply couldn't see why anyone would choose to do it.

But then I became pregnant, and discovered what a magical experience it was to listen to my unborn child, and to be open to her wisdom. This is the story of how she chose to be lotus born.

I have a very close relationship with my cousin, Kd; and she offered to come over to the UK from Australia for a few weeks to help out towards the end of my pregnancy. I think we both harboured a secret hope that she'd be here for the birth too, but as she could only come for three weeks, we knew that that would be in fate's hands. The week before she was due to fly over, she was leaving her yoga class, in a suburban town hall in Melbourne, when she heard voices from down the hallway, and felt called to investigate. There was a 'Women's Mystery' workshop in progress, and one of the women caught her eye, and invited her to join the circle. After some enlightening conversation and sharing, the circle came to a close, and a raffle was drawn for a copy of the book, Lotus-birth, by Shivam Rachana, who happened to be one of the women leading the session. Kd won it, and had it signed by Shivam as a gift to me.

The following night, two days before she was due to fly out to the UK, I started having contractions. As my partner, Rae, started blowing up the pool, transforming our lounge into a birthing room, and called my sister, Alice, to head over, I moaned down the phone, and around the world, to Kd. She told me about the women's workshop, and the book, and within a few hours my contractions had come to a stop. They didn't come back. We deflated the pool, my sister went home, and before long, Kd was with us, and had given me the book. Something about the serendipitous circumstances made me feel as though I'd been given it for a reason, as though our child had chosen not to be born until I'd read it; so read it I did.

Through the book I learned a lot about the physiology of the baby and placenta; about the changes in the baby's blood flow before and after birth, as the source of oxygen and routes for waste disposal shift from the placenta to the baby's own organs; and about how uncut cords heal nearly three times faster than those cut immediately at birth. It was all fascinating, but what the book did more than anything else, was to awaken me to the deep connection that my unborn child, that any unborn child, has to their placenta.

Some nine months previously, my precious child had been one tiny, miraculous cell. This cell had split into more cells, some of which had gone on to become her body, her organs, her skin and her hair; and others had become her life support system, her cord and her placenta, but they all had come from the same place, the same one cell. They were all her. Her placenta was as much a part of her as her heart or her hands.

Equally, for her entire existence so far, she'd shared her world with one thing: her placenta. She'd snuggled against it, stroked it, and enjoyed its companionship. Its sounds had lulled her to sleep. The cord connecting her to it had been her friend and plaything. Birth was going to take her from that world and into a new one, a transition that, no matter how peaceful her birth, was bound to be an overwhelming experience. If we were to cut her cord, we'd be severing her one last connection to her pre-birth world, to her sole friend and companion in her life so far. If we left her cord uncut, she could let go of her placenta when she was ready, and her transition to the outside world would be more gentle, and as much as we could make it, on her terms. Once I'd begun to look at the placenta and our child's relationship to it in these ways, I couldn't help but question why we thought we had a right to cut her cord, to dictate when she should be ready to let go of her placenta. Our journey towards Lotus-birth had begun.

I still wasn't ready to go all out and say "Yes, we're having a Lotus-birth." This was in part down to the trepidation I still had about how to care for the placenta, and also due to the late pregnancy aversion I had to making any kind of definite plan. Rae was equally unsure, but having had me ramble at her about much of the content of the book, she was equally willing to keep an open mind about it. We decided we would simply not cut the cord until it felt like it was the right time to do so. Over the next week or two I casually collected together a few extra items, just in case: a colander, a bag of sea salt, and a bottle of lavender essential oil. I also found a use for the beautiful yarn made of recycled sari silk I'd picked up in Australia the year before ~ I began to crochet a placenta bag.

The days rolled by, and the time for Kd's departure began to get closer. One evening, she cooked us up a feast of vegetarian sushi, and we then stayed up late, talking until the wee hours, whilst I crocheted away. I finished the bag at 1:30am, and we finally went to bed. At 3am I was woken by a contraction, followed by a trickle. My waters had broken. Our baby had decided it was time to be born.

Some 27 hours later, our daughter, Ember, was born at home into the waiting hands of her other mother, Rae, and our independent midwife, Olivia. She was a little limp, initially, but due to her continued connection to her placenta, and the oxygen it was providing her, she soon perked up. Her cord wasn't very long, but it was long enough for her to reach the breast, and we settled in for a cuddle and a breastfeed, and waited for the placenta to arrive. Five hours later we were still waiting, after having tried various positions, a bath and a selection of homeopathic remedies. Olivia was getting a little concerned, as she couldn't responsibly leave us until it had arrived, despite the fact that I'd had very little blood loss. The prospect of a trip to hospital for a manual extraction was beginning to loom. By this time, all the blood vessels in the cord had completely closed off ~ it was like a tube of white jelly ~ so we decided to give syntometrine and cord traction a go. Fortunately this worked, and out popped Ember's placenta, all warm and soft and beautiful.

After it had been checked over, we placed it next to Ember in a colander over a bowl, to drain ~ and settled down to cuddle together. It felt like a completely natural thing to do, and even the GP that came around to do the 'new baby' check that afternoon, was quite accepting of it, at least to our faces. But by the time evening came we were beginning to wonder what to do next, as we tried to work out how were going to manage our new baby, as well as her placenta (still currently in the bowl), in the bed with us. We talked it through, ummed and aahed a bit, then decided we would cut the cord. The moment the decision left our lips, Ember, who had been completely calm and contented up to that point, let out her first real cry. Rae and I just looked at each other, knowing without needing to speak, that Ember had just made her own decision. Her cord would remain intact.

So we washed her placenta under running water in the bathroom sink, removing the excess blood and clots, then we patted it dry and coated it in sea salt, to help to preserve it over the coming days. We then wrapped it in a bamboo nappy, and then wrapped Ember, and the placenta, up together. As it turned out, the ongoing placenta care was incredibly simple. Every morning and evening we removed the old nappy, and replaced it with a fresh one, adding some more salt and a few drops of lavender oil. There was no unpleasant smell at all, and it very quickly felt completely normal.

The day after she was born, Rae's parents came over to meet their new grandchild. We weren't sure how well the idea of a Lotus-birth would go down with them, so we just put Ember and her nappy-wrapped placenta into a gro-bag, together, and neglected to mention that there was more than just a baby in there. We nodded in agreement when they commented on her healthy weight (she was 4kg without her placenta, anyway), but to this day they have no idea they were cuddling her placenta, too.

After a day or so, Ember's cord began to go brittle and turn a dark brown colour. Then, two and a half days after she was born, she was in my sister's arms when she began to become quite fractious ~ something that was unusual for her up to that point. Alice looked inside her blankets, and saw her cord had come away, neatly and completely. She was lotus born.

Throughout the days that Ember and her placenta remained joined, she was calm and content, and seemed quietly aware of all that was going on around her. On an energetic level, it felt as though her placenta was acting as a shield between her and everything else, allowing her to transition from unborn to born, slowly and gently. She has remained a very relaxed and happy baby. Maybe she was always going to be that way, but I can't help but feel that the fact that she was able to transition gently, and that she knew from the start that she would be heard and her choices would be respected, have played a part. Having a Lotus-birth was, for us, a beautiful, spiritual and deeply loving way to welcome our child into the world. We may or may not have more children, but if we do, my wish would most definitely be to let them be lotus born, too.

Placenta ~ Latin, from the Greek plakous ountos, meaning flat cake
From root: plax plakos, meaning flat plate
"Each year on the anniversary of our birth ~ our birthday ~ it's customary in Western culture to have a cake, served on a flat plate, decorated with lit candles. We have a birthday song sung to us, we blow out the candles, we're clapped and cheered, we stab the cake, we cut it and we share it with others to eat.
Even in our modern culture, so devoid of ritual, we enshrine a sense of devotion to and celebration of the sacred placenta through these customs."
Rachana, 2000, p1.

The time it takes for the navel to heal:
[] When cut at birth, 9.56 days
[] After the cord has stopped pulsing, 7.16 days
[] Later, 3.75 days

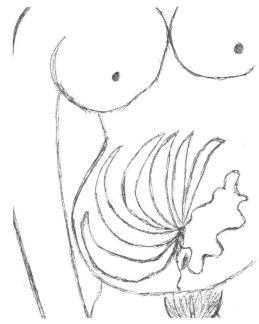

Illustration by Bethany

Once upon a Winter Sunset
The birth of Rocco Bello Benjamin Morfea
As told by his mother, Liz Walkden Morfea

Sunday 16th January, 2005

The tale starts at the beginning of January. I would wake suddenly, feeling a strong contraction that would last for half an hour, until sleep would prove the more attractive option, and I would wake the next morning still pregnant. I joked with my husband, Peter, that I was going to experience labour a bit at a time, in nice manageable chunks, spread over a few weeks, until finally the baby would just pop right out. As it happened, that was not too far from the truth.

On Tuesday, 10th January, my sister, Sarah, flew from Scotland into New York, during a snowstorm. Driving at 15mph in frightening weather to meet her at the airport, my belly very full and hard, I mused that my dream birth did not happen on the hard shoulder of the Bronx River Parkway on the back seat of a Toyota (however spacious).

A jet-lagged Sarah proved to be the perfect companion during my 3am forays in the kitchen. I'd read that during the last few weeks of pregnancy one should eat as though each day could be the big one. I was taking no chances, devouring an entire fresh pineapple and tub of trail mix every night.

Friday 14th, I felt an overwhelming desire to mop the kitchen floor, which really isn't me. I ought to have recognised this as the bizarre and telling nesting instinct, but instead I polished up a shine, and then slept until Saturday afternoon. When Peter came home from work that evening he brought me a big bunch of beautiful, tightly closed irises. The next morning they were in full bloom; and, unable to tolerate any more nocturnal pineapple, my baby was ready to be born.

Sunday 16th January: Taking my morning pee, I felt a strange popping sensation. I couldn't be certain that it was the breaking of the waters rather than yet another weird thing that happens during pregnancy, like itchy tummy skin, or gaining a big Moon face, or the ingestion of excess tropical fruits. I fried myself a couple of eggs with soldiers, and monitored the plumbing situation. When I phoned our midwife, Connie, she said, with a big smile in her voice: "Congratulations, today is your baby's birth day!" "Crikey," I thought, "I'd better get some rest." I wasn't entirely convinced, but after a couple of hours with my hypnosis CD, I was ready to share the news with my 11 year-old daughter, Polly, and Sarah.

Polly broke into a hysterical whirling dervish of a dance on the sparkling kitchen floor, and slipped, almost breaking her ankles. I had visions of us in the emergency room, rushing to get back in time to give birth at home. Polly embraced my belly, and firmly instructed the baby to "pick an exit and make sure it's down".

Much excitement followed. Peter cooked a hearty soup and the girls prepared *limoon*: the Arabic lime drink that I had requested for labour. After lunch I needed to move around a lot, and so, stylish even in labour, I paired wellies and a bobble hat with pyjamas, and walked with Peter out over the crispy snow in our garden, stopping occasionally to go with a contraction. As we talked about our plans for the garden I lost focus, and became disinterested in conversation ~ I was turning inward, leaving this world of intellect and reason for the primal, the animal; the unconscious place. I was now entering Labourland.

At 2.15pm, Peter called Connie to come over to our house. I went upstairs to take a shower. I then needed to lie down, so I took a bath, and with each contraction I just breathed out. So this breathing thing does work, I thought. As the contractions got stronger I began making this noise. It just came from deep within me, a noise I've never made before, but that I maybe recognised from a CD of New Age whale music.

It's when I get out of the bath that things really kick in. The contractions are so close together that I cannot get up off the floor. So there I am on my hands and knees ~ fortunately, Peter thought to put towels under me, or I would be forever arthritic ~ on the bathroom floor; and believing this was still only the beginning, with many hours to endure, for a second I doubt that I can do this. Childbirth without drugs...was I totally out of my mind????

But I see Peter, who has made himself comfy on the toilet. He looks so calm and believing, and just nods every now and then. Later, I see Connie's feet. She's wearing black slippers that I haven't seen until now, and I realise these must be her special birth shoes. I will have my baby soon. I keep making the whale noises.

I am transfixed in this position, so heavy on the floor. Now Polly, Sarah and birth attendant Judy are also with me. I ask for silence, I need to be free from distraction.

I feel the immense power rushing through me, my whole self contracting for three minutes, then resting for 30 seconds, although time has lost any true meaning. Each break I take a long drink, and everyone encourages me lots, and this is how it happens, this is how I get through.

There finally comes a rest, and Connie asks me if I would prefer to have my baby in the comfort and warmth of my bed. I say yes, but can't imagine how I'll ever get up off the floor. Team UK/USA managed to pick me up and support me to my never-so-welcoming bed. The room is peaceful and beautiful. I have a little stone lion next to me. Late in pregnancy I'd found a painting of a half woman, half lion giving birth. And now here I was, on hands and knees, birthing my own cub.

My baby inherited the rather large Walkden forehead from my Dad's family (which 31 years before, at my own birth, had resulted in a very difficult labour for my poor Mum, with much struggle and intervention).

For me, being at home and unhindered by machinery, monitors, wires, strangers, routines, bleeping, ticking and interference, I was able to tune in to my body, and adopt the optimal position in which to birth such a big, brawny baby. It's truly awesome that the body knows; that when we shut out the din of life, out of the silence comes this ancient knowledge that we all possess.

Judy applied pressure to my hips, pivoting the bones of the pelvis to further ease the passage of the baby. She asked for some oil for massage, and Sarah dutifully returned from the kitchen with a five gallon bottle of extra-virgin olive oil, though thankfully not the contraband liquid gold Calabrese olive oil, hand-pressed by my in-laws. Only in an Italian home!!

The Winter sunset illuminated the bedroom, beaming light onto my pillow, which was decorated with animals. Through each contraction I made these loud noises, becoming the lioness; and between them I felt the wonderful rush of endorphins, and smiled at the animals.

I was suddenly struck with this incredible clarity, consciousness and enlightenment ~ that this was life, Nature, trust, in all its raw, sweaty, Earthy, elemental beauty. This is what we are capable of when we trust in life, give in to instinct, and let Nature do her work. This was intense, but not suffering. I felt as if I'd been let in on life's greatest secret.

As the baby's head appeared, everyone cooed about his thick hair. Then, a few more pushes, assisted by the baby, who was using me as a springboard, kicking so hard it hurt!

At 4.39pm I gave one last push, and out he tumbled into his Daddy's waiting hands. It wasn't until I heard a baby crying that I realised he was actually born. Those endorphins are pretty damn good, and in my valley-of-the-dolls state I went to sit back on my heels, inducing a moment of panic for Peter and Connie, who were passing the baby, still connected by the umbilical cord, underneath me to my front side. Ooops!

Once in my arms, he started feeding instantly, like a crazed, starved thing. We all adored our beautiful, perfect baby, with his Dad's cleft chin and Mum's giant forehead. After a few minutes, Polly checked the vitals and announced that we had a boy. With his broad shoulders, big manly chest and strong neck, he looked like he was ready to get up and crawl away.

We revelled for hours in the magic feeling birth brings; holding our precious boy, taking photos. Connie made a print of his placenta ~ the tree of life ~ and we laughed, talked and felt amazed at how quick it had all been.

For the next week we mostly stayed in bed, resting and falling in love with Rocco Bello Benjamin. Peter, Sarah and Polly kept me well fed with nutritious foods, juices and treats, and Mamma Morfea came and fed our souls with her Italian recipes. Outside, the snow fell fast and deep, and it was such an enchanting feeling to be snowed-in in our house filled with cards, flowers and our new baby, safely wrapped up in birth energy.

When it comes to having a baby, there really is no place like home.

*"Epidurals rip
women off
of an opportunity to
experience themselves as competent adults."*
~ Margaret Egeland, CNM

Birth and Bonding
by Joseph Chilton Pearce

Joseph is the author of Magical Child; From Magical Child to Magical Teen; The Crack in the Cosmic Egg; Evolution's End; The Death of Religion and the Rebirth of Spirit.

Shortly before scheduled to speak at a conference on birth-bonding, I received a lengthy form from The American College of Obstetricians stating that I had to disclaim any conflict of interest I, as a presenter at said conference, might have with the practices of said college, my signature of agreement being required. In the ensuing paragraphs, I was warned that my failure to comply would result in said college informing the audience attending my talk of such perfidy on my part. That college, consisting of some forty thousand obstetricians, had just passed a resolution that any woman desiring a c-section could have one without any medical reason, simply her own whims. Both hospital and obstetrician make far more money on c-section than ordinary vaginal delivery; birth accounts for some two-thirds of all hospital revenue, and a majority of hospitals are owned by large corporate chains.

Documentation for the following short essay is in the common domain, but for the sake of brevity is largely left out here. I also leave out reference to the epochal work of James Prescott and Michel Odent. My intent is to cover aspects of birth-bonding not ordinarily addressed.

A Conflict between Nature's Intelligence and Human Intellect
Recall the triad of interdependent needs Paul MacLean states as imperative:
audio-visual communication
nurturing
play

All are established by mother-infant bonding at birth, and stabilised through breastfeeding in the first year of life. Deprived of bonding and breastfeeding, all subsequent development (of both infant and mother) is compromised.

Years ago, Muriel Beadle asked, "Why is it that the human infant seems born in a state of alert excitement that quickly reverts to distress, followed by conscious withdrawal?" (This withdrawal lasts for ten to twelve weeks on average.) Answering Beadle's query leads to a richly woven fabric of Nature's proposing and man's disposing.

First, most mammals, on preparing to give birth, seek out the most hidden, preferably dark, quiet and safe haven available. At the first sign of any intrusion ~ even the snapping of a twig in the wilds ~ the creature's natural intelligence slows, or even stops, birthing, waiting to make sure the setting is safe. We humans' mammalian instincts are in charge at birth, interpreting and responding to environmental signals.

If safe, supported and secure, in touch with herself and Nature, human mothers have given birth in as little as twenty minutes. But at the first sign of interference of any sort, regardless of the nature or reason for it, the birthing process will be disrupted, slowed down, or even halted, by these ancient and powerful intelligences within.

If disruption does occur, a mother's smooth muscular coordination of resonant responses can be lost, and chaos can reign within her ~ muscle fighting with muscle, instinct with instinct, inner-knowing confused by outer intrusions, Nature's intentions clashing with culture's attentions, mother and infant losing on all fronts. Sadly, this has been the norm for the majority of modern women, and a primary cause of our ever increasing personal-social turmoil.

Nikos Tinbergen (Nobel laureate in ethology) studied the metabolism of the early infant, and determined that a human newborn needs to feed about every twenty minutes in its early days, the periods between growing progressively longer as the months go by. Mother's milk, it seems, has few fats and proteins, but is, instead, as Israeli doctors termed it, a rich cocktail of hormones. This rather thin diet requires that the infant feed quite frequently ~ which is the whole point. Some mammals, rabbits for instance, produce a milk so heavy with fats and proteins their offspring need only feed once or twice a day, allowing mother's forage to make more rich milk for that next powerful wallop. One might wonder why Nature didn't make a similarly handy arrangement for us humans, instead of a procedure so inconvenient, particularly to us modern people. Look a bit further, however, and we find that Nature did this on behalf of an intricately interwoven fabric of interdependent needs, rather exclusively human, and absolutely critical to being fully human.

No Digestive Juices?

First, hydrochloric acid ~ found abundantly in other infant mammals, since necessary for the digestion of fats and proteins, is not found in human infants in the same quantity, since so few fats and proteins are found in human mothers' milk. Some nine months after birth, however, hydrochloric acid spontaneously appears in full flow. Remember this nine-month marker in what follows here:

Just as it took Nature nine months to grow that infant in mother's womb in the first place, it takes another nine months in the <u>arms</u> of that mother to firmly establish the infant in the matrix of its new world, continue the growth of the infant's brain, stabilise its body functions, particularly the heart; and Nature does what she can to keep that infant 'in-arms' for that period. Audio-visual is number one in MacLean's Triad of Needs, and a rudimentary hearing develops early in-utero. If the foetus has normal hearing and a speaking mother, language development gets underway in the second trimester, through muscular responses the infant makes to phonemes, those foundational units of words in the mother's speech. This language foundation builds in successive stages until birth, and leads to speech.

Vision, however, while it occupies more of our brain than all other senses put together, obviously can't develop in-utero (though visual sensitivity appears early on, as seen in an infant's aversion to bright lights should we shine them directly on the mother's belly ~ which prompts the infant to turn its head away). Visual development, though, and the audio-visual communication that accompanies it, must await birth, to unfold. (There is a vast difference between stimuli and communication.)

And at birth, if given a face within six to twelve inches away, two immediate responses take place in the newborn: its initial excited alertness (noted by Muriel Beadle long ago) stabilises, and visual, and audio-visual, development begin. That close-up face literally turns on the infant brain, its conscious awareness, and keeps it turned on. For the infant is born with a preset neural pattern for cognising-perceiving a face, and will lock eyes on a face if one is given at that required distance, and hold that face in focus. Perception-cognition automatically begins, activating the infant's entire body-brain system. Focus is immediate so long as a face is there to focus on; parallax (muscle coordination of the eyes) forms within minutes (so the infant can even follow that face around should it move about), and a construction of knowledge of a visual world begins ~ a world based on this stable foundation of a face.

Before long, other objects in the mother's immediate vicinity are registered, and, through processes of association, corresponding new neural patterns form, and a cognitive field of recognisable objects grows exponentially (as does the brain itself) ~ so long as that face-pattern remains the <u>stable point</u> of reference. Although any face will work at birth, face constancy, and all that goes with it, is the critical factor in this early infant movement from known to unknown, and is vitally necessary for a stable and stress-free development.

Should a face not be presented, along with all the attendant functions accompanying it (to be described shortly), distress takes over, and conscious awareness will fade within about 45 minutes, and does not ordinarily reappear, as mentioned above, for upwards of some ten to twelve weeks on average.

Bonding as a reciprocal function between mother and infant is then fragmented, and the ongoing nurturing instincts, which bonding awakens and locks into the mother's responses, aren't there. Most infants then receive only sporadic exposures to a face or faces, and by then, consciousness largely retreated, the awareness needed for such cognition to take place and be stabilised is missing. Nature will compensate as best she can, but under these conditions, her capacity to compensate is diminished and slow.

Nature arranged that this magical face-trigger be some six to twelve inches from those equally wonderful mammary glands from which flows that life-giving fat-and-protein-free nurturing-nourishment. Frequent nursing assures a frequent reinforcing of the stable face pattern on which vision and awareness are based. 'Object constancy', as Piaget called it, the stabilisation of an object-world of vision, occurs around the ninth month of this busy construction period. Among the many facets of this ninth-month milestone, myelination of the neural patterns of this primary visual world takes place, making the neural foundations permanent and cheap to operate, the ongoing expansion of the visual world automatic and effortless. Now Nature can turn her world-building energy to other developments, which open around that pivotal ninth month. (Any society separating mothers from infants at birth will have a disproportionately large population with impaired vision. The United States, for instance, is virtually a nation of eyeglasses. (We ignore and/or forget that pre-literate, primitive people have far more accurate and extensive vision than we have ~ some of those people can see the rings of Saturn with their naked eye.) Far more seriously, for those willing to look, note how many of the infant-toddlers we see, pushed about in various wheeled devices that keep them separate, out of the way and helpless, have strangely vacant, barely-focused eyes, and vapid, nobody-at-home expressions ~ as though a light were blown out in their brain, or rather, never ignited.

Some forty years ago, Whittlestone, at The University of Adelaide, pointed out that the mother's heart is a most critical factor from conception through birth. This has been well established. Now we know that her heart is every bit as critical a part of the next nine-months in-arms. Over half a century ago, researchers found that a heart cell could be removed from a live rodent's heart, put in an appropriate nutrient to keep it alive, and, when examined through a microscope, would continue to pulsate, expanding and contracting regularly, according to the rhythm set by the donor-heart. After some time of this separation from the heart, however, that rhythmic pulsation would deteriorate until collapse, and that erratic jerky spasm called fibrillation, precursor to death of the cell, would set in. If two heart cells are placed on the slide, however, separated from each other, when fibrillation begins, through bringing the two cells into close proximity with each other (they do not have to touch and can be separated by a tiny barrier) they both stopped their death-spasms and re-established their co-ordinated pulsation, in sync with each other. Each cell had 'lifted the other' out of that fibrillation that leads to death, into the shared rhythm of life. This miracle occurs, it turns out, through bringing into spatial conjunction the electro-magnetic fields that arise from, and surround, each heart cell, a phenomenon only recently discovered. These electro-magnetic (EM) fields are not affected by ordinary physical boundaries, and when the fields come into contact, their waves entrain, go into the same coherent pattern (and coherent wave-forms reinforce each other). This coherent resonance, in turn, lifts those cells out of chaos into order. Cells and their EM fields mutually give rise to and/or influence each other, and the same phenomenon occurs, on a far larger and far more serious level, with infant-mother hearts at birth: a major, but largely unrecognised factor, in bonding.

The heart itself produces a very powerful EM field, in three successive waves: the first and most powerful surrounds the person's body, flooding every cell and neuron of that body; the second extends some three feet in all directions and interacts with other heart fields within that proximity, a principal ingredient of emotion and interpersonal relationships; the third extends indefinitely, for all purposes universally (possibly a factor or aspect of the human spirit). So at birth, following separation, infant and mother's heart must be brought into immediate proximity, wherein they confirm and stabilise each other or 'lift each other' into their familiar, stabilised order. Again, that six-to-twelve inch distance of the mother's face, giving immediate proximity to those nurturing breasts, vital to the ongoing awakening experience of the newborn, assures a return to and ongoing stabilisation of the infant's heart given by the mother's heart, to which resonance the infant had imprinted on it at a cellular level from conception. This order must be continually reinforced through that warm proximity for about a nine month period. By that time the infant heart has matured enough to 'stand on its own' without so frequent a stabilisation by mother's heart. Thus here we have another critical ninth-month milestone marker.

Newborns and mothers wired up for heart and brain wave recordings (electrocardiograms and electroencephalograms) show coherency and entrainment (matching of the wave frequencies) when infant and mother are together. Both systems become incoherent (chaotic) if prolonged separation takes place, whereupon cortisol is released by both mother and child systems, and general stress takes place. Remember our two heart cells on that microscope's slide, and remember that excess cortisol is quite toxic to neural systems, particularly new ones.

(Remember, also, that any society interfering with natural bonding at birth will have a corresponding increase of heart trouble. When primary heart connections fail to take place, heart development in the infant is immediately compromised, and a 'wounded heart' trauma takes place in the mother, whether she is aware of it or not. The post-partum blues that often follows birth-separation can be a devastating experience, affecting the health of both parties thereafter.)

Years ago, biologist-anthropologist Ashley Montague wrote a now-classic work called Touching, and recently Mariana Caplan wrote a similar work called Untouched. Both are well-documented studies showing the critical necessity of infant skin-stimulus at birth. For at birth, the newborn's nervous system is quite undeveloped, since the millions of sensory nerve endings distributed over the body can't be activated or developed in-utero. In that water world the infant's body is protected by a waterproof coating of a fatty substance called vernix caseous, the protection of which also insulates the myriad nerve endings. So at birth, all mammalian mothers vigorously lick their infants off and on for many hours, even sporadically for days thereafter, to activate the dormant sensory nerve endings and the peripheral nervous system, which is, of course, a primary extension of the brain.

Failure to activate these nerve endings results in a de-sensitisation affecting the reticular activating system of the old brain, where all sensory stimuli are collated or organised into those resonant patterns which are then sent on to higher cortical areas of the brain for world-making and experiencing. Touch deprivation results in a compromised and diminished over-all neural growth, sensory system and general conscious awareness in the infant, as well as affecting inner ear development, balance, spatial patterning and so on, later. (Mothers separated from their infants at birth obviously can't provide this touch-stimulus, nor are they stimulated to do so later if the separation is prolonged. Mother, too, has a critical window of opportunity for activating those ancient nurturing responses, considered by Paul MacLean to be our species' survival instincts. These instincts are activated by her skin-to-skin contact with her infant, making bonding a reciprocal dynamic of awaking and discovery.)

Language learning, as mentioned, begins late in the second trimester as muscular responses the infant makes to the phonetic content of the mother's speech. This dynamic continues after birth, if the appropriate model-stimulus is provided ~ a speaking mother in close proximity. And, recall, during that initial nine-months of continued language learning and phonetic completion, speech preparation takes place. Around the ninth month after birth, the average infant's speech preparations have led into lalling or infant-babbling, and even the first words ~ if, and only if, of course, the appropriate model-signal-stimuli are provided in that critical second-matrix period, a provision made by simply nursing the infant and speaking. (Infants separated from their mothers and confined to various forms of ongoing separation thereafter [as most modern infants are ~ through cribs, bassinets, carriages, playpens, strollers, etc., or that most immediate and thorough devastation called day-care], are denied all these responses, and their development is correspondingly compromised. Nature will compensate as best she can ~ but compensation is always a poor substitute for natural, spontaneous mimetic growth.

We live in a compensated society, however, where the abnormal has been sustained until it has become the norm ~ we citizen-victims none the wiser.)

Finally (in this brief survey), but perhaps the most important of all these ninth-month-markers, we come to the prefrontal cortex, a major neural system which cannot unfold in-utero (except in a most rudimentary form), and must await birth to begin its full cellular growth. If conditions are right, it will develop into the largest neural lobe.

During the in-arms and early crawling period, the primary phase of prefrontal growth takes place, completing in that significant ninth month. (A second growth spurt, equally 'experience dependent', is designed to begin at mid-adolescence. This later prefrontal growth-spurt is critically dependent on the successful completion of the first one, years before.) Since the mid 1980s, the prefrontal cortex has been the subject of intense investigation, and is now recognised as the latest evolutionary neural system to develop (it is probably less than 50,000 years old, compared to millions up to hundreds of millions of years behind the older lobes and modules of our brain).

This latest and greatest of Nature's neural achievements proves to be the executive brain, able to moderate and control all responses, reactions and instincts of those older animal brains, with their sensory-motor, defensive, sexual and instinct-bound patterns, as well as the neo-cortex giving us speech and a vastly higher intellect.

Only this newest prefrontal system can organise the entire brain into a smoothly synchronous attention or intention, link all our lower instincts, as well as thinking-feeling, with higher fields of intelligence, and translate all the higher human attributes such as love, empathy, care, and creativity, into daily action. The prefrontal cortex gives us what Elkhonon Goldberg rightly calls 'civilised mind' ~ if developed.

But, as Allen Schore's research makes clear, the genetic structure of the prefrontal cortex proves to be the most 'experience-dependent' of all brain systems, that is, those genetic systems are critically dependent on appropriate environmental feedback. This feedback is given through the multi-levelled functions of infant-mother bonding and ongoing relations, and the overall positive emotional environment that should result. This feedback includes nurturing through breastfeeding, sufficient movement and sensory stimuli, immediate proximity to the mother's face and heart, the continual coherent resonance between mother and infant heart fields, language and speech stimuli, and so on.

Failure to provide this overall emotional support inevitably means a compromised prefrontal cortex. It literally cannot grow sufficient cellular structures and make the necessary neural connections with the rest of the brain for full operation. And a compromised prefrontal cortex results in an impaired 'emotional intelligence', with a corresponding difficulty in relating with others or controlling our ancient sexual-survival reflexes, with a corresponding tendency toward apathy, hopelessness, despair, and/or any of the many forms of violence.

Just as it took Nature nine months to grow the basic 'triune brain' unfolding in-utero, this prefrontal growth takes the nine months following birth, with all the attendant developments which centre around the heart. Thus all these strands, briefly sketched in the above, gather to completion around this ninth month milestone. Then, if the necessary foundations are in place and functional, from the ninth to twelfth month another major neural structure grows to connect this new evolutionary executive brain with the ancient limbic or emotional brain, which older system has direct unmediated neural connections with the heart (through the ancient amygdala which is as much the top part of the defensive hind-brain as lowest part of the emotional brain). Thus this orbito-frontal loop, as it is called, a large bridge between old and new, proves, as the research of Allen Schore clearly shows, the most decisive factor of our life, and is, again, critically experience-dependent.

If emotional nurturing is lacking, this bridge will be compromised and/or largely deconstructed in the little development made. At this ninth-month point, when the orbito-frontal loop begins its massive growth, the ancient cerebellum, in the back of the brain, undergoes a corresponding growth spurt. The cerebellum, rudimentary until this time, since only sparsely employed, is involved in all speech, walking, coordination of muscular systems and much more. (This muscle coordination takes place through the muscle spindle system, tiny neural extensions found on each striation of muscle tissue throughout the body. These spindles played a major role in the uterine infant's physical response to those phonemes underlying language, literally 'embedding' language in the body.)

So, at this ninth-month period, as Nature prepares to organise the entire forebrain into a single coherent whole, the cerebellum readies the infant body for that upright stance we humans enjoy, which will be followed by walking and talking, displayed in that excited exploration of 'building structures of knowledge' of our physical world. Infancy comes to an end, and the early child or toddler appears.

To prepare for the toddler's excited charging out to explore all aspects of the world, (equally dictated and orchestrated by Nature's agenda), the child will not only touch, but taste, every item of interest in that world; and to prepare for the new diet-world opening, which will no doubt contain fats and proteins, the appropriate digestive juices are forthwith provided. Nature dutifully turns on that long-absent hydrochloric acid in the child's metabolic system. Hydrochoric acid simply wasn't needed ~ at least not according to millennia of genetic encoding ~ in that critical 'in-arms' period, for which Nature provides a vastly superior food, and supreme method of dispensing.

So we have now come full circle in this brief sketch of birth and bonding, its ways and means and whys, from the initial enigma of no hydrochloric acid to its grand entrance as cued by Nature, when the curtain rises on a new stage of development, ushering in an ongoing series of new bondings with new matrices, over the years ~ the family, the Earth itself, society, the pair bonding leading to species renewal, bonding with one's own offspring, with the spirit within and universal without, and so on.

Marshal Klaus spoke of an interlocking cascade of redundant patterns Nature has built in to assure this critical first bonding between mother and infant, which meets the threefold need MacLean referred to, truly an 'eternal golden braid' (to steal Hostadter's phrase). Marshal Klaus calls bonding the establishment of the greatest love affair in the Universe, on which this wondrous unfolding of human life depends. Now we can see the astonishing and thorough intelligence and careful planning, the intricate interweaving of myriad critically-timed and interdependent responses which Nature evolved over eons of time, and invested in this birth-bonding process entrusted to us. And now, more than ever, we can see the astonishing extent to which modern practices have by-passed, compromised, or outright eliminated, virtually every item on the agenda of this incredible architectural design. Now we can understand why our medical interferences with birth ~ taken as axiomatic and unconsciously accepted as the norm by virtually the entire globe ~ are proving to be our global undoing.

You cannot do to a living organism what we are now doing to the vast majority of human infants (and the ongoing spill-over into the general abandonment and neglect of children taking place world-wide), without paying a price.

The ruinously expensive takeover of all birthing by hospital-medical procedures, has brought into play an equally huge and expensive cradle-to-grave therapeutic operation, undertaken in our efforts to repair the damage we are blindly causing at the same time. We witness the strange contradiction of being madly caught up in patchworks of healing and hoped-for wholeness, while blindly allowing a radically damaging, unnatural birth practice to continue unquestioned and unchecked. Our contradiction overwhelms us, neutralises our very effort at recovery, and breakdown is widespread.

Child abuse and child suicide are but the most blatant signs of the breeding ground for violence our interventions are spreading worldwide.

There may never have been a 'golden age' of birthing and child rearing (the closest being the Yequanna, Jean Liedloff wrote about), but also there are no historical precedents for a species abandoning its own offspring, as witnessed today, worldwide.

There is a direct correlation between the final abolition of breastfeeding through an insane birthing, and day care culture. Day care, now so massively present, is but cosmetically camouflaged abandonment, and a direct result of failure of bonding. A bonded mother does not abandon her infant, no matter how socially sanctioned such behaviour might be.

Hospital-medical childbirth, now made sacrosanct, and unquestioned on every hand, is a more insidious and devious danger than atomic bombs or germ warfare, since unrecognised and even unrecognisable for the demonic force it is by the public at large. Taking away a woman's rights over her own reproductive process has been a disaster, but intervening in, and all but abolishing, the bonding of mother with infant at birth is a devastating crime against Nature: perhaps the most criminal and destructive act on the planet today, and an ultimate, if slow but sure, instrument for species' suicide.

Until we get medical-hospital interference completely out of birthing, and put birth back into the hands of women and the mother herself, as Nature intended, we will continue to decline as a species. Surely, the 'collective cultural imperative' for medical intervention is enormous and powerful. And surely, our entire culture promotes the medical myth through film, literature, the daily news, schooling, on and on.

But, no organisation has as yet really set about exposing the medical myth of birth, and at least trying to awaken the general public to the outrage. The focus must be put on prevention of the travesty, not therapeutic patchwork after the fact.

Surely, the medical-myth is woven into every fibre of the social fabric, but that fabric is becoming our shroud. We can awaken in future mothers the ancient intelligence of the heart; de-condition her culturally-imprinted self-doubt and fear; and restore in her the knowledge and power of being the mother of our race, with the courage to act accordingly. In undertaking such a restoration, we will unfold an ongoing educational agenda not only for survival, but for a higher, nobler, more compassionate way of life.

You cannot do
to a living organism
what we are now doing
to the vast majority
of human infants
(and the ongoing spill-over
into the general abandonment
and neglect of children
taking place worldwide),
without paying a price.

Reaching the Light:
Gabriel's birth story
by Anna Packham

I'm in our tiny bathroom, talking to myself in the mirror. "Can this be?" I'm asking, and still rocking with the tide. I nod back at me. I've never given birth before, but I'm starting to understand how this goes. It's like they all said, you just have to go with it.

I knew it would happen today. We even left our artful pregnancy photos until this afternoon. One final hour of intimacy, the two of us for the last time like this. Laughing at the ridiculous sheet we picked to make it look discreet, when my ripe fruit roundness was perfect as it was. Trying out stupid poses, and making shadows on the wall with the bump. By the time we got bored, the twinges had already begun.

We took a final walk to the park behind our flat. The sea glistened in the distance, the sunset-coloured leaves shone in the Autumn Sun, dogs ran, the homeless man with his hundred black sacks caught my eye, and smiled, as I carried my shifting secret inside. We'd never see any of this with the same eyes again. Tomorrow, we'd be parents. I'd be a mother. I'm ready. Or at least I think I am.

It takes time to find the rhythm that holds me true ~ keeping it is trickier. I try to relax my mind, unplug it from the planet, and trust this clever body instead. I can do it. I know I can do it.

Deep in the night, I've created my space in the bedroom. The streetlights stream through the gap in the curtains, over my bare body, and I sway at the end of our iron bed. I keep the world out by closing my eyes. Images stream behind them instead: the sea blasting at rocks, castles, forests, long stone corridors, white sails ~ could be curtains, could be people in white robes ~ flowing at either side of me. If feels like my time could be near, but, instead of letting it happen, I escape to the bathroom. The contrast of the overhead light, the grey tiles, the grasping hold of the cold towel rail, bring me out of myself to the decision that this hurts; stings like salt water. The thinking and deciding make it hurt more.

The thoughts come thick and fast now, can't stop them. Can't stop myself grabbing my phone to see how long this has been going on (12 hours and counting), wondering what Dom's doing (filling the birth pool with the kettle). I stumble back to the dark bedroom, still niggling at myself ~ I just need another pillow, another sip of water, another remedy, another way to avoid this ~ the raging rapids of the life force. But as someone once said: this is not Disneyland. And the ride ain't gonna stop for me, no matter how hard I swim against it. I think I'm getting it now.

I reach for a touchstone. I think about all the women birthing now, those who birthed before me. I think about letting birth work through me. I think about a cave, and the sea whooshing through it, and "Ah, ok, there it is," and I flow with that. And that's how it goes. The flowing, the feeling, the far-seeing mixed with cold moments in the bathroom ~ struggle, fight and fear. But the night beats on regardless, and my body beats on, and my baby beats on. And soon, I will meet him.

I become focused,
bring my hands to prayer,
squat down into the water
like a pregnant Buddha,
and appear to go
inside myself completely.

The long night disappears somewhere. Morning is here, but the baby isn't. "Ok sweetie?" Dom asks me. No, I'm not. I sob sorry, salty tears. I'm beat, and I don't want to be a birthing goddess. I want my mum. I beg the hospital on the phone to please send the reinforcements. But the hospital isn't interested. "It's not time dear. Get in the pool. Get some sleep."

I slide into the simmering water for the first time, and 'Mercy!' I experience the most gratifying relief of my entire life. I'm held up, the liquid absorbs my tensions, soothing heat caresses my swollen body. I gratefully surrender to it, and begin to cry. Wail, really. Letting go of myself. That's when it finally happens. I forgot what they told me about the inland sea. The waters come rushing down, and with them, my baby's head: hot and sharp and ready to be born. But I'm not ready. I cling to one last shred; hold on by my fingernails. I tell myself I need to wait for the midwife. It's an eternity before she arrives and says what I already know ~ it's time to push. Now. But even when I try, something holds me back. I may not be on the planet, but I clearly hear her say, "You've got ten minutes, and if he's not out, you're going in an ambulance."

I think not.

Me, the one I really am, steps up now. Dom tells me afterwards I become focused, bring my hands to prayer, squat down into the water like a pregnant Buddha, and appear to go inside myself completely. I am not aware of this. All I know is that at this moment there is nothing. There is no me. There is no pool. There is no body. There is just everything. The Whole. The One. The All. Light. Exploding. And then, there is him. The sleek pup plunging into the water below me, shimmering to the surface, into my arms, fleshy and luminous, and real. And the world rushes back again, and I soar in behind it, incandescent with my joy.

Soon, it is quiet in the sunny bedroom, and I am smiling like a proud fool, as he latches on and feeds from my left breast. He is perfect and plump, downy and delicious. I hold him close to my heart. I am all heart.

It was the 27th October, 2006. The day I came into my birth right. The day Gabriel was born. He, the light bringer. Miracle maker. Life never has been the same. It just gets brighter and brighter and brighter, day after day after day.

Birthing and Saying the Great 'Yes'
by Georgina Kelly

In order to give birth and in order to passionately say "Yes", we need to open ourselves up wide. Our womb, the repository of life, needs the door unfastened to give birth. Our heart, the core of our being, needs to be unlocked to say a heartfelt "Yes".

Recently, I read the phrase 'saying the Great Yes' in a poetry book called "Women in Praise of the Sacred", and I experienced deep feelings of resonance. Jane Hirshfield[1] writes that the poets included in her book all shared themes evocative of a "spirituality of affirmation" ~ releasing their hearts in a trusting gesture to others and experiences. I thought at once of women birthing; and the times when many spoke or moaned "nooooo" when the sensations intensified and became seemingly overpowering. As a midwife I would, at this point, encourage the woman to welcome these rushes ('contractions'), to say 'YES!' as they approached, to meet them with appreciation. There is such a shift in every way when a woman manages this. There is a release; the energy changes. If anyone else is present, they are simultaneously inspired to echo the 'YES' in their own heart. There is a revival.

A Spiritual Practice

I believe 'saying the Great Yes' is indeed spiritual practice, a spirituality of affirmation, especially in our lives as women. We women can open our hearts and greet the opportunities for enlarging and knowing found through a connection with our cycles, our pregnancies, our birthing, and our mothering. It's in these times that we can become more self-aware, enjoy a heightened consciousness, and transcend our familiar experience of self, the new understanding being linked to changes in our female bodies.[2] Through the initiation of childbirth particularly, many of us are lifted up high on the powerful wave of Nature, dumped and churned about, then, still breathless, thrown upon the shores of a new and glorious land. For some women, it's a wonderful, fulfilling and intense pathway where subsequently our eyes see everything in a new way ~ above all, our selves. Our transformation, however we birth our babies, is inevitable. No matter how we experience the journey, there is the promise that we can discover our potential for growth and maturity when we dismiss our expectations, and embrace the uncertainty that Nature and life offer. I believe in the intrinsic Mystery of Birth; a place beyond rational understanding, where knowledge about ourselves and existence may be made known by revelation, an epiphanic experience. Through a spirituality of affirmation, we women are capable of intimacy with the sacred deep in our wombs, and can begin to appreciate the interconnectedness and the aliveness of everything.

Saying 'No' to a Gift

In our society when we talk about birth, we talk about 'pain relief'. I would like to offer a different perspective inspired by the language of the Spirituality of Affirmation and 'saying the Great Yes'. We have an aversion to pain, and an aversion to the very thought of pain. We don't see it as positive or helpful or necessary; and are fearful it will lead us to suffering. As Kabat-Zinn explains, it's not always pain, per se, that can create suffering; it's the way we see the sensations, how we judge them, and how we react to them that determines our experience.[3] Many pregnant women in our society dread the pain that they may experience in birth, and fear that they'll suffer, 'lose control' and be unable to cope. The options our culture offers are an attempt to eradicate or lessen the pain through pharmacological means; or to deny them through forms of distractions. Distraction may work as a coping mechanism in the early part of labour, yet, in the midst of birth, the power that rises up in the body refuses to be suppressed. Our body demands that we take attention so we can enter into a relationship with it. Furthermore, deadening or relieving the physical sensations of birth may steal from the riches gained in passing through the rite of passage to motherhood. Our culture informs us that the pain of birth is pointlessly brutal. Fairy tales symbolise this phenomenon where many characters reject what they mistake as repulsive or insignificant. This is because it appears in a form that isn't easily recognised. They are not aware that they are saying 'no' to a meaningful gift or profound secret.[4] If our pain is perceived as an unwelcome curse, we will gladly have it taken away. When we do, we can't fathom what our body is doing, as her voice is silenced. With our pain numbed or gone, we lose the cues and the simultaneous know-how to birth our babies. Without our pain, our teacher, we must depend on our attendants to tell us what to do. We can't entirely reach down into our core and summon all our potency. Resultantly, we don't have the chance to explore this wild land, and discover how resourceful and creative we can be. This gift, the opportunity for self-knowledge, is rejected along with our pain.

Sensational Birthing and Mindfulness

A Spirituality of Affirmation would encourage us not to try to relieve the pain, but to fully engage with it. This encompasses the practice of mindfulness, which is developing awareness of the physical and emotional experience. We need to 'put the welcome mat out'[5] for the sensations we experience in birthing; to be receptive to its teachings; to discover what is actually happening; to know what positions or movements are needed and how we should be. Mindfulness in birthing will lead to revelations about our body and our self which distraction or pain relief can never do.

The inherent preparation for mindfulness in birth is initiated in pregnancy. Whilst pregnant we are reminded that we are in our body; the dramatic changes and physical sensations grab our attention deliberately. When growing our babies, our body tells us when to rest, when and what to eat and drink; what environment to avoid and what to seek. We need to take heed for the well-being of our baby and our self. Thus, we reconnect to our body, our Earth nature, and modify our behaviour to grow our babies lovingly. Many women come into a new and confident relationship with their bodies during this time as they witness their physical transformation with wonder. Pregnancy is the time to become more acquainted with our inner voice or subjective knowing ~ an imperative preparation for birthing and mothering. In birth, more than at any time, we cannot afford to override our body's messages to us. It teaches us what to do to get our babies born. The sensations we feel whilst birthing our babies ~ the twinges and niggles, the tightenings and throbbings, the stretches and openings, the thrusts and bearing down, the burning and power and pain, the rushes and urges and energy ~ these are the words and poems of birth ~ the body language. We need to listen actively, and respond; to join in the conversation and be connected. Our body and our baby become other aspects of our selves, along with our mind. We work together in unity, prompting each other in harmony ~ a trinity of sorts.

Mindfulness is about being attuned to the very present, moment by moment. We avoid clocks and watches and counting how long the birth is taking, or worrying about how we'll cope with the next phase in the journey. We only know in that very instant what we need to do ~ we may want massage and touch one minute, the next minute touch seems excruciating, and all we want is solitude. Therefore, we can have no real plan except to welcome the moment.

Larry Rosenberg writes that mindfulness is a practice of intimacy: of being one with what we are observing or watching.[6] We are not objective observers of our experience: we are 'fully living out our lives, but are awake in the midst of it'. With mindfulness we don't make judgements about what is being experienced. We don't evaluate thoughts that arise, or our selves ~ it's simply about being watchful and saying 'yes'.

By doing so, we affirm the experience and we affirm birth. We give birth. The giving is an act of creation and an act of offering. When we give, we let it pass out of our hands. It's not an act of handing over responsibility to someone else. It's simply saying that we let go of expectations and control, and let the birth force pass through us.

In transition, as the neck of the womb is nearly fully open, and the baby is soon to commence travelling through the birth canal in the 'second stage', it can seem to some women like they're 'splitting in two', or 'going to rip apart'. To connect with this intensity is to allow oneself to be ultimately vulnerable ~ to permit an emotional and psychic rupturing that lays one bare. Out of this experience, a woman is able to metaphorically die to her old self and life, and embrace and affirm the new.

When the widest part of the baby's head stretches the perineum and vaginal opening to its utmost, we say that the baby is 'crowning'. This is the widest and most open we women can naturally be ~ a majestic instant before our baby is at last fully visible; the pause before he or she is birthed along with all our anticipation, hopes, and love. The supreme 'Yes' moment.

Consequences of Saying 'No'

In our lives, we don't find satisfaction when we attempt to be in total command of our situation, avoid fears and pain, or make everything safe and comfortable. When we spend our lives saying 'no' to what life offers, our creativity dries up and we become stilted and one-dimensional. Saying 'no' causes us to close down, to be in opposition, and to resist. We can not birth our babies this way. When we resist sensations, we tighten up our muscles instead of 'letting go' in surrender. We slow down the process of birth. When we are fearful, our shoulders hunch, affecting our breath and causing rigidity in the rest of our body. The energy is trapped in our chest and throat.[7] When we are saying 'no', we hold our breath or hyperventilate ~ causing the sensations to be perceived much more intensely and painfully.

When the baby has entered our birth canal, we need to have a relaxed and open throat to allow our baby to be born, as tightened throat muscles correlate to tightened pelvic floor muscles. Therefore we can begin by saying the Great 'Yes' through making lots of instinctive and sonorous sounds, chanting, humming, deep sighs, or by literally saying 'Yes'. If we say 'no' when our baby is in the birth canal, we develop resistance, and our pelvic floor muscles and perineum tense up and delay our baby's appearance.

Whilst birthing my first child, I spent over four hours in the second stage, with very little progress. The energy dissipated, my rushes finally rushed off, and I didn't feel like I was any longer in labour. I had lost the urge to push ~ which was the phase I had been dreading without properly addressing, all through my pregnancy. I made token efforts to push ~ but felt like my baby was stuck. I said 'no' to the impulse to push; so it vanished. Fortunately I was at home with my partner, and my closest friend, a midwife. They both gave me the time and the freedom to work out my fear. I ultimately became conscious of my need to confront my anxiety, and trust myself to push my baby out. I chose to whisper an intense 'Yes', the 'Great Yes' in my heart, and instantly the rushes returned with power. Tilda was then born very quickly after this, into the hands of her father.

Saying the Great Yes to Life

In a general sense, opening up, saying 'Yes' in a deep and heartfelt way, and 'giving birth' to that which is new, describes a development of transformation common to us all. I would describe them as conterminous; that is, they share a common boundary and co-extend in space, time and meaning. This process of transformation through the act of opening/affirming deeply/changing evolves into a transcendental process when applied to childbirth. It's the most sublime example, or the apotheosis of the Feminine. Through understanding the process of birth, and loving and trusting our bodies (which takes a lot of unlearning for many of us women), we allow ourselves to open up, to be vulnerable, and yet not to fear. When we experience the sensations, we don't try and stop them or relieve them or have them taken away from us. We acknowledge our feelings, remembering that it is the power of our own bodies, the power of birth, and the power of being a woman ~ and we say in affirmation, the 'Great Yes': 'yes' to being a woman; 'yes' to the mystery we enter into; 'yes' to the pain of transformation and change; ''yes' to the wildness of our bodies and birth; 'yes' to moving deeper and deeper; 'yes' to meeting with our innermost nature and giving it a voice; 'yes' to the triumph of nurturing and birthing our creations; 'yes 'to the birth of a new relationship with ourselves and with our babies; 'yes' to taking responsibility for our birthing and our babies and our lives.

Saying 'the Great Yes' makes us accessible and available to life, in the present moment. It's a spirituality of affirmation. It requires the practice of mindfulness so that we may be truly present to the experience. Out of this flows our confidence in pregnancy and the birth process, and our faith in ourselves. When we speak out the deep 'Yes' from our hearts, we are celebrating our existence and all its light and shadows.

References

(1) Hirshfield, J. ed. (1994). Women in Praise of the Sacred – 43 Centuries of Spiritual Poetry by Women. Harper Perennial: New York, pg 2.
(2) Rabuzzi, K.A. (1994) Mother with Child - transformations through childbirth. Indiana University Press: Indianapolis.
And
Davis, E. and Leonard, C. (1996) The Women's Wheel of Life – 13 Archetypes of Woman at Her Fullest Power. Hodder & Stoughton: Sydney, pg 2.
(3) Kabat-Zinn, J. (1990) Full Catastrophe Living – How to cope with stress, pain and illness using mindfulness meditation. Piatkus: London.
(4) Rabuzzi, K.A. (1994) Ibid.
(5) Kabat-Zinn, J. (1990) Ibid. pg 295.
(6) Larry Rosenberg, L. (1998) Breath by Breath. The Liberating Practice of Insight Meditation. Thorsons: London.
(7) Davis, E. (1999) Heart and Hands – A Midwife's Guide to Pregnancy & Birth. Celestial Arts: California.

The Doula
by Keeley Farrington

In times gone by, pregnant women and their families would have lived surrounded by their tribe or village: their own parents, siblings, extended family and community. At transitional times in life, such as pregnancy, birth and new parenthood, they would rarely have been short of a willing pair of hands or some practical advice when it was needed. Many would have seen birthing or labouring women, and helped out with new babies in the family or community before they were even old enough to have their own children. Birth was an everyday experience, a sacred part of life.

Modern life is very different, and so is the experience of birth and motherhood for many. Women are more likely to be living away from their own family, cut off from the natural support network of 'tribe'. For many modern women, having our first child can be the first real contact we've ever had with a baby. I know that was certainly the case for me when I had my first child ten years ago. Given the limitations of modern-day nuclear families, and the culture of fear and medicalisation that has grown up around birth for the majority of women, it's no wonder that the doula is a concept whose time has come.

A doula is a holistic birthing partner, someone to journey with you and support you, your partner and family through your pregnancy, birth and those vital early hours, days and weeks of new parenthood.

In today's society, we've lost sight of birth and motherhood as a rite of passage, but that is exactly what it is. It's an immensely important time, one of unparalleled joy and excitement, but it's also a time of transition ~ that is, a doorway from one stage of life to another for all concerned: expectant parents, siblings and the babies they are welcoming. With this in mind, caring support and nurturing are vital for the well-being of all, at every stage.

I always try to remind women that although pregnancy and birth are monumental events in their lives, they're also just the start of a much larger adventure! If you can start your journey well nourished in body and spirit, how much better for you!

I've experienced the wonderful role of a doula from both sides of the equation. I've been a doula for three years, and have also had the joyful experience of having a dear friend, who is also a trained doula, fulfill that role for me at the birth of my daughter, last August.

It truly is a magical path. One of the first things I remember from early in the training was that "doulaing is a way of being, not just something that you do".

I understand this to be true in many ways, but especially in that this isn't a job that you start and finish at set times, within set parameters. To do justice to the sacredness of attending birth, and to give of your best to the family, it's not something that you can look at in those terms. I feel that being a doula is both an immense honour and an unrivalled opportunity. It allows me the opportunity to serve, and enrich the experience of the families I work with, as well as chances for personal and spiritual expansion every day. I don't look at it as a job I do, but as an extension of who I am.

I think that therein lies the beauty of this path. We each bring to it our personality; a good strong measure of heart and soul; and our own eclectic (and ever expanding) medicine bag of skills we've picked up along the way. These things are unique to each of us, and I feel that it's these gifts above all that are of value to birthing women and their partners.

Preparing for birth
A doula usually has had children herself, and will have a sound (though not clinical) understanding of the anatomy of birth and how labour unfolds under different circumstances. I often find that women are hazy on these specifics, and that this can cause a lot of anxiety and also unnecessary embarrassment. If I suspect this is the case I always address it, as it can otherwise be quite a mental roadblock. I will (if they wish) go through this briefly with them to satisfy the intellectual need-to-know part of the mind, whilst also gently reinforcing that you don't birth with your brain but with your body. Letting go is the main function of the conscious mind during birth. In order to balance and engage both sides of the brain, in the same session as we cover the physical process of birth, we use this knowledge to build beautiful, vivid mental pictures of the best birth imaginable. I encourage them to dream their birth.

I once heard a saying, which I remember as, "that which you would have, must first be dreamed"; and I've found this to be a profound truth at work in so many aspects of my life. Put another way, it's the law of attraction ~ you attract what you think about. It's such a powerful maxim to share with the women I work with, and it really is one of the cornerstones of my work. It's led me to working with birthing affirmations, visualisation, relaxation and hypnobirthing techniques as the core of my birth preparation work.

It's important for women to move beyond the rigidity and 'structure' of birth plans, with their implicit illusion of control. I try to help them to find the essence of the birth that they want, rather than the form. Once the essence has been felt and spoken, we can work together to prepare for birth.

The role of a doula is not to advise you or make decisions for you. That's not usually in anyone's highest interests. I see the role almost as that of a good, non-judgemental friend ~ and we ALL need at least one of them (pregnant or not!).

When I'm working with a couple, I make sure that I'm available to them to speak to by telephone or in person as much as they need. This varies from person to person, but usually in the final months we'll speak at least weekly, sometimes more frequently, depending on circumstances.

For me, and other doulas I know and love, working with a pregnant woman is like welcoming in another member of the family for that stretch of time. We support them in the way you would a dear friend or sister. Making time for them is vital, and good listening skills are essential. When you're truly listened to in a loving, supportive way, you can access your inner wisdom. You may find that you had the answer all along and just needed clarity, or that your fears have less power over you once they've been heard. We all know the negative effects of fear on childbirth, and talking through your worries with someone who will not judge, belittle or immediately try to put a band-aid on them is one of the most important things you can do to diminish their shadow.

And so to birth...

The birth environment and communication therein should be as non-verbal as possible, so during antenatal sessions we'll have worked through preferences for comfort measures and positions during labour. Of course these can all change once labour commences, and this is where the good working relationship you've built up comes to the fore. We can work together to help you realise the labour and birth of your dreams.

I always try to make sure that whilst I never leave a mother once labour has started, I do leave spaces for her and her partner to be together in the moment, unobserved. It's an intense and intimate experience for a couple, which can strengthen and deepen their bond. Often the rite of passage of birth can extend to their relationship, too, moving it onto another level. It's so important to honour, respect and allow for the father's role in the birth of his child.

In the course of a birth, I may rub backs (dad's as well as mum's!); run baths; massage hands and feet; help mum to get around, change position, etc.; comb hair; provide drinks and snacks; administer homoeopathic remedies, flower essences, essential oils and reiki; as well as performing any number of other tasks, however seemingly small, that may come up ~ I've even been known to hold a sick bucket! (Anyone who knows me will recognise what a personal triumph it is each time that happens!)

I'll support a birthing woman in every way that I can ~ practically, emotionally and spiritually. During labour, I'll hold the vision for her of the birth that she and her baby are creating. If needed, I can remind her to keep the connection with the soul that's arriving, and to trust that bond. I can help her to refocus if events or energies disrupt the rhythms of her birth, and to go within to find the strength that she needs. Once in labour, I won't leave her until mother, babe and family are happily resting, uninterrupted on the other side of birth, and are ready for me to go.

In the bubble...

Usually, in the magical bubble that follows birth, the only priority is that the new family be allowed peace to bond and fall in love all over again. The importance of this time can't be overstated, and I ensure that I do all that I can to protect the bonding space. I'll give as much space or help as is needed at this time, including help with breastfeeding, and getting mother and baby settled.

I'll always encourage a Babymoon. The birthing bubble doesn't (or shouldn't) just go pop after 48 hours. Many women and their families expect a lot of themselves very soon after birth, but rest and recuperation are paramount. The intense energy of birth, with all its gifts, should be allowed to gradually integrate into the heart of your family. Let your bubble dissolve slowly, rather than go pop!

Don't have a house full of visitors if you don't want to; take things at your own pace. It's about listening to yourself, and being clear about your needs. This is a good habit to get into early, as many women will fade into the background of family, swamped by the needs and desires of everyone else. I'm as guilty of this as anyone, at times, and it always helps me to remember that if mum is happy and healthy, then so is everyone else. You must meet your own needs before you can spread yourself around, and although this always applies, never is this more apparent than in the post-natal period. You'll never get this precious time back again, so protect and cherish it.

It's useful to encourage mothers to think about the post-natal period beforehand. What support network do they have already in place? What can they grow or develop to help them? People are often happy to help out with other children, a meal rota and even housework, if you're able to ask. Sometimes this takes more courage than we realise. I believe that our strength always comes from within and from knowing ourselves. By looking within gently and honestly, we can ask for and graciously accept what we need to nourish ourselves and our families.

One expression I often hear applied to the work of a doula is that of "mothering the mother", which I feel needs some clarity. I don't see the work as mothering in a sense that would imply helplessness on the part of the mother. I feel it's one of many pure threads of mothering; a doula's intent is to nurture a woman by loving, accepting and being present with her fully at this vital time.

In some ways, a woman who births with a doula does rely on her, but this isn't in a disempowering way. In the relationship that you create, you trust your doula to be there for you, and you rely on her to hold many aspects and details of your birth for you in order that you can fully inhabit your birthing self. You can let go, and rise up to meet your child knowing that the Earthbound details are in safe hands.

"A birthing woman is both vulnerable and powerful, human and Goddess. When lost in her human fragility she may sometimes need the 'Presence' of another to help her re-member all that she is, all that she can be." ~ Olivia Seck, Birth Creation.

Birthing women are Divinely powerful. I want nothing more for them than that they believe this, and believe in themselves; for it is they who will bring their babies Earthside, no-one else. I want to show them what Birthing Goddesses we all are, and support them that they may remember this aspect of themselves. I aim to inspire trust in themselves and their bodies, and to create space in which they can listen to their inner voice, and access their innate feminine wisdom.

I'm humbled and grateful to be a doula and a mother. May your births be all the colours of your soul.

I would like to dedicate this article to my soul systers and dear friends ~ Sonya; Olivia Seck, with whom I trained; and of course, Veronika, who continues to light the way for so many with The Mother. Blessed Be.

Breastfeeding

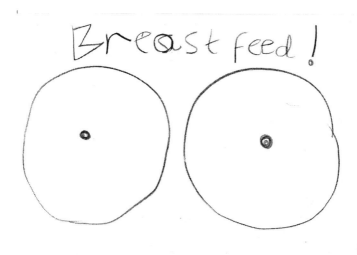

It's simple: BREASTFEED! By Eliza Robinson

Intraductal thrush and breastfeeding
by Karen Arnott

Karen Arnott is The Mother magazine's web mother. She's married to Bob, and they have two children, Audrey and Finlay. www.arnottdesign.co.uk

While I was pregnant with Finlay, I was adamant I would breastfeed. To me, there was no other choice. However, I gave up exclusively breastfeeding him when he was just three months old. I still wince with guilt about this. Why did I give up? We developed intraductal thrush. This painful condition resides inside the milk ducts, rather than being exclusively contained on the skin.

Most people, myself included, have never heard that thrush can get into the breasts. I ended up in A&E, and the attending nurse confirmed that it is one of the most painful conditions you can have. Unfortunately, by this point, I was so broken I just couldn't carry on. I couldn't lift or cuddle Finlay. Wearing him in the sling was impossible; I could only hold him sideways, resting in between my breasts. I sacrificed breastfeeding him because I was desperate to mother him in every other way.

One of the reasons many people don't hear about thrush and breastfeeding is because it's incredibly difficult to get rid of. I was met with incredulity that I didn't just want to give up straight away. I was in excruciating pain from when Finlay was five weeks old. All day, every day ~ all night, every night ~ I spent most days in tears.

How did we get thrush?

Finlay's birth was a relatively straightforward (drug-free) hospital birth, but fast and quite traumatic. Finlay was desperate to feed straight away, and this caused him to suck so hard I ended up with blood blisters covering my entire nipple area. These scabbed over, and refused to heal for several weeks while we got to grips with correct latch. A friend had also given me the (misguided) advice to wear a bra all the time (including in bed) to prevent stretch marks. After five weeks, my nipples had healed, but I was experiencing hot stabbing pains that extended all the way through my breasts and radiated across my back. My lovely husband, Bob, spent many nights gathering wet flannels to use as cold compresses. I desperately searched my books and websites to find answers ~ I started to match my symptoms with thrush. I wasn't altogether surprised; I had taken antibiotics throughout my teens for acne, and as a result, suffered from vaginal thrush on a regular basis. Antibiotics are well-known for destroying the healthy bacteria in the gut, and causing vaginal thrush. I used to collect a prescription for Canesten with my antibiotics! But, I hadn't had it for years. The repeatedly unsuccessful courses of antibiotics for the acne had made me lose my faith in the medical profession. Unfortunately, the only concrete advice I could find about thrush and breastfeeding was to 'see your doctor as soon as possible'. There was also little advice about dietary changes. I remembered much of this from my teenage years: avoid sugars, avoid yeasty foods, etc. I also started to find information about natural supplements which are useful for preventing and treating thrush.

I went away and religiously stuck to the sugar- and wheat-free diet, and took probiotics every few hours. After a couple of weeks, the pain was still so bad I went to see the health visitor. I was in such a state she didn't recognise me as one of her 'ladies'. She persuaded me to go to A&E. There I got sympathy and understanding, as well as a prescription for a week's worth of fluconazole, and some gel for Finlay's mouth. They didn't explain that I needed to go to the doctor for more as they had only given me a week's worth (you need to continue treatment for at least ten days after the symptoms have gone). After a couple of weeks, the thrush came back. What ensued was a back-and-forth of repeat prescriptions. This was against what I really believed, but the diet changes just weren't working quickly enough.

I was broken, and couldn't cope with such excruciating pain on a daily basis. I desperately tried to express, and tried every breast pump on the market, but just couldn't manage more than a couple of ounces. On the insistence of well-meaning family and friends, I started introducing formula. Finlay and I did carry on part-time feeding for another couple of months, until he just lost interest in breastfeeding (I wish I'd known then about re-lactation!).

I've since had Audrey, and we started getting the symptoms of thrush a few days after her beautiful home waterbirth. We treated it naturally, and are still happily breastfeeding at sixteen months.

What is thrush?
Thrush is a yeast (fungal) infection, often referred to as

Candidiasis. Candida albicans is the most common of the species. Good bacteria on the skin and throughout the body normally keep overgrowth in check. There are extreme ranges of thrush infection, from the relatively superficial skin and mouth infections that cause inflammation and discomfort, to complete systemic infection. Candida lives in the mouth, which is why correct latch is critical: babies can pass thrush from their mouths into the breasts via cracked nipples. Thrush infection in the milk ducts (intraductal thrush is a systemic infection) is a huge threat to breastfeeding because of the almost continuous excruciating pain deep inside the breasts, and the length of time treatment can take.

How can you prevent thrush?

During pregnancy, avoid sugary and yeasty foods. Thrush thrives in sugary, yeasty conditions. Avoid the following: refined sugar, refined flour and all wheat products; and any foods containing yeast (including soy sauce, mushrooms, marmite, etc.), as well as fruit. Include plenty of fresh vegetables, sea vegetables, nuts and seeds (nuts and seeds should be well within their shelf-life, otherwise they can harbour yeasts). Taking a probiotic supplement may be beneficial ~ this is especially important if you have a history of thrush or antibiotic use.

Read everything you can about breastfeeding, and attend local breastfeeding classes. Correct latch is vital to prevent cracked, sore nipples, which can let infection into the breasts. Once baby's born, if you do have a few problems with correct latch, see a breastfeeding counsellor as soon as possible. There are usually local groups, and the NCT and ABM have great telephone services ~ some counsellors will be more than happy to visit you if necessary.

When you start breastfeeding, avoid wearing a bra all day, and certainly not in bed at night. Let the breasts breathe. Change breast pads after every feed; use natural, washable pads.

How do you know what you've got is thrush, and not something else?

Thrush can be distinguished by one or more of the following symptoms in the mother:

[] Itchy, puffy, dry, flaky nipples and areola. Often, the areola will appear tight and shiny, and may have clusters of tiny white spots.

[] Nipples may have small cracks that remain even if the latch is correct/ed; these cracks may appear with a white discharge.

[] Deep, stabbing, hot pains (like a hot poker!) that seem to penetrate from the nipple and radiate through to the back/shoulders ~ these pains usually start half way through a feed, and can continue for hours (very different from the tingling sensation of milk let-down).

[] The absence of lumps, red patches and a temperature associated with mastitis.

And in the baby:

[] Discomfort while feeding; clicking noises; coming off the breast; wriggling.

[] White spots inside the cheeks and on the roof of the mouth.

There is disagreement about a white coating on the tongue, but all I can say about this is that both my babies had a thick white coating on the tongue that disappeared once we'd got rid of the thrush.

[] Possibly also discomfort in the digestive system, accompanied by unexplained, prolonged crying, and drawing up of the legs.

[] Nappy rash and/or spots around the genitals/bottom area.

As with other aspects of parenting, trust your instincts, and do plenty of research. Google: thrush and breastfeeding.

If you do get thrush, how can you treat it naturally?

Research anti-candida diets online or in books. Eat a clean, high-raw diet containing absolutely no sugars, no wheat products, and avoid dairy and other acid-forming foods. An abundance of green vegetables is crucial. Prebiotic foods, such as raw oats, chicory root and Jerusalem artichokes may also help re-establish healthy digestive flora.

Supplements for the mother:

[] Grapefruit seed extract

This should not to be confused with grape seed extract. Personally, I found this the single most effective treatment. This is available in independent health food shops, and online in capsules and as a tincture. Build up to the maximum dose of the capsules daily, as well as a few drops of tincture in plenty of water throughout the day.

[] Caprylic acid

This is a fatty acid found in coconuts (and breast milk!) that is an extremely effective anti-fungal. Available as tablets in health food shops and online. Raw, virgin coconut oil/butter can also be used as a dietary supplement.

[] A high quality probiotic. Threelac contains three types of lactic acid-producing bacterial strains, and is one of the most effective candida treatments. Also include acidophilus and bifidus to replenish the good bacteria.

[] Superfood powder. A freeze-dried green vegetable powder, such as Nature's Living Superfood (available from www.detoxyourworld.com). This will alkalise the body's system (Candida thrives in a high acid environment). This food supplement also contains probiotics.

[] Colloidal silver

This can be taken orally, and is also useful for applying directly to irritated, itchy nipples.

[] Digestive enzymes. For chronic, long-term, systemic thrush infections, these may be worthwhile.

A quick die-off effect (extreme pain, fever and aches) can occur with high doses of any of the above. If this happens, reduce the dose and build up again slowly. Continue to take the supplements, and follow the anti-candida diet for at least three months after symptoms have abated.

Some women report success with homeopathic treatments, but you'll need to see a qualified practitioner, who will carry out a thorough investigation of your personal history to diagnose and recommend specific treatments for your situation.

For baby: your breast milk is full of pro and prebiotics, but if the thrush is severe, a probiotic supplement such as BioCare Bifidobacterium Infantis is specifically formulated for babies, and is vegan. This is a pleasant-tasting powder you can apply to baby's mouth with your finger. A few drops of colloidal silver in baby's mouth may also be beneficial.

General advice:
Wash all bras, breast pads, towels and bed linen, using a cup of distilled vinegar. Don't share towels with other members of the family, in order to avoid cross-infection. Line dry them to take benefit of the Sun's natural anti-fungal properties. Don't use any detergents (even natural ones) when washing your breasts, as this will destroy the beneficial bacteria; a quick splash of lukewarm water is sufficient. Expose breasts to fresh air and sunshine as often as possible, and go

bra-less if you can (if you feel you still need the support, cut holes around the nipples to let this area breathe).

If you're trying to treat it, but nothing's working, what are your options?

Bear in mind the above treatment can take weeks and months to take effect, rather than days, particularly if the thrush infection is intraductal. However, there are extra steps you can take to speed up the process:

Express your breast milk, and feed baby alternately from the breast and using a cup/syringe/bottle (you may need to increase the number of expressed milk feeds if alternate feeds are too frequent, to prevent baby passing the thrush back and forth).

As an absolute last resort, you may need to consider anti-fungal drugs on prescription. It's important to get the correct length of the course to halt the infection once and for all, or you risk becoming resistant to the anti-fungals, and get into a repeat-prescription cycle.

You could also consider donated breast milk. Fresh milk from someone you know is preferable, so you can be sure of the mother's health and diet. Or you could request milk from your local hospital's milk bank, if they have any spare. However, this is from numerous women, and is pasteurised (heat-treated) to destroy bacteria (unfortunately, this also destroys many essential nutrients and all the vital enzymes), but it's still better than artificial dried milk from another species!

Keep up at least two feeds a day to maintain a little supply and prevent engorgement, and to help your baby maintain his sucking reflex. Once the thrush symptoms have gone, increase your feeds, drink plenty of fennel and raspberry leaf tea, and your milk supply should increase with a little perseverance.

Editor's note: Both olive leaf extract and propolis will kill off candida. Propolis can be taken internally, and applied to the nipples.

Useful links
www.citrosept.co.uk ~ Grapefruit seed extract
www.thinknatural.com ~ Caprylic acid
www.detoxyourworld.com ~ ThreeLac, Nature's Living Superfood and Colloidal Silver
www.positivehealthshop.com ~ Biocare Bifidobacterium Infantis (INT B1)
www.kellymom.com/bf/concerns/thrush/thrush-resources.html ~ Tons of information about thrush and breastfeeding.

Breast milk and the human brain
by Tish Clifford

Recently, my five year old son became utterly connected to my breasts and nipples. He wanted to feed again and touch them, and rubbed his face over my shirt against them in a slight state of ecstasy. I felt waves of sadness descend, knowing that ultimately he would have fed until about seven, and I had, in effect, cut his need for breast milk and sensual contact short.

When Veronika and her family appeared on the amazing documentary *Extraordinary Breastfeeding*, I was stunned by some of the reaction from my alternative friends, which was outrage and disgust. Although I had never particularly enjoyed breastfeeding (more on that later), I knew from the bottom of my heart that every child has a need to breastfeed full-term, and I personally think full-term would be around seven years.

When I first started my breastfeeding 'career', with my firstborn, Lexi (now 9), I thought breastfeeding beyond one and a half was a bit weird; my conditioned mind was still very dominant, and although I was connected to being a more 'natural parent' than my own mother, feeling instinctively that I needed to sleep with my baby, and hold her close at all times, responding to her needs instantly, I still hadn't connected with full-term breastfeeding.

Although there was no way on Earth I was not going to breastfeed for the intended one and a half years, I found I didn't enjoy it. Particularly at the beginning, every time Lexi would latch on an intense feeling of depression would come over me. Being into personal growth at the time, I wondered what was happening, but I was working on a more intellectual level and the best I could come up with was that it was connected to not having been breastfed myself, as well as some verbal sexual abuse connected to my nipples at the age of 10. I certainly wasn't able to heal it, and although the sensation eased off slightly after a few months, it was there to some degree throughout the whole time I breastfed both my children.

I breastfed Lexi for about one year, whenever she made a peep. My breasts were large for the first time in my life, and I allowed her constant access. In this time I had come to realise through my own internal questioning that breastfeeding should be done way beyond my original belief of one and a half years. I realised that if children were meant to have milk, then they were definitely meant to have the milk that was designed for them. At the time, I had a suspicion that this would be until around seven, the main reason being that 'milk' teeth fall out around this time.

Not really knowing many natural mothers, and certainly none who had fed for so long, I wasn't able to get much collaboration for my suspicion, but being on a quest to research biological truths, I soon discovered a wealth of information that led me to continue to believe that the full-term age would be around seven. In some cultures I discovered that their children would have flasks of breast milk up to the age of 10, and the worldwide average age for weaning is four years. Considering that the average weaning age in the West is six weeks, it doesn't take a genius to work out that that must mean that there are many mothers around the world feeding for much longer than four years.

I breastfed Lexi for three and a half years. She weaned when I became pregnant with my second child, Jago. This seemed to happen naturally, but I felt like I wanted her to stop. I'm sure she picked up on this energetically, and it influenced the situation. When Jago came along, I'd decided that although I wanted to feed longer than three and half, I wasn't going to feed him as much as I had with Lexi. She'd had milk for every emotion she felt, and in hindsight I feel I wasn't completely connected to her variety of needs, and used milk as a constant way to meet most of them.

Jago wasn't as settled as Lexi; he suffered from colic, and for the first three months would cry in gassy pain. I feel now, again in hindsight, that I pulled back too far and didn't feed him enough. Not that I can do much about it now, but it does make me feel sad to think that I still wasn't tuned in enough to get it 'right'. He continued to feed until he was nearly four, and was weaned somewhat artificially when we both got sick in Thailand, and I just felt unable to feed him for a few weeks. This break forced weaning when really I had wanted, at least intellectually, to continue. I can't say I missed it, but having developed a greater understanding of brain development I feel that I didn't meet his biological needs. After some weeks, I decided that I would try to encourage him back on and was able to do so a little, much to Jago's delight. But it never really went anywhere, as it appeared to some degree he had lost the sucking reflex. For children who are allowed to feed full-term this doesn't appear until nearer the seven year mark ~ something else I find inherently biological.

It's said that when children are left to wean naturally, it happens between two and seven. And although I understand this has been the experience of many, I have to wonder whether our inherent cultural conditioning around weaning earlier than might be natural, energetically influences children's desire (or the mother's) to wean before full-term.

The human brain has its most intensive growth period for the first seven years. The first year is proportionally the largest, but it still continues up until around seven. The 'milk' teeth also start to fall out around this time too. The larger-brained primates in the wild don't wean until they're around five and beyond ~ and our brain is larger still. Considering breast milk is vital for the correct neurological development of the brain, and that creates the very structure that directly affects our sense of self, one could say this is crucial to creating a world of sane individuals.

That primates, with smaller brains than ours, breastfeed for so long uninhibited by social madness, is as shocking as it is telling.

The human brain is made up of 80% DHA. The limited amount of fatty acids (particularly DHA) in man's evolutionary frugivorous diet (and a diet that the larger-brained primates still eat) has led many to believe that our large brain has to have been a product of time living by the coast where there is an abundance of DHA-rich food. Interestingly, science has been unable to explain how the relatively large ape brain evolved in the forest, and subsequent pollen analysis at famous savannah hominid fossil sites has clearly indicated that the habitats were wooded or forested. Other species that eat a diet rich in fruit also have larger brains than their insect eating cousins, e.g. bats. Could there be a connection?[1]

Breast milk has abundant DHA ~ freshly made each day, full of antioxidants to protect the delicate structure of the fat, and therefore the delicate structure of our brain. How the human brain could be created with anything less than the fat in human breast milk is incredibly short-sighted. Considering the majority of brain growth happens in the first seven years, and the human brain needs DHA, to be created, and maintained correctly, then is it so difficult to see that it would make perfect scientific sense to grow it on human breast milk, that is made with an abundance of raw unprocessed fresh DHA?

The woman's diet is also, of course, of crucial significance. If it is deficient in EFAs, then her own reserves will be sucked dry, and it can lead to a whole host of problems, including depression. I personally prefer using clean sources of raw hemp milk made fresh daily, as well as high quality raw linseed oil (Stone Mills is an excellent brand and is pressed daily on demand)[2].

As I lie each night to cuddle Jago to sleep, and he snuggles close to my body, I get the sense somewhere he still yearns to be at my breast. It's biological, and I personally don't separate what is biological from what is spiritual. I think the main reason that people are horrified in Western culture that a child would feed naturally for so long is because we associate breasts so heavily with sexual contact. Surely it's close to 'incest' that a woman would desire to feed her child for 'so long'? It's a sad reflection of the current state of affairs that this fear is so present in our society. Children yearn for skin contact as deeply as all mammals. That it could be pleasurable for both mother and child is seen as wrong, and yet body contact with another human being raises oxytocin levels in the brain, which increases our ability to love and be happy; this is not about sex, it's about sensual contact that is normal and natural. If more children and mothers were given the support they needed to be able to carry out this biological and natural process, I predict that we would see a radical change in human behaviour.

I don't write this article in a judgmental way towards either myself or others for not breastfeeding to what I believe to be the true full-term age of around seven; I write to help bring light to a taboo that needs dismantling if we're to help humanity reach its full potential. Science is proving, without doubt, that the human brain is a most complex organ, and getting the correct bio-chemistry flooding it is essential for creating a healthy and happy sense of self; and although I write about a few components of breast milk that are vital, one would need a book to speak of them all.

Recently I watched a programme on gorillas. A women researcher was saying how the gorilla is just like the human and takes nine months to grow in gestation, and breastfeeds for seven years ~ showing some footage of a gorilla of seven feeding off its mother. It was beautiful to watch and I couldn't help but wonder how my friends would react to this footage. Would they also think that the gorillas were disgusting? Somehow I doubt it...

1 *For a more comprehensive investigation into the connection between fruit and our neuro-endocrine system and how they may have affected the growth and expansion of the human brain, please see www.kaleidos.org.uk*
2 *This product can be found at www.funkyraw.com*

The Mother magazine's guide to
ethical sources of DHA / EPA & essential fats
for non-breastfeeding humans
by Veronika Robinson

Although the human body can't make essential fatty acids (except in the creation of breast milk), it does require them, as they're absolutely necessary for building the brain and supporting the nervous system. When we consume omega 3 and omega 6 fatty acids, our body converts them to EPA (short for eicosapentaenoic acid) and DHA (short for docosahexaenoic acid). Our cell membranes are made more flexible, allowing both the releasing of toxins out of the body, and the taking in of nutrients.

Our body converts the omega oils into what is known as long-chain polyunsaturated fatty acids. Commonly referred to as omega 3, this fatty acid, otherwise known as alpha linolenic acid, becomes EPA and DHA. Fish is normally recommended; however, all we have to do is consume the EPA and DHA through algae-based foods and we too can obtain the essential fats directly. During pregnancy it is vital we eat foods rich in DHA so our baby has the optimal chance of developing its nervous system and brain.

Linoleic acid, known commonly as omega 6, is required to balance female hormones, among other things. This is converted in our body to arachidonic acid (AA). In our culture there is a danger of consuming excess, as it's readily found in dairy and meat. Over-consumption of AA has been linked to cardiovascular and arthritic complaints ~ again, another reason to consume plant based omega 6.

Some people have difficulty converting EFAs because of a health condition, such as an atopic allergy (eczema, hay fever and asthma) or diabetes. It's recommended they purchase an EPA/DHA algae supplement.

Reasons not to obtain your essential fatty acids from oily fish:
    * Ethical sources exist in the plant world
    * Toxicity (dioxins, mercury, PCPs) found in fish
    * Commercially farmed fish require antibiotics etc., because of the unnatural conditions in which they live, and the processed foods which they eat. There's no proof that they're able to convert omega oils in this environment from the foods they eat.

Lifestyle changes to increase your absorption of essential fatty acids.

Your ability to convert EFAs to EPA and DHA is affected by smoking, alcohol, viral infections such as herpes, animal fats and trans fats in processed foods, stress, excess vitamin A, caffeine (coke, coffee, chocolate, tea) and excess copper.

Include in your meals, each day, the oils from nuts and seeds, as well as eating them whole. Try having spirulina smoothies, chorella or Nature's Living Superfood every other day. To be able to convert EPAs ensure your diet is rich in vitamins B3 and B6, zinc, biotin, vitamin C, calcium and magnesium. Omega 3 and omega 6 oils need to be balanced. Commonly, people have far too much omega 6 because sunflower oil is used in abundance in processed foods. Have about 1 part of omega 3 to 3 parts of omega 6.

If you need oils for cooking, the best two are coconut oil and cold-pressed olive oil. All other oils should be kept in the cold in dark glass containers.

Omega 3
Flax
Hemp
Pumpkin
Walnuts
Green vegetables

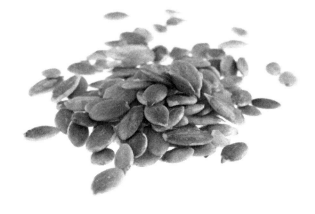

Omega 6
Hemp
Flax
Sunflower
Sesame
Nuts
Borage
Blackcurrant seeds
Evening primrose

Breastfeeding Your Premature Baby
by Veronika Sophia Robinson

In January 1998, my husband Paul and I spent a few long days (literally around the clock) in a neonatal intensive care unit watching over our newborn baby.

From memory, there were about ten other babies in that ward. Each of them was deliberately isolated from human touch by the plastic cribs which held them.

My own daughter weighed 10lb 4oz and looked like a whale in comparison. All the other babies were premature; some so tiny they could nestle into the palm of an adult hand.

In their brightly lit, sterile environment, attached to man-made machinery, and nursed in incubators, they were ALL missing something modern medicine could never give them, and could never hope to replace: *their mother*. During my round the clock vigil I saw only one mother come to visit her baby (and that was just once for a few minutes to put some milk down a tube).

"Where are all the mothers?" I kept asking the staff. They told me many times to go back to my ward because "there was nothing I could do."

They confirmed that this was the instruction they gave to every parent of a babe in Neonatal Intensive Care. No matter what medical help a baby or child might need, they *always* need their mother. And if she can't be there then the baby's father should be. There is always something you can do when your baby is hospitalised.

The touch of a hand, the familiar smell of a mother, her voice... these may not register in the world of medicine, but in the life of your baby it's priceless. Babies don't talk, so we don't know what they're feeling or thinking in terms of the way we relate as adults, but they're *always communicating*. The intuitive and bonded mother knows that her presence, her being, is very much needed by her infant. The first nine months of life outside the womb are very much a gestation period. Nature designed us to be held in our mother's arms, to suckle on her breast without crying or begging for a feed. When a baby is born before he or she has completed a full gestational term, we owe it to them to put this continuum into practice immediately. Even babies who are strapped to machines can still be touched.

The Mother magazine urges all parents of premature babies to remind staff that the role of a mother is every bit as important as the job of the medical profession. There are many things a mother or father can do to help their baby thrive and bring 'going home' day much closer.

A baby is considered premature when it hasn't fully developed in its mother's womb, and is born at 36 weeks or earlier. In terms of breastfeeding, premature babies fall into two categories. Those who can nurse at the breast or a bottle from birth, and those who will need to be fed via tube.

For the baby who can not nurse:

These babies NEED you more than ever, mother. Your breast milk is vital. The colostrum in your breasts contains nutrients especially for this preterm baby. Ask the hospital to provide you with an electric breast pump ~ ideally, one which is hands-free, and does both sides at once (a double pump).

Begin expressing as soon as possible, and insist that your baby be given your milk straight away, and <u>not</u> mixed with formula or heated in any way.

Colostrum
is
Nature's Biotic.

Colostrum is thick and rich, and it's the birthright of every baby on the planet to have it from its mother.

Some mothers freeze their breast milk to create a bank of milk for their baby. If you're with your baby around the clock and parenting naturally, you'll probably find this unnecessary.

Milk can stay refrigerated for up to a week. Don't process or heat your milk above 48 degrees Celsius as this will kill vital enzymes. Persevere with expressing, for soon you'll be able to put your baby to the breast. In the meantime, hold your baby as close to you as possible. Many babies can be nurtured through what is known as Kangaroo Care. If your child can't be held close to your breast for any reason, try and maintain physical contact as much as possible. Hold hands, rub feet or back. Rescue Remedy rubbed into the soles of a baby in NICU can be very helpful. Talk to your baby. Sing to your baby. Express your breast milk into a cloth to leave near your baby's face so s/he can smell you. The breast milk of a mother who births early has more antibodies and nutrients than a full-term mother's (see, Mother Nature was watching out for you after all!).

Remember, when staff offer to 'top' your baby up with formula, they're not doing either of you any favours. Your breast milk is easier for your baby to digest. The more time and energy the body has to spend on digesting, the less healing energy is available for recovery and growth.

Although formula has proteins and fats, they're not able to be assimilated in the same way by your baby as your own milk.

Your breast milk has been perfectly created for your baby. No medical labouratory or scientist in the world will ever be able to replicate it. Think about what that really means: your milk is, and will always be, unique. Nature designed it especially for your baby. Breast milk always changes in composition throughout the day, and from day to day. It's designed to provide what your baby needs, depending on his age and stage. A baby at day one receives different milk than at day three or week thirty three or year three.

Expressing
When expressing for your baby (this goes for any mum having to express for a newborn) you need to mimic the feeds of your baby. One, two, three or four times a day is *not* enough. A naturally-nurtured breastfed baby can easily feed every twenty minutes in the early days and weeks. Some feed more, some feed less. There's no right or wrong in their needs. Express hourly, at least ten to fifteen minutes to ensure you get both the foremilk and the hind milk. Try and express where you can see your baby. Expressing takes practice, and is an emotional and physical activity. Try to approach it with pleasure. Touch your baby as you do it. If you have to be in another room away from your infant, nurture yourself with some peaceful music, a cup of chamomile tea (relaxant), and shut your eyes!

Premature babies who can bottlefeed will need to develop strength in their jaw when graduating onto the breast. The sucking action is different. Milk flows out of bottles and doesn't require any effort on the baby's part. This can make it difficult for mums trying to establish breastfeeding. I recommend cup or syringe feeding, rather than a bottle.

Nature meant for us to work at breastfeeding. All that jaw work and sucking is to enhance our orofacial development. It will enable us to talk better, and have a stronger jaw.

Don't give up if your baby prefers your breast milk in a bottle. He is not rejecting you! Make sure you're both relaxed and comfortable. Let breastfeeding be a pleasure, not a chore.

If your baby is able to go on the breast immediately, feed her on cue. Don't wait for her to get agitated and cry. Lying down might be the best position if you have a lot of milk coming out. She needs time to get used to sucking. Your baby may not have the strength of a full-term newborn, so be patient.

The truth about iron and breast milk
The continued undermining of the qualities of breast milk
and the push towards the inappropriate,
premature introduction of solid foods.
by Emma Lewis

One of the most frequently asked questions amongst parents of babies from about four months of age is when to begin introducing solid food. One of the most common points of concern, in my experience (and reported by other LLL and ABA leaders), is the iron issue.

The WHO guidelines recommend babies are exclusively breastfed for the first six months of their life. That means, no solid food before six months [***see below]

This is a very conservative, standard guideline. Health Visitors, Plunket Nurses, Maternal & Child Health nurses (or the equivalent in other countries) and parenting publications are supposed to recommend six months as the very minimum age at which to begin introducing solid foods. Often, however, it appears such health 'professionals', and indeed parents themselves, find this open to personal interpretation!

The iron status of formula-fed infants has always been ~ and still is ~ a valid and significant cause of concern for healthcare professionals. With artificial feeding, too little iron results in anaemia and an increase in infections. Too much iron also causes anaemia, along with other problems, such as zinc deficiency, which can result in retardation, failure to thrive, skin disorders (Lonnerdal 1983; M.K. Hambridge 1977) and a compromised immune system.

These are well known, recognised and documented Formula Mishaps (Breastfeeding Matters: Maureen Minchin 1998).

The experience of babies receiving artificial milk with synthetic iron led to recommending the introduction of solid food prematurely, and is possibly appropriate for babies receiving inadequate early nutrition (i.e. formula). However, this is NOT the case for breastfed babies.

Sadly, the assumption was mistakenly made that breastfed babies were the same (as their formula fed peers), and that the smaller amounts of natural iron in breast milk were an indicator that breastfed babies would not be receiving enough iron. This is not true.

The meat and milk marketing boards, and baby food manufacturers, have done a magnificent job of promoting this myth; and providing and pushing supposed full, unbiased, scientifically sound (?!) information about iron stores in babies ~ and encouraging mothers to compromise their babies' optimal nutrition, by consistently and inaccurately undermining breast milk.

There are the provocative and emotive posters of a big man holding a small baby, and stating that the baby needs more iron than the man, and the continual references to the lower amount of iron found in breast milk in comparison to artificial baby milk.

Although the amount of iron in breast milk is small, it's well absorbed and utilised, and the high lactose and vitamin C levels in human milk ensure its optimal absorption.

Babies absorb between 50 and 70% of the iron in breast milk. This is compared to only 4% of the synthetic iron in formula. Artificial feeding also commonly causes intestinal fissures, which result in the baby losing iron through the bowels. This doesn't happen with breastfed babies.

A healthy, full-term baby has sufficient iron stores at birth, and these, combined with the iron from exclusive breastfeeding, are ample for a minimum of six months. (Krebs 2000; Engelmann 1998; Makrides 1998; Pisacane 1995; Duncan 1985; Siimes 1984; McMillan 1976.) Paediatrics 1976 advises that "breastfeeding maintains excellent iron status for 6-9 months".

In fact, it has been shown (Pisacane 1995) that babies who receive iron supplementation or iron-fortified cereal before SEVEN months have a high rate of anaemia in their first year ~ those who received breast milk exclusively showed no anaemia! A similar study found that babies exclusively breastfed for seven months absorbed iron more effectively for life, than their counterparts who received food prior to seven months.

ABA Topics in Breastfeeding set VIII, Dec 1996, LRC (Dianne Carroll) shows that the longer a baby is exclusively breastfed, the less likely they are to have anaemia.

One of the most significant reasons for actively discouraging the introduction of solids before six months (yes, even "just a little taste"!) is because the presence of other foods decreases the availability of nutrients in breast milk by interfering with enzymes and transfer factors that make breast milk uniquely well-absorbed (Minchin 1998).

Giving iron-containing foods can also result in iron deficiency (Lawrence, op.cit.,p.64). Cereals, and particularly breads, are notorious for compromising iron absorption.

It's ironic (no pun intended) that the countries whose population eats the largest amount of meat (and, we would therefore be led to believe, an appropriate volume and source of iron) have the highest levels of anaemia. The conditions for iron absorption need to be optimal within adults too ~ for example, if the vitamin C level is compromised, iron absorption can not occur effectively.

It's also important to note that the iron levels in a mother's milk are not affected by the amount of iron in a mother's diet or by any iron supplements she may take (Vuori 1980).

Other points of reference, and (importantly) non-profiteering information, are available from: La Leche League (LLL) International http://www.kellymom.com/nutrition/vitamins/iron.html

...babies exclusively breastfed
for seven months
absorbed iron
more effectively for life,
than their counterparts who received food
prior to seven months

The yoga of breastfeeding
by Jamie Abrams

Jamie has been sprinkling her yoga bliss globally for ten years, having worked with the best in the business and taught in the US, New Zealand, Australia, the UK, and, recently, Costa Rica. Between bending, breathing and stretching, she shares her time with her homebirthed, breastfed, unvaccinated, co-sleeping, raw-vegan, sparkly three-year-old boy, and hunky hubby. She teaches in the London area, and can be contacted via www.RawYogaTeacher.com

I don't think many people see the deeper connection between yoga and breastfeeding, or that many people associate a successful breastfeeding relationship with having a supple, strong body and peaceful mind.

Even though I was in reasonable shape when my breastfeeding career began, I was utterly surprised by how physically taxing breastfeeding could be on my muscles. In the early days, when my babe seemed to suckle for what felt like hours on end, I would wind up with achy arms, shoulders and back. My legs would feel restless, like I'd just been sitting on an aeroplane for 12 hours without moving. I laugh now at my initial weakness of body.

Not only was I tackling the purely physical side of nourishing my buttercup, I was grappling with my cerebral thoughts. During those long feeds, or those times when I felt like all I did was have my ta-tas hanging out all day, my mind would alternate between the ecstatic bliss of what I was doing, and the monotony of it all.

Even with my many years of familiarity with meditating and yogic practices of softness and mindfulness, I still struggled with the monkey living in my mind. I was/am still working at entering my own silent abyss with ease.

The stillness of breastfeeding could rattle up my monkey, causing me to feel trapped or like I was being held hostage. When it got all too much for me I couldn't transport myself out with mind-dulling TV, and my head generally was too full of fogginess to comprehend a good book. My self-love and yogic practices were being put fully to the test! [Personal note: I don't feel that self-love and yogic practices can be separated.] While I can't speak for every lactating mama, I can only assume every mum has had instances during nursing that weren't all filled with creamy hues and rosiness. Fortunately, Mother

Nature designed us perfectly to, by and large, experience enormous ripples of satisfaction and love while we nourish our cherubs. While it could be very easy to blame my modern, Western lifestyle for any shortcomings, and all the counter-intuitive messages it gives me every day about raising my child, I would rather not squirt my precious breastmilk on the antagonist. Instead, I tried (I use that word because, after all, I'm human, too!) to tap into that peaceful space that dwells within me at all times, and not allow myself to be totally consumed by the guilt of feeling bored, or wondering when my nursling would ever release my breast.

For me, this is where the ability to utilise yogic thinking truly ups the anti. My interpretation of the meaning of yogic thinking is just that it's another phrase for positive thinking and affirmations, believing in something greater, the law of attraction, meditation, mantra japa, etc. Basically, if I remain calm, allow positivity to abound, it's the natural order of the Universe to sort the rest of it out. If I was really in a mental tizzy, it became paramount for me to find a mantra to soothe my soul, and begin deep yogic breathing. This would eventually bring me back to a euphoric equilibrium.

Of course, I can't possibly leave out the importance of proper breathing or yogic breathing on my triumphant breastfeeding passage. Like many women in modern society, I'd never seen a baby breastfeed (although I was breastfed), and had very little practical knowledge. Everything I knew about breastfeeding was theoretical, from books. Although I was aware that I might have a slight disadvantage for not having practical familiarity, it wasn't enough to prevent me from doing everything humanly possible to make the breastfeeding relationship with my angel work.

In the first weeks after birth, I battled to get a proper latch-on. My nipples were severely cracked. I cried at nearly every nursing session. But in my heart I knew I had to march forward ~ for me there was NO other way to feed my baby. While my midwives and my LLL leader patiently helped us, I would begin deep, three-part breathing, fully oxygenating my body, and then I would get on with it. As with any relationship, there is ebb and flow; so later, when things became awkward due to teething, toddler titty twirling, tot boobie gymnastics, or my own restlessness, I would call in the goddess of yogini breathing to get me through.

Not only had yoga been a crutch for me pre-pregnancy and during my son's birth, it helped me create a magical breastfeeding bond between us. You don't have to have years of experience on a yoga mat to benefit from its healing powers, just a little faith and motivation. I also think it's worth mentioning that it doesn't matter where you are in the spectrum of life ~ now is as good as any time to breathe more deeply and realign your body and mind. So lactating or not, mama or papa, old or young, the following yoga postures (asanas), yogic affirmations (mantras), and yogic breathing (pranayamas) will manifest a more easeful body, peaceful mind and blissful life. While I can't make any guarantees, you don't have anything to lose unless you call spontaneous laughter a side-effect.

Yoga asanas to nurse a woman's body into a full-time lactating queen
Eagle (Garudasana ~ just the arm position)
Cow Face (Gormukhasana)
Wide Legged Forward Bend ~ variation with hand interlaced behind back and moving towards head (Prasarita Padottanasana)
Cat-Cow, Cobra (Bhujangasana)
Camel* (Ustrasana)
Fish (Matsyasana)
Downward-Facing Dog (Ardho Mukha Svanasana)
Thread the Needle
Rag Doll
Sun Salutations (Surya Namaskar)
Half Locust ~ Superhero variation (Ardha Shalabhasana)
    As with any yoga postures, proceed with care, listen to your body, and if you're a complete newbie, seek the advice of a qualified yoga instructor. *Camel ~ the beginner's variation ~ is suitable for new mamas. Wait until at least six months postpartum to enjoy the full pose (hands to feet), to ensure your uterus has returned to its pre-pregnancy position. [Psst…go to www.yogajournal.com ~ most of the above poses are pictured and thoroughly explained.]
    Yoga mantras (affirmations) to quieten your inner-monkey
~ *I am at peace with myself and my surroundings.*
~ *I breathe in the serenity of my beauty.*
~ *I am peace (use any descriptive word such as love, happy, exuberant, etc.).*
~ *Om Shanti.*
~ *Om Tat Sat.*
~ *Om Mani Padme Hum.*

There's a boundless number of mantras/affirmations that can be used to transmute the negative mind-chatter. They don't have to be cheesey and New Agey either! The key is to use one that feels delightful to your soul, and just keep repeating it (in your mind or vocally ~ your darling will love to hear such positive vibrations exiting your mouth). Eventually, the constructive thoughts will prevail!

Yogic Breathing ~ Pranayama

Hands down, my favourite pranayama is deep three-part breathing. From this base of expansive breathing all other breathing techniques become possible, and it allows your body to fully unfold in any yoga asana. Safety note: yogic breathing should never be forced or laboured. If at any time you feel shortness of breath, dizzy or faint, discontinue the practice, and resume your normal breathing.

Start by sitting in a comfortable position ~ any position that allows your spine to be long and expanded (you can lay supine on the floor). Place your right hand on your abdomen, and your left hand on your chest. All exhalations and inhalations happen through the nose. Begin by inhaling through your nose, drawing the breath down to your belly. You should feel your right hand expanding out as the air presses the abdomen out. Continue to draw the breath up through the diaphragm into the lungs, and then into the chest/heart. You should now feel your chest expanding into your left hand. Continue the breath up into your collar bones and throat. Now, slowly exhale through your nose in reverse order ~ chest, lungs, diaphragm, and abdomen. As you exhale, you should first feel your left hand soften on your heart, and your right hand on your abdomen. With each inhalation you're working to expand, and each exhalation to naturally contract and relax. Eventually, each one of these parts will flow one into the next, making it a seamless breath. Continue breathing wholly and completely.

This should be our natural breathing pattern, but stress and modern life have shifted us into shallow chest-breathers. If this three-part breath is practised often enough, it will eventually become your natural breathing rhythm. If you're lacking in inspiration, watch any sleeping baby to see how they entirely employ their full lung capacity.

I extend special kudos to every goddess mama who embarks on a yoga journey at such a precious time in her life. Conceiving, birthing, breastfeeding and raising aware kiddies is a monumental task, and by inviting yoga into your family's life, you're coming one step closer to relishing more moments of infinite bliss.

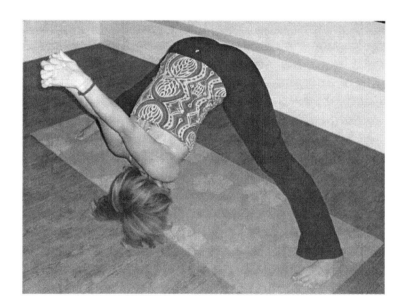

When to start solids, or when not to?
by Emma Lewis

I dislike the standard guidelines of: if a baby is sitting up, has teeth, is interested in or grabbing food, appearing more fussy or hungry...

Babies around six months are generally interested in everything they see happening around them. They learn through copying and mimicking. They often grab things (anything!) and put them in their mouth, as this is one of the ways they learn about their world. It doesn't necessarily indicate a readiness for food.

If a parent were to smoke, drink alcohol, write a letter, drive a car, knit a jumper, sew a shirt, stir a pan of hot soup ~ a baby of this age would want to mimic, and probably reach out for the cigarette, glass, pen, steering wheel, needles or spoon. This does not mean that they're ready to smoke, drink, write, drive or cook ~ or that it's safe or appropriate to do so.

I would suggest, in the above scenarios, most parents would provide a protective role, redirecting a baby towards more appropriate activity. I believe we, as parents, need to play a more protective role towards the inappropriate introduction of (often substandard) food.

A baby becoming fussy and appearing hungry doesn't necessarily mark the need for solid foods to be introduced. Babies have growth spurts. A baby may well be indicating the desire for more nutrition. So, as with the six week, three month or other growth spurts, this is a time to slow down, take things a bit easier and ensure baby has free and easy access to the breast ~ to increase their optimal nutrition: breast milk.

Yes, the optimal nutrition for baby is still your breast milk. Despite all attempts to undermine its gifts, never underestimate the magical, mysterious properties.

One of my observations has been that my (eight) babies naturally began to spread out their breastfeeds between the ages of about six to ten months, having longer spaces between feeds. Some of them began to sleep for longer periods around this time, too; and even started to nap for a bit during the day, without needing to be held for the duration. When this occurs, many mothers attribute it to the fact that the baby is eating solids. However, at this age, none of my babies had anything other than breast milk.

The thought of their baby sleeping for longer, motivates many parents' choice to introduce solids, often prematurely. Two studies that compared sleep patterns of babies receiving solids with those who did not, found no difference in sleep patterns. (Macknin 1989; Keane 1988).

Another important factor to keep in mind is that women, throughout time, have masticated food for their babies. This wasn't done whilst waiting for the food blender or processor to be invented. This is an essential part of introducing food to babies. Babies don't have the full range of enzymes available for optimal digestion. The mother passes them on in the masticated food.

I've received plentiful feedback on this comment over the years, due to concerns about the passing on of gum disease and other problems caused by our inadequate Western diet. I've noted valid and convincing arguments on both sides of this discussion. However, gums and teeth in a state of dis-ease don't make sense in evolutionary terms, and have never before been at such epidemic proportions. I would urge mothers to investigate the dis/advantages of a compromised digestive system versus compromised gum/tooth health, and use it as a prompt to be particularly conscious and mindful of the foods they allow past their babies' (and, indeed, their own) lips. I think the advice a midwife passed on in an antenatal class was just perfect. If we culturally begin to look at introducing solids in this way, I believe more optimal health would be achieved, and much stress would be removed from the food journey, both in the beginning and through the passage of time.

She suggested that breast milk be the baby's sole (soul) source of nutrition for their first year, and that full weaning be child-led (the world average being about four years). It is then appropriate to introduce tastes of single foods in an unprocessed state (i.e. as close to its natural [raw] state as possible) in the latter part of that year.

The key factor for consideration is always that, whatever we offer a baby as food, we ask: IS IT WORTH REPLACING BREAST MILK WITH THIS?

I would also suggest that the most important factor in the decision for beginning solids is to let go of noting prescribed, external behaviours and observations that would be pretty common in all babies around that time, whatever their circumstances. Carefully consider the political and financial profiteers behind any supposed advice; ignore what the health nurse or I or any studies report.

Begin to look within. Hear the messages your individual, unique baby communicates to you. Listen to them. Hear your heart. You and your baby already have the answers.

Bovine messages
In TM9 (p. 49) Eva Tombs-Heirman asked readers
"When is the right time to stop breastfeeding?"

Rae writes: There's no 'best time to wean'. Anyone looking for a textbook answer to Eva's question is grossly misguided; there's only one expert on the right time to wean your child: your child.

Within the tiny, seemingly 'helpless' body of your child is all the wisdom s/he needs for a richly fulfilling life. It's up to you to open your heart to the wisdom of your child, and they'll let you know all you need to know about caring for them, including when they're ready to wean. We're too eager in this society to allow what others think to overpower what we feel and know to be right. We're so conscious of 'fitting in' that we'll make decisions to the detriment of ourselves and our children. We constantly look outside ourselves for the answers to all of life's questions, preferring instead to relinquish our power to 'the experts', refusing to take responsibility for ourselves. We don't give credence to our hunches or intuition, we dismiss these as 'New Agey', and set about destroying our most precious gift with our logical and rational minds.

Fearful of what others might think, we rush our children to grow up and conform, beginning with early weaning. We're driven by fear: fear that our government, medical profession, friends and family instil into us; fear that we cannot nutritionally satisfy our child; fear that our child will be 'one of the clingy ones'; fear that we will be a social outcast; fear that we will in some way 'fail'; fear that we will lose our place in the rat-race if we don't hurry and get back to our career; fear that our partner will cease to find us attractive. Breast milk isn't merely nutrition that can be replaced by some other 'food'. In my experience, breast milk is nurture in its purest form ~ unconditional love, spiritual bonding, the wise healer (to my mind and heart, it's exactly the support our children need when they experience the 'consciousness jolting experiences' that can be traumatic or painful.) To see our child to go through the pain of teething and to stop breastfeeding seems in some way barbaric.

More importantly, it's a birthright, and every child should be able to benefit from this for as long as s/he desires.

If you're serious about finding the answer to this, look into your child's eyes the next time you're breastfeeding, and ask them the question 'When is the best time to wean?'

Beth writes: I feel that the lazy approach works best for our family. When my babies can feed themselves, it's then the perfect age for starting on solid foods. Why mess with the pureeing? It goes into baby's mouth and comes right back out. I prefer to toss a few tidbits onto my baby's plate, and see the joy in that little face of having them choose which bit, reach out and try to land it home. Then seeing a big grin of accomplishment.

Kirsten writes: I've been pregnant, breastfeeding or both for about eleven years now, and the children soon show me when they're ready to slow down or stop breastfeeding, and also when they want more. It's the children who've shown an interest in eating other foods other than breast milk in the same way as they soon let you know what foods they like and those they don't. Breast milk is so much more than food: it's food for the soul, and nurtures all a child's senses. Taste: sweet. Smell: the smell of a warm mum. Her smell is unique. Touch: the soft touch of a breast. The poking of the other nipple. Sound: the sound of the mother talking. The body sounds of the mother that the child has been used to in the womb, the recognition of the nurturing that began inside the womb and now carries on externally. Sight: recognition of mum and other family members, and recognition of the mum, so she doesn't pick up the wrong child. Is it just coincidence that mum's face is about the distance a new baby can see when at the breast? I doubt it. All this can take place alongside the beginning of trying new tastes and textures, and is a journey we never finish, as all through our lives, with luck, we find different foods we've never tried before, and of course, those we never want to try again!! Rice pudding, yuk!

Stephanie writes: Do you think your readers would be freaked out if I shared that my son didn't receive any solids until he was fourteen months old? And only then because I was pregnant and thought I'd best get started. He only breastfed at the breast, never from a bottle.

Veronika writes: My own breastfeeding practice is that of child-led weaning. When a child no longer feels the need to breastfeed, she'll stop. It's that simple. Who are we to determine or quantify what that need might be? Each child is unique. Toddlerhood is such a turbulent time, and what better 'Rescue Remedy' than to snuggle up into mum's lap and breastfeed? The eruption of teeth doesn't seem to me to equate with being a time to force a child off the breast. In fact, quite the opposite. The pain of teething (remember the last time you had a toothache? It's damned horrible!) is soothed so much by breastfeeding. We're physically unable to eat food with two top teeth or even four teeth. It takes a few years for all our teeth to come down. It would seem that if teeth were the indicator of when a child needed to cut back on breast milk, then after the eruption of the molar teeth (for chewing our food) would make more sense than in the first year. Looking globally to our systers who live more naturally than us, their babies breastfeed till well into toddlerhood, indeed early childhood. These women need no textbooks, gurus or clairvoyants. They follow their intuition ~ the ultimate guide for what is best. Their pregnancies and breastfeeding play a large part in when they'll conceive again, also. Their lives are in more balance than ours. When is the right time to stop breastfeeding? When your child no longer needs or wants to be at your breast.

Elizabeth writes: What happens when we put diesel fuel into a petrol engine car? It might run, but not very far, and not very well, and it will create a terrible mess along the way.

Following the thought of "you are what you eat", a baby until six months old is pure milk. It's the only food they've ever eaten, so it's easy to know what has made them what they are, and who they are.

The baby's body, mind and spirit grow and develop following the genetic codes and information received from human milk. If we're giving our babies bovine codes and messages from fast-food style "convenience" milk, what effect will they have on their little bodies?

It's not to say that they'll grow four legs and a long tail, but cows are ruminants with two stomachs; they have a different metabolism to that of a human, and humans think, have feelings and talk ~ whereas cows don't talk, or at least not in the same way as humans.

We are the mothers who are feeding the generation of people who won't be trashing the planet, so we need to make sure that all our children's components are given the optimal fuel to enable them to function in the correct manner. So, if the messages that make those developments evolve are for the wrong species, what will become of humanity? After all, you really wouldn't put diesel into your two-stroke now would you?

We're physically unable
to eat food with
two top teeth or even four teeth.

It takes a few years
for <u>all</u> our teeth
to come down.

It would seem that
if teeth were the indicator
of when a child needed to cut back
on breast milk,
then <u>after</u> the eruption of the molar teeth
(for chewing our food)
would make more sense
than in the first year.

NOT the mama
by Lynda Cook Sawyer

The loves of our lives ~ those wonderful creatures who love and support us…the ones who watch in awe as we blossom larger and larger with our pregnancies ~ be they spouse or brother or mate or partner, or even our own fathers, these humans, the adult male, mean the world to us. However, in all of their wonderfulness, there are just a few things they cannot biologically do, nor were they meant to. They cannot be pregnant. They cannot give birth.

And, they cannot breastfeed. Well, not easily, and certainly not gracefully.

If they cannot do these things, just what exactly CAN they do for our babies? (Believe me, they're wondering and worrying about this, too.)

Could we invite, welcome, entice, plead, threaten, force (?!) them to our births? Check. We've done that.

Could we offer, tell, instruct, teach, and allow them to catch our babies at birth or at least, "let them" cut the cord? Check. We've done that.

Could we offer to express our milk into bottles, or convince ourselves that "just one or two bottles" of artificial milk is okay for our babies so that "Dad can feed and bond with the baby, too?"

Aaaaaahhhh, the artificial baby milk companies would really like it if you did that. They would like it very much. They really want everyone, especially dad, to think that this is the only way dad/mate/partner/friend/grandparent can "bond" with a new baby ~ they must feed them!

After all, it's the way YOU do it. Right? There you sit, 10 to 12 times a day, with your nursling snuggled up to your chest, gazing deeply into his/her face, stroking this newbie's body as they frantically search for the breast, and finding it, nurse hungrily for a while, then deeply for a while, and eventually, he/she/you doze off into some netherworld sleep or haze. Total bliss for 15 to 30 minutes. These must be the essential bonding moments! Of course they are.

But, they are breastfeeding bonding moments. Nursing a baby and feeding a baby are two different functions. (Shhhhh, the ABM companies don't want anyone, especially the father, to know this.) To the babe, it's not just the milk that's important ~ although the human milk produced by the mother's mammary glands is exquisite ~ the act of breastfeeding is finally being noted as vital to all involved.

Feeding a baby merely provides sustenance. Nursing a baby, the actual act of suckling at the breast, however, provides so much more: warmth; comfort; safety; security; ever-changing food tastes; smells; protein and vitamin amounts that change in accordance to the baby's age and health; the smell of Mama, her heartbeat and breathing patterns; environmentally-correct live cells and antibodies to combat the bacteria, viruses, and allergens in your own home and village. In addition, the breast conforms to the infant's developing jaws and palates so as not to misshape the facial features as these structures continue to grow and harden.

The suckling infant/child is able to stabilise their body temperature, their breathing patterns and their heart rates. Their oxygenation rates (the ability to intake oxygen, exchange it in the lungs, and disburse it to the body) soar to nearly perfect levels as their breathing, in relation to suckling, becomes optimal. In fact, in the April 2003 issue of <u>Pediatrics</u> (a journal of medical research for paediatricians), recent research on the act of breastfeeding only confirms what mothers have known for years: that a suckling infant experiences a substantial relief of discomfort/pain, and nursing may, in fact, block the sensation of pain altogether.

For mum, the act of infant suckling at the breast provides sufficient releases of the hormone prolactin to produce copious amounts of milk around the clock, virtually non-stop, until directly nursing the infant at the breast is interrupted ~ sleeping through the night, back to work/school, starting solids early, weaning. Prolactin provides a sense of well-being in the mother's body which promotes rest, relaxation and sleep: and erects a hormonal barrier in her brain that suppresses the likelihood of postpartum depression. When nursing occurs frequently and regularly in response to the baby's cues, high prolactin levels are effective at preventing ovulation, thereby delaying the opportunity of a closely-spaced follow-up pregnancy.

The regular release of another hormone, oxytocin, which occurs in the mother when the nipples and areola are suckled, ensures the current pre-made supply of milk is delivered in full (let-down), and that as much as baby wants or needs at this particular feeding is manufactured, fresh, on-the-spot. Oxytocin also provides regular contraction stimulation to the uterus to control postpartum vaginal bleeding, and promotes quick involution of the uterus to its more normal resting state.

So, with all of this mounting factual evidence that it's the act of feeding at the breast, not "just the milk", that provides the Madonna-like bonding scenario for mum and babe......what information do dad/friend/grandparents need to understand that feeding the baby ~ even with our own milk in the bottle ~ is NOT the bonding moment for them that they've all been led to believe? That the bonding that occurs with breastfeeding is a culmination of all of the aforementioned points? The most glaring aspect of which is that there are no hormones, live cells, breathing recognition or regulation involved with bottle-feeding. In fact, none of the aforementioned aspects of breastfeeding are involved when feeding an infant with a rubber teat.

How, then, will anyone else bond with the new baby?

Let's revisit the biological determination of roles, and assuage all of their fears with truthful insight, rather than million dollar marketing schemes of artificial baby milk manufacturers.

Let's start with the equally vital "other adult" in your child's life: the adult male. While these men are not able to conceive life in their non-existent wombs, nor are they able to breastfeed naturally from their hard, tight, furry and oh, so sexy chests, they are very capable of bonding with their infants. In fact, it's vital that they do so.

Our children need a man and a woman to be conceived, for a reason. It takes both to provide the love and dichotomous emotional environment for the optimal growth of a child. This starts at conception, not at 12 years old.

Men are biologically designed to protect, commit, nurture, and to provide. They're masters of decision making in the moment, anger management, and great feats of strength and adventure. Their ability to imagine the wondrously impossible is glorious. (The Eiffel Tower? The Golden Gate Bridge? A trip to the Moon?) These are the attributes that adult men bring to the table.

Of course, we can reject these attributes and the men to which they're attached, and pretend they're not necessary; but then, what are we left with? A lonely and overworked mother; a lovely, cuddly mother-held-only infant; toddler and preschool children who have no concept of self-control, and the absolute inability to accept the answer "No" without incessant whining or a major tantrum; and pre-teen and teenage boys who seek the camaraderie and male edification of gangs of other teenage boys, and have no limits to their anger and to their death-defying senses of adventure; or adolescent girls who are craving the love of a man, and thinking whatever they're getting from their boyfriends is "it".

These children, boys and girls, have no basis for their roles in an adult relationship because neither had ever seen it modeled in their home. They were deprived of the opportunity of seeing an adult male treat their mother or young siblings kindly, gently, and with tenderness; they were not rough-housed and tickled and told when to "stop" ~ so they've no idea what a boundary is; and they were never told, in a voice only a man is capable of "Your mother said NO, and that's the answer."

They've never viewed their mother's role or any authority figure's role with respect, because no one was there to model respect, and command that it be shown ~ whether they felt it or not. Mothers model the art of mothering, and respect for their mates. Men model respect for all wombyn, small children, animals, and for the importance of the role of mothering.

The child's sense of adventure and imagination is distorted. It's the adult male who encourages adventuresome play with wild abandon and realistic physical limits, not the mother.

Mothers/adult wombyn are softly designed to teach love, nurturing, and patience; provide life and sustenance; and are to be protected when they're birthing, recovering and establishing the newborn's food supply. Fathers/adult men are strongly designed to teach self-control, duty, honour, respect, and through their guidance and modeling ~ nurture and protection of the mother, the young, the small, weak, and/or infirm. Men are built for fun and games, and endurance, as well as for family protection. In harmonious combination, these very beautiful qualities, innately biological to two genders, come together to make a whole and complete child.

All of this to say: men are important in the lives of babies and children, and they need to know it. If the father of your baby is not or cannot be involved, hopefully there are other men in your life that would be willing to be a close and involved surrogate. It is vital.

Embedded learning of life-values is best taught from the inside of a trusted and bonded relationship. For humans, these bonds are most easily formed with infants. A bond is simply a "uniting or binding element or force: tie <the bonds of family and friends>. (Webster Unabridged Dictionary)

But, what facilitates these so-called bonds? These uniting or binding elements in a family? Time.

What facilitates the intimate, knowledgeable, trusting bonds of a close and involved family? Time, togetherness, sweet and tender interaction, caring, empathy, support, and a full history of shared moments.

Biologically-driven to establish their milk supply, newborns will nurse 10 – 15 times in 24 hours ~ Mama-time. They'll also sleep, nuzzle, gaze interminably, eliminate more than five to ten times, need to be held throughout the day ~ even when sleeping, and in addition to nursing, enjoy a bath in the tub laying on their back on someone's legs, in a few inches of warm water, so they can splash and feel the sensation of it drizzling over their skin; will like to feel the breeze on their face and the sights and sounds of birds and the trees' leaves twinkling in the outdoors; they innately love the sound of music and laughter, and the lulling rumble of an auto's engine; they may even enjoy being read to, and learning to ride atop a man's shoulders is an adventure infants love! All of this is: NOT-the-Mama time.

These are all opportunities of sweet and tender interactions that lead to shared moments, and all too quickly become memories of your child's infancy and youth ~ a bond is formed with the person most often in attendance to share them. A kid's first choice would always be dad, but any loving person, really, will be welcomed.

Time spent in interactive companionship is what creates bonds. Adult men, securely providing their time in interactive and tender companionship with their infants and young children, establish amazing bonds that last a lifetime. And, other than a secretly shared ice cream cone for breakfast when mum is sleeping late, feeding need not have a thing to do with it.

Why breastfeeding mothers are important
by James Prescott

James W. Prescott, PhD. is a developmental and cross-cultural psychologist. His work centres on the affectional bonding between mother and child (through breastfeeding and baby-wearing) as the most effective way to prevent violence and addictions later in life. His research findings have the potential to change our culture. Eds' note: we highly recommend his DVD The Origins of Love and Violence: Sensory Deprivation and the Developing Brain. Research and Prevention with James Prescott and Michael Mendizza.

The greatest terror a child can have is that he is not loved, and rejection is the hell he fears. I think everyone in the world, to a large or small extent, has felt rejection. And with rejection comes anger, and with anger some kind of crime in revenge for the rejection, and with the crime, guilt ~ and there is the story of mankind.
John Steinbeck, *East of Eden*, 1952

Breastfeeding bonding and baby-carrying bonding are the first events of life in which the newborn/infant/child first learns about love and non-violence. Love is first learned at the breast of mother, and by being carried on her body ~ like in-utero, where the first lessons of being connected with mother are learned. Baby-carrying is the external umbilical cord that assures that the baby is connected with mother; and breastfeeding bonding for 2.5 years, or longer, has been found to be essential to optimise brain-behavioural development for the prevention of depression and suicide, and makes peaceful, harmonious and egalitarian behaviours later in life possible. Baby-carrying bonding was found to predict with 80% accuracy the peaceful and violent behaviours ("killing, torturing, mutilation of enemy captured in warfare") in 49 tribal cultures distributed throughout the world. (http://www.violence.de)

How the developing brain of the infant/child and teen is encoded with pain or pleasure experiences will determine whether a life-path of peace, harmony and egalitarian relationships will be followed, or a life-path of its opposite, of depression, alienation, anger, rage and violence (homicidal and suicidal) will be followed. Culture shapes our brain biology for peace or violence, where pain and pleasure are the formative life experiences that shape our two cultural brains for either peace or violence. In many cultures throughout the world, the first painful experience imposed upon the infant/child (male and female) is genital mutilation, a practice that many organisations and individuals seek to abolish. See http://www.montagunocircpetition.org for one such effort. The inflicting of pain on the child, as a form of punishment for wrongdoings, is legendary throughout human history. The punishment of children and teens for masturbation is a prime example of how pleasure is discouraged, and pain is emphasised, in the moral development of the child. Pain is moral and pleasure is immoral. Pain (physical and emotional) is the foundation for war and authoritarian relationships; pleasure is the foundation for peaceful and egalitarian relationships. These biological experiences influence not only the subcortical emotional-social-sexual brain, known as the limbic system, which is the first to form in evolution and development, but also the neocortical brain, which comes later in evolution and development, where values of what is good and evil are formed.

The first brain (olfactory-limbic system) encoded with pain or pleasure and their associated neural networks, informs the second brain (the neocortical brain) and its associated neural networks, whether pain or pleasure becomes the dominant influence that structures behaviour. The neocortical brain, through a complex feedback system, informs the subcortical brain which sensory experiences of pain or pleasure are acceptable. Thus, the neurointegrative and neurodissociative brains are formed, which yield the cultures and behaviours (peaceful or violent).

The ultimate value of breastfeeding bonding during the first three years of life is the sculpting of the developing brain for peaceful and egalitarian relationships where pleasure is the central experience, which is mediated by the complex biochemical nutrients of breast milk not found in infant formula milk, and the rich sensory experiences of touch, smell and body movement of mother involved in breastfeeding. Infant formula feeding robs the developing brain of those essential biochemical nutrients, particularly the essential amino acids tryptophan and tyrosine, that are necessary for the normal development of the brain neurotransmitters serotonin and dopamine, which mediate the emotional behaviours of peace or violence, of happiness or depression and suicide. These are only two of the many brain neurotransmitters involved in the development of our emotional behaviours.

Infant formula feeding also robs the developing brain of the rich sensory experiences that can only be realised through the intimacy of breastfeeding, which also translates into the coding of the developing brain for peaceful and egalitarian behaviours. Imagine this process of breastfeeding for the first three years of life and the rich sensory stimulation that continues to bathe the developing brain with pleasure ~ the glue of affectional bonding.

For these reasons, I have stated that it would be a rare event to find any murderer, rapist or drug addict in any of our prisons who has been breastfeed for two years of age and beyond, a time period recommended by WHO/UNICEF (1990), a viewpoint shared by Ashley Montagu.

In The Natural Superiority of Women(1952/1974) he stated:

"Women are the bearers, the nurturers of life; men have more often tended to be the curtailers, the destroyers of life." (p. 241).

"Women must be granted complete equality with men, for only when this has been done will they fully be able to realise themselves." (p. 242)

"Women are the mothers of humanity; do not let us ever forget that or under-emphasise its importance. What mothers are to their children, so will man be to man." (pp. 247-248)

"Women are the carriers of the true spirit of humanity ~ the love of the mother for her child. The preservation of that kind of love is the true function of women. And let me, at this point, endeavour to make it quite clear why I mean the love of a mother for her child, and not the love of an equal for an equal or any other kind of love." (p. 248)

"Woman knows what true love is; let her not be tempted from her knowledge by false ideas that man has created for her to worship. Woman must stand firm and be true to her own inner nature; to yield to the prevailing false conceptions of love, of unloving love, is to abdicate her great evolutionary mission to keep human beings true to themselves, to keep them from doing violence to their inner nature, to help them to realise their potentialities for being loving and cooperative. Were women to fail in this task, all hope for the future of humanity would depart from the world." (p. 250)

"Human societies must be based on human relations first, and economic activities must be a function of human relations, not the other way round." (p. 243)

How can human societies develop those cultural conditions that make the vision of Ashley Montagu possible ~ truly, a mission impossible? There are so many first steps to be taken it's difficult to know where to begin. What we do know is that the primary affectional bond between mother and infant/child must be developed and maintained where pleasure, and not pain, are the primary life experiences of the infant/child. This is dramatised by the cover image from John Bowlby's book on attachment. It's perhaps surprising that the two most outspoken leaders of the 20th Century supporting mothers and children were two Englishmen ~ John Bowlby and Ashley Montagu, who were born at the turn of the 20th century.

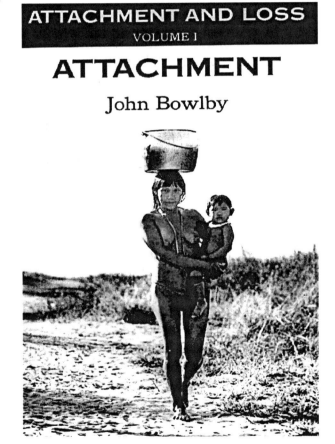

The first step is accomplished by breastfeeding bonding for 2.5 years or greater (data obtained from tribal cultures), and by baby-carrying throughout the day during the first year of life; no intentional infliction of pain on the infant/child; and freedom to naturally explore one's own developing sexuality where no harm or injury is inflicted upon others. We have learned that pleasure is not only moral, but morally necessary if we are to become moral persons.

Aristotle (384-322 BC) observed "Therefore, the highest good is some sort of pleasure, despite the fact that most pleasures are bad, and, if you like, bad in the unqualified sense of the word."

(Nichomachean Ethics, Book 7)

These peaceful cultures are readily accomplished in matrilineal/ matrifocal tribal cultures, but not in patrilineal/patrifocal tribal cultures, where the wisdom of the ancient African proverb prevailed: "It takes an entire village to raise a child". Unfortunately, the cultural evolution of Homo sapiens has resulted in the domination of the patrilineal cultures, with the accompanying extinction of the wisdom of the matrilineal cultures. As a result, America and the modern human culture have unfortunately lost the tribal village and the kinship relationships that made these child-rearing practices possible.

In the United States, The Third National Health and Nutrition Examination Survey, 1989-94, gives the following estimates for duration of breastfeeding. For all children, 6.8% were breastfed at 12 months; 2.7% were breastfed for 24 months or more; and 1% breastfed for 30 months or more. The Center for Disease and Control (CDC) National Vital Statistics Report does not include the weaning age of every child born in the United States, like the reports on infant and child mortality rates. This is a glaring deficiency in the keeping of health records in the US, particularly given the vital importance of breastfeeding bonding for the mother's and child's physical, emotional, social and sexual health. No modern state, unfortunately, keeps record of the weaning age of every child born in their country, which should be a part of their immunological record, and reflects the indifference and neglect to this most important measure of the mother-infant/child relationship, and the future health of the child.

I have evaluated the suicidal behaviours of 26 tribal cultures with a weaning age of 2.5 years or longer, as given in Textor (1967), A Cross-Cultural Summary, and found that 77% (20/26) of these cultures were rated low or absent in suicides. Eighty-two percent of these cultures were rated low or absent in suicide when support of youth sexual activity was added to the predictive equation. Punishment of pre-marital sex was found to predict 69% of "killing, torturing, mutilation of enemy captured in warfare" in 35 of the tribal cultures studied.

Barry and Paxon (1971) provided the ranges of weaning age for 186 cultures, among a number of other behavioural codes on infancy and childhood, which I utilised to extend my studies on weaning age and lack of suicide.

The average weaning age of each culture was calculated from the range scores given that permitted the statistical studies on those cultures whose weaning age was 24 months or less v 30 months or more. These data were added to those reported by Textor (1967), which yielded 65 cultures where information was available on both weaning age and suicide. It was found that 64% (23/36) of cultures were rated low or absent in suicide with a weaning age of 30 months or greater; 62% (18/29) of cultures with high suicide rates had a weaning age of 24 months or less. This difference was statistically significant ($p < .05$).

These findings suggest that a formative period of brain development exists between 2.0 years or less, and 2.5 years or greater that would account for these results. It should be noted that "no breastfeeding" does not exist in tribal cultures, for obvious reasons. The obvious comparison group is a "no breastfeeding group", available in modern human cultures, to compare with those who breastfeed for 2.5 years or greater. Despite repeated requests to the National Institutes of Health (NIH), these studies have yet to be conducted.

Modern MRI, fMRI and PET brain scan studies permit a level of sophistication in the measurement of brain development and function not previously available, and there's no excuse for such studies not being conducted. Similarly, for the evaluation of the perinatal trauma of circumcision, that would most certainly adversely affect the developing brain in structure and function. These studies have also yet to be conducted.

Unfortunately, the World Health Organization (WHO), the National Institute of Health (NIH) and the many international research organisations concerned with the health of mother and child, have not recognised the urgency of the issues raised by this data. Mothers, by breastfeeding their children (male and female) for 2.5 years and beyond, can radically alter human societies, reduce depression and violence by over fifty percent, and pave the way for true human equality.

The elimination of intentional pain in the rearing of infants and children, and supporting youth sexual affectional expression, are critical factors in this developmental continuum for creating peaceful cultures and egalitarian relationships. The benefits of breastfeeding assume that mothers are well-nourished, an unrealistic assumption in this modern world of continual warfare and poverty. Gender equality in sexual expression is also a condition of the peaceful, egalitarian and harmonious culture, where sexual expression is too important to be made a prisoner of marriage, and marriage is too important be a prisoner of sex.

Depression, suicide, homicide and rape are the leading emotional, social, sexual and mental health problems of the world, as the human atrocities against women and children escalate worldwide; and war, genocide and religious/ethnic conflicts continue without end. In America, school violence goes unchecked, where the recent attack of Seung Hui Cho, who fatally shot 32 students at Virginia Tech on April 16, 2007, is a continuing reminder of the previous massacres at Columbine High School in Colorado (April 20, 1999), and the eleven female Amish students (October 6, 2006), where five children were killed and six children critically injured. All were murders followed by suicide. The sexual assault of these Amish children was the intent of the killer, where condoms and lubricant were found in his possession.

The social isolation, alienation and rejection by the social group, and the failure to establish social and intimate relationships by the killer ~ the "loner" syndrome ~ is well established. The roots of this social-sexual dysfunctional relationship can be traced back to parental and childhood life experiences.

An interesting event occurred after the Columbine Massacre. Parents thanked God for saving their children, and other parents asked why God did not save their children. A number of atheists were born on the fields of Columbine that day. The same question should be asked following the Virginia Tech massacre, and particularly for the Amish children. Where was God when he was needed the most?

The difficulty that mothers have in breastfeeding their children in public is legendary. Charges of indecent exposure and "why don't you breastfeed elsewhere" are commonplace. A number of US states have had to pass laws protecting the right of mothers to breastfeed in public. Breastfeeding is a continuing struggle, when it should be the most natural event in the world, private or public.

School educators need to be educated. Maria Glod, in a story in The Washington Post, reported on a school policy of "NO PHYSICAL CONTACT!!!!" (June 18, 2007):

Fairfax County middle school student Hal Beaulieu hopped up from his lunch table one day a few months ago, sat next to his girlfriend, and slipped his arm around her shoulder. That landed him a trip to the school office. Among his crimes: hugging.

All touching, not only fighting or inappropriate touching, is against the rules at Kilmer Middle School, in Vienna. Hand-holding, handshakes and high fives? Banned. The rule has been conveyed to students this way: "NO PHYSICAL CONTACT!!!"

All mammals need physical contact ~ touching and body movement ~ from birth throughout adulthood, to assure normal emotional-social-sexual development. Species survival depends upon it. Our school systems should not be engaged in teaching and promoting those very life events that end in school violence, but teaching life events that promote affectional bonding and peaceful behaviours.

Holding hands while walking with your boyfriend or girlfriend, carrying her books, a peck on the cheek, are all time-honoured customs in any civilised society. I have a suggestion to the Fairfax County School Board to promote affectionate relationships in children. Beginning with kindergarten, and with the beginning of each class, each child is greeted with a hug by another child. The next day a different child is given a hug. Eventually all children get a hug from every child in the class. Next year, it is kindergarten and first grade; next year kindergarten, first and second grade, and so on. By high school, all children will feel more or less comfortable with getting a hug. The hostility to such a program can be anticipated in our touch-deprived cultures.

Gender equality is fundamental to achieving the goals of the natural family, as Ashley Montagu has emphasised. There's not a single millennial theistic religion on this planet that has recognised equality between the feminine and masculine. Fifty percent of the species, Homo sapiens, has been disenfranchised by just being born female. Women are morally and socially inferior to the male, the property of males and the source of moral evil. "Woman is the origin of sin, and it's through her that we all die." (Ecclesiasticus 25:24).

A partial political solution to this intractable human inequality is to demand gender equality in the legislative bodies of the world. This thesis was advanced in an essay in The San Diego Union Tribune, entitled The challenge: achieve gender equality.

Without this international voice of gender equality, the equality of the feminine with the masculine will remain the unfulfilled dreams of the poets and philosophers of the world, and breastfeeding bonding will become a relic for the future. Women are defenceless against the despotism of male-dominated legislatures, and must reclaim their right to full human equality, if they are to assure their future and that of their children.

References

AAP (1997). Breastfeeding and the Use of Human Milk (RE9729) Pediatrics 100(6). December. http://www.aap.org/policy/re9729.html

AAP (2005). Breastfeeding and the Use of Human Milk PEDIATRICS Vol. 115 No. 2 Feb pp. 496-506. http://aappolicy.aappublications.org/cgi/content/full/pediatrics;115/2/496.

Barry III, H., Bacon, M.K. and Child, I.L. (1967). Child, Definitions, Ratings, and Bibliographic Sources of Child-Training Practices of 110 Cultures. In: Cross-Cultural Approaches. (Clellan S. Ford, Ed). HRAF Press. New Haven.

Barry III, H. and Paxon, L.M. (1971). Infancy and Early Childhood: Cross-Cultural Codes 2.

Ethnology X(4):466-508.

Bowlby, J. (1953). Child Care and the Growth of Love. Pelican/Penguin. Baltimore/London.

Bowlby, J (1969/1973). Attachment and Loss. Vol. I & II. Basic Books. New York.

Cook, P.S. (1996). Early Child Care: Infants & Nations At Risk. News Weekly Books Melbourne.

Fazzolari-Nesci, A., Domianello, D., Sotera, V. and Raiha, N.C. (1992). Tryptophan fortification of adapted formula increases plasma tryptophan concentrations to levels not different from those found in breastfed infants. J. Pediatric Gastroenterology and Nutrition. May. 14(4): 456-459.

Hardy, S.B. (1999). Mother Nature. A History of Mothers, Infants, and Natural Selection. Pantheon Books. New York

Montagu, A. (1952/1974). The Natural Superiority of Women. Collier MacMillan, New York, London.

Montagu, A. (1971). Touching: The Human Significance of the Skin. Columbia University Press.

Montagu, A. (1995). Mutilated Humanity. The Humanist. 55(4):12-15. July/August.

Prescott, J.W. (1975) Body Pleasure and the Origins of Violence. The Futurist April.

Reprinted: The Bulletin Of The Atomic Scientists (1975) November.

Prescott, J.W. (1977). *Phylogenetic and ontogenetic aspects of human affectional development. Progress In Sexology. Proceedings of the 1976 International Congress of Sexology.* (R. Gemme & C.C. Wheeler, Eds.) Plenum Press, New York.

Prescott, J.W. (l979): *Deprivation of physical affection as a primary process in the development of physical violence.* In. Child Abuse and Violence (Gil, D. G., Ed). AMS Press New York pp 66-137.

Prescott, J.W. (l990): *Affectional bonding for the prevention of violent behaviours: Neurobiological, Psychological and Religious/Spiritual Determinants.* In. Violent Behaviour Vol. I: Assessment and Intervention. (L.J. Hertzberg, et. al., Eds). PMA Publishing NY pp. 110-142.

Prescott, J.W. (1992): *Consequences of Perinatal Trauma - Genital Mutilation / Circumcision - and Somatosensory Affectional Nutrurance Upon the Adult Brain: Nuclear Magnetic Resonance (NMR) and Positon Emission Tomography (PET) Scan Evaluations of Brain Structure and Function.* http://www.violence.de/archive.shtml

Prescott, J.W. (1995). *Violence Against Women: Philosophical and Religious Foundations of Gender Morality. New Perspectives.* (March/April). Hemet, CA.http://www.violence.de/prescott/women/article.html

Prescott, J.W. (1995). *OPINION. The challenge: achieve gender equality. The San Diego Union Tribune.* December 10. http://www.violence.de/politics.shtml

Prescott, J.W. (1996). *The Origins of Human Love and Violence. Pre- and Perinatal Psychology Journal.* 10(3):143-188. Spring http://www.violence.de/prescott/pppj/article.html

Prescott, J.W. (1997). *Breastfeeding: Brain Nutrients In Brain Development For Human Love And Peace Touch The Future Newsletter,* Spring http://www.violence.de/archive.shtml

Prescott, J.W. (1997). *The Ashley Montagu Resolution to End the Genital Mutilation of Children Wordwide: A Petition to the World Court, The Hague.* In. Sexual Mutilation: A Human Tragedy. (G.C. Denniston & M.F. Milos, Ed). Proceedings of the Fourth International Symposium on Sexual Mutilations. Plenum Press, New York and London.

Prescott, J.W. (2004). *The Origins of Love. How Culture Shapes The Developing Brain and the Future of Humanity.* Byronchild. Byron Bay NSW Australia. March-May.

Prescott, J.W. (2005): *Prevention Or Therapy And The Politics of Trust: Inspiring a New Human Agenda. Psychotherapy and Politics International.* 3(3):194-211 John Wiley & Sons, http://www.interscience.wiley.com http://www.violence.de/prescott/politics-trust.pdf

Prescott, J.W. (2006). *Breastfeeding and Intelligence Not Demonstrated - Rapid Response. BMJ,* October 27. http://www.bmj.com/cgi/content/full/333/7575/0

Salk, L., Lipsitt, L.P., Sturner, W.Q., Reilly, B.M. & Levat, R.H. (1985). *Relationship of maternal and perinatal conditions to eventual adolescent suicide. The Lancet March 15.*

Textor, R.B. (l967): *A Cross-Cultural Summary.* HRAF Press. New Haven.

WHO/UNICEF. (1990). *Innocenti Declaration. Florence, Italy.*

Insufficient Milk Syndrome:
the greatest let-down of all
by Veronika Sophia Robinson

Humans, like other mammals, have breastfed their young since the beginning of their species' evolution. Indeed, without breastfeeding, they simply couldn't have survived.

The consequences of little or no breastfeeding are manifesting all around us, and the Great Bottle-feeding Experiment has shown us quite clearly how quickly mind, body and soul deteriorate without the milk of human kindness. The tragic story of thousands of babies in China suffering from infected artificial milk is a symbolic tip of the iceberg of what we're doing to our babies by not feeding them naturally.

We pay lip service to the ol' mantra: breast is best, but have you ever noticed how quickly even the strongest advocates of breastfeeding follow it up with 'but of course not all women can breastfeed'? Even my Oxford dictionary states, under breastfeeding: breastfeeding is not always possible. It's this latter statement that lets every mother and baby down, for it adds to the Cultural Soup which denies our mammalian nature. And it is the complete lack of understanding of a woman's whole being that lets us perpetuate the myth that some women with healthy, intact breasts, can't make milk.

Insufficient Milk Syndrome (IMS), contrary to popular opinion, is not an incurable medical ailment, but a man-made invention. How do we know this is true? Because for millions of years, humans have successfully breastfed their children. IMS began at the very time when breastfeeding was considered unfashionable ~ the 1940s, when women were encouraged to join the workforce because men were 'at war'.

Breast milk is made in the alveoli ~ large numbers of sac-like structures, and taken to the nipple via milk ducts. If you can imagine a bunch of grapes, with the woody bits in-between being a bit like tunnels, or ducts, which transport the milk out of the grapes, you can get a visual image of how it works. A nipple is sensitive because of the number of nerves it contains, and it's stimulation of the nipple which is an important part of making milk. But this isn't the only important aspect in breastfeeding.

The milk-secretion reflex involves the baby sucking at the breast, which in turn sends a message to the pituitary gland, which then produces prolactin. This then sends a message to 'make milk'. At the same time, the infant's sucking causes the pituitary gland to send oxytocin, the love hormone, into the blood. Once this message arrives in the breasts, the milk lets down. This is commonly known as the let-down reflex. Some women feel this quite distinctly, others always have milk leaking and rarely experience the sensation of letting-down. Let-down is susceptible to things such as anxiety and fear, and is certainly not a happy bed-fellow with strict breastfeeding routines a la Gina Ford and other childcare advisors who aren't in alignment with a child's needs.

We have to question why malnourished women, living in a state of poverty, are capable of creating nutritious milk for their babies, but well-nourished Western women have a mysterious ailment that snatches away their milk-making ability. How have we, as a culture, come to accept this without questioning if this is really possible? One of the biggest culprits is the artificial milk advertising machine, which will state their formulaic 'not intended to replace milk, but if you can't breastfeed we're here'...and ready to make a bundle from you. But we do it to each other, as well: woman to woman, mother to mother. We repeat the myths over and over again. If we had no other option but to feed our children naturally, from our breast, IMS would disappear overnight.

Some women try desperately to get their milk down by using a breast pump, but lactation consultants, in general, seem to omit an important piece of information: pumps are NOT efficient in getting the milk down and stimulating supply. They can only achieve about 20% of what a suckling baby can. Don't ever believe your pump.

The emptier the breast is, the faster it tries to refill. The breasts are never really empty. If milk is regularly and thoroughly removed from the breast, more will keep being produced. This is the wonderful breastfeeding law of demand and supply. The physical reasons for slow or no let-down can include:

[] when there is a retained placenta
[] contraceptive pills disrupting the hormones
[] breast surgery
[] baby sucking on dummy rather than breast
[] baby being supplemented with formula/water
[] some sort of latch-on problem

But if none of the above is accountable for lack of let-down, what else would a mother or lactation consultant look for? One of the things I hear over and over again is women saying they tried 'everything' and still didn't make milk; that they must be one of the unlucky ones with Insufficient Milk Syndrome. And yet, when I start talking with them, the story that always emerges is that 'everything' actually only looked at the physical side of their being.

We're multi-dimensional beings, with other aspects to us which can impact on how we live our lives. We have an emotional self, psychological self and spiritual self (amongst others).

If you've got breasts, and they've not been damaged in surgery, it's physically impossible to not make milk. We're mammals. We make milk. It's possible, however, to 'withhold' the milk.

Indigenous cultures don't have such a thing as Insufficient Milk Syndrome. This mysterious affliction is unique to cultures with ready access to infant formula and advertising to match. This fact alone should have us questioning why we believe, and wrongly perpetuate, that some women can't make milk. Whether a woman chooses to release that milk for her child or not, is a psychological/ emotional matter, not physical, though it manifests that way.

One analogy that can help explain this is to compare letting milk down as equivalent to the female orgasm. Unless you've been the victim of female genital mutilation (clitoridectomy), then you are capable of orgasm, physically.

Some women go their whole sexual lives without ever experiencing the intense and indescribable pleasure of this climax. And other women can have multiple orgasms in one sexual encounter, either with a partner, through self-stimulation, mechanically, or while dreaming. Why would one woman be able to experience this, and another not? Quite commonly in our culture, we suggest that the sexual partner was not 'skilled' enough to bring his/her partner to orgasm. This is simply not true. No-one can make you have an orgasm. It's something you give to yourself. It happens when a woman allows herself to surrender fully to the experience: when she can let go of control and become one with the sensations. And the same happens with the let-down reflex of breastfeeding. We have to be able to trust the sensations, and let it all hang out, so to speak. One of the things that tends to happen with breastfeeding mothers is a sense of fear or emotional discomfort if breastfeeding is pleasurable. Because breastfeeding is something we don't readily or easily discuss in all its fine details, women don't share with each other that it is natural and right for breastfeeding to feel good and pleasurable. Nature designed it to be so. Culturally, we associate pleasure with sexuality, and because the cultural mindset has them inextricably linked, we therefore assume it must mean that a woman is having taboo sexual feelings for her breastfed infant/child. And what greater taboo than incest? No wonder we dare not talk about pleasure and breastfeeding in the same sentence!

I watched a TV documentary recently called Other People's Milk (about wet nursing). A woman was trying to explain about these sexual/sensual feelings, and it was completely misconstrued by the presenter. It was such a wonderful opportunity to educate. Sadly, it only furthered people's fears and ignorance.

The same hormones are used in birth, breastfeeding and making love ~ we must learn not to be afraid of the power and pleasure of the female body. We were designed to enjoy being in our skin. Women have been left with such a hideous legacy: the burning of nine million witches is etched into every cell of our being. They were burned for knowing women's craft, like birth, herbs, dreams, etc. No small wonder that we don't physically celebrate our femininity as Nature ordained it. Instead, we run from it, scared it might show us something within ourselves. We engage in superficial femininity, rather than allowing it to emanate from within.

Letting our milk down is about surrendering, which is a pretty apt description of mothering in general. We need to surrender to our body, and to our dependent child. For many women, the breastfeeding instinct is triggered during birth. Others have had birth engineered, and the job to discover their instinct has been sabotaged to a greater or lesser degree by hormonal interference. Other women <u>unconsciously</u> withhold their breast milk due to sexual abuse in childhood, or withheld mother love in their own infancy/childhood. Some women find breastfeeding painful or irritating, and wrongly assume it has something to do with the baby or feeding, when actually (assuming the baby is latched-on correctly) it's a physical reaction to emotional discomfort. As in childbirth, fear and tension lead to pain.

Sometimes the confusion of puberty brings new beliefs about one's body, which, if not celebrated by those around us, go on to have a negative impact on one's beliefs about sexuality, and this can manifest in difficult birth and/or breastfeeding experiences.

Daily, we're bombarded by visible and invisible cultural messages of breasts being for sexual purposes only. The messages are subliminal, and go to the core of our subconscious. Who are we when we lift our shirt to breastfeed? Mother or slut? Nurturer or sex-kitten? Breastfeeder or boob exposer? Why do we allow ourselves to feel intimidated about breastfeeding our children whenever and wherever they need to drink or have physical comfort? We allow it because we've been assaulted by the invisible field of our culture, that says artificial milk is normal, and that breastfeeding is unnecessary; because, at some level, we believe it; because the invisible field is strong, and tells us breasts exist only for men's sexual pleasure, and that, by breastfeeding in public, we're flaunting ourselves. The vast majority of women were taught as little girls not to express sexuality in any shape or form. Sexual energy is creative energy. Why do we see it as so shameful? Sure, it can become sordid, violent and abusive. But at its most honest and beautiful, it's deeply inspiring and creative. We can choose to see and express sexuality in all its glory.

We can't do much about culture, but we CAN take charge of our own mindset and fish out debris in the subconscious. And in the end, that's all that matters: that you, and your child, know without a shadow of a doubt that the milk from your body has been uniquely made for your child, and it's designed to be consumed at source, not pumped out to be served in a bottle or cup. Breast milk is perfection in action.

If I'm working with a woman who believes she has no or low milk, I encourage her to go inwards and ask herself why she's withholding love from her child. Withholding love? On the surface it can seem rather rude, or even cruel, to suggest that is what a woman is doing. Clearly it requires empathy, compassion and an awareness on the part of the lactation consultant to know how far one can go when exploring this aspect of breastfeeding. But let's think about it for a moment. Breast milk is LIQUID LOVE. It's created through the love hormone, next to our heart: the love organ. Sometimes it takes the bold suggestion that a mother is withholding love, for her to go searching her own heart. I can't answer it for her, only she can, if she has the courage. I can, as a lactation mentor, hold her hand, offer support and love, and be with her when she comes out the other side. When a woman is willing to go the distance and ask the big questions, a breakthrough occurs on her breastfeeding journey.

Visualisation

Many pregnant women, when asked if they plan to breastfeed, say that they'll 'try'. What sort of a culture have we created that women believe it might not be possible to do something as innately mammalian as breastfeed?

It sounds simplistic, but in order to breastfeed, you have to want to ~ not as in a conscious thought, but a deep, inner yearning. It has to come from a place of wanting to become one with your child through breastfeeding. Visualising the body making milk, and the messages going to the pituitary gland and sending the message to 'let milk down', brings the emotional self into alignment with the physical self. Visualising the milk coming out of the breasts, directly into the baby's waiting mouth, helps a woman to connect with the experience in a way she can't when she's focused on pumping breast milk or desperately trying to get a newborn to latch. Visualising herself as a breastfeeder is vital.

In the field of sports psychology, self-hypnosis is well-known for helping sports people achieve their goals. Breastfeeding is no different. Unfortunately, very few lactation consultants consider the whole woman, and until such time as they do, their work at the front line is limited.

I ask a mother not only to visualise milk-making, I encourage her to 'travel to her heart' and imagine her spiritual self being made manifest through the physical. Women who've never had children are capable of spontaneous lactation. They're not freaks of Nature, but women who've opened their hearts to children. These women show us what is possible.

For some women, it's particularly helpful to look at the spirituality of breastfeeding and how it impacts on their physical selves. Ancient cultures teach about the seven centres of life and consciousness, in the spine and brain, called chakra (chakrum = singular). They begin at the base of the spine and can be found along its length, up to the head (see picture on page 208). The process of aligning and awakening a chakrum is very much holistic, taking in our whole being. It happens spontaneously and naturally throughout our childhood development if our biological needs have been met through a mother's affectionate bonding ~ a gentle birth, unrestricted breastfeeding, co-sleeping and baby-wearing. The unfolding of our physical development reaches through into our spiritual unfolding. The development of the chakra mimics child development.

The first two chakra represent our physical self ~ our base survival and reproductive needs.

Three and four are to do with how we relate, and are connected to the mammalian brain. The green chakrum, our breastfeeding one, next to our heart, is where we let through peaceful feelings, love and harmonious energy into relationships. A closed or undeveloped heart chakrum leads to reluctance in letting milk flow for our baby; rigidity in love; lack of compassion; anger; health issues to do with the heart; and immune-system stress. Chakra five and six correlate to the neocortex, our new brain. And the seventh, known as the seat of consciousness, or crown, has no connection to the brain at all. Indeed, to reach this state of consciousness or enlightenment we need to leave the brain (ego) well behind.

The heart chakrum teaches us that love can't be contained. We surrender ourselves into this bond; and in giving ourselves up to our children, we're returned to our self in even greater form. The more we give, the more we're enhanced. Despite our cultural messages to the contrary, it's not a sacrifice to be a bonded mother. We forfeit great jumps in our personal evolution by avoiding being fully committed to mothering.

When humanity's heart centre closes down, the human race will be unable to exist. We simply can't live together with closed hearts indefinitely. Because this syndrome of closed heart chakrum is so widespread, it's now considered normal to be distrustful and unloving. Normal, in this case, is not natural. Seven million people in Britain live alone. That is, more than one in eight people. This isolation and alienation is an example of the closing down of the heart centre.

Breast milk is, in many ways, a link for the child to Cosmic Sustenance: compensation for incarnating Earthside into this world of limitations. Breastfeeding is the birthright of every baby, and what's good for the baby is good for the mother.

We can offer herbal, mechanical and psychological support to new mothers, but while we have artificial milk readily available and heavily advertised, and a culture which screams out that breastfeeding is obscene, there will always be women who claim they can't make milk. The cultural tide has engulfed them. IMS is not a mysterious ailment, and it isn't a situation that can't be remedied. The greatest gift we can give to such women is to educate them that every mother with intact breasts can produce milk, and breastfeed, if she wants to. The power to let milk flow comes from within, and does so when we open our heart.

Tools to bring breast milk down:

Herbal teas: Starflower; red raspberry leaf; fennel; goat's rue.
Flower essences: Starflower, Nui, Watermelon
Aromatherapy oils: Jasmine, Fennel

Mechanical
. Nipple stimulation by baby, or if not possible, the mother's partner or self-stimulation
. Breast pumping (not as effective as a baby suckling)
. Massage with warm oils

Psychological
. Visualisation
. Meditation
. Breathing/relaxation
. Hypno-breastfeeding

Resources:
Maggie Howell's Breastfeeding CD www.natalhypnotherapy.co.uk
Starflower tea & Starflower essence from <u>www.starflowerpress.com</u>
International Flower Essence Repertoire

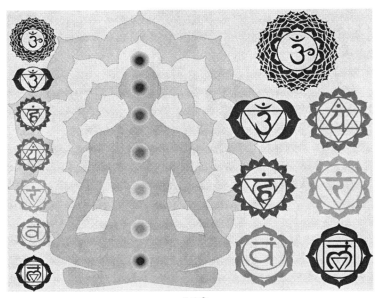

But It Hurts!
by Lynda Cook Sawyer

One of the leading reasons for choosing not to breastfeed a baby is because "it hurts". If you do choose to nurse your baby, the leading remark, storyline or question is always, "But, what about the PAIN?" (said with grizzly emphasis on the word pain).

Well, it would be easy for me to tell you to tell "them" to just keep their knowledge deficit to themselves, but it would be too late. They've already planted the seed that "Breastfeeding does hurt". And that seed, mixed with the fertiliser of routine isolation, common sleep deprivation, and a healthy dose of ongoing, conflicting breastfeeding commentary, is capable of growing into a huge and scary whomping-willow tree (a-la "Harry Potter") that will indeed sneak up on you in the middle of one of those early nights and cause your nipples and/or breasts to become engulfed in blinding pain!

And, then, of course, all prophecies will have been fulfilled. "They" told you it would hurt.

So, let's grace ourselves with the intuitive knowledge that's available to everyone. 1) If breastfeeding hurt like that all the time following the birth of each baby, then our human race would be extinct, because no foremother of any of us would have put up with it. They were very strong and busy wombyn. 2) There's a kind, loving and gentle God/Goddess (insert the name central to your belief-system) who would not form a life-creating being, you, and then cause you to essentially walk over cut-glass and razors with bare feet (my description of nursing pain) to ensure that the new little life-creating being: your nursling ~ survives their first year and beyond with exquisite nourishment! That would be silly. 3) If breastfeeding was supposed to cause this described damage and blinding pain each time a baby is born, and mouth-to-breast milk removal is initiated, then we would have already created a far superior method of extracting milk from the breast, and providing it to our offspring; or at the very least, we would have abandoned the whole idea of providing nourishment from our own bodies, and created an incredibly more nutritious substance. After all, we are wombyn. And, none of the above, by the way, has occurred.

Breastfeeding is not supposed to hurt.

The horror stories that are told of terrific nipple damage that led to a debilitating breast infection and was followed by a three week spree of a rabid, undiagnosed thrush, are not "common ailments of breastfeeding".

These types of stories are most often repeated as if each additional problem were individual and unique; as if they were unrelated to the last, and occurred simply because the mother has bad luck, bad breasts, a bad baby, bad karma, no spousal support, no insurance, etc... And, just because this exact scenario happens so often in our culture, the implication with which the listener is then left is: "this is what happens if you breastfeed".

This snowball of problems is the culmination of waiting too long to seek assistance, unknowledgeable assistance, misdiagnosis, and/ or unhelpful treatment plans.

As a matter of fact, the first twinge of discomfort is your first caution signal that "something might be wrong". At the first signs of "hmmmmm, this is feeling uncomfortable", nursing mothers should be thinking, "Maybe something is wrong" versus our trained thoughts of, "Uh-huh. Here we go. They told me it would hurt."

Even worse than the scheduled response above, is the response that goes something like this, "Oh, this isn't so bad. I'll wait to see if it gets better" It's been my experience that nipple or breast pain when nursing doesn't "get better". On the contrary, it gets worse ~ over time, of course, but worse.

So, here's Lynda's Primer for Recognising and Reversing Pain Associated with Breastfeeding.

Lesson One: speak the same language. There is a left breast and a right breast. The breast can be any size. It can be any shape. It can be different sizes and shapes from left to right. The mammary gland (the organ inside the breast responsible for milk production and delivery) is basically the same size regardless of the breast size or shape. Really, really voluptuous breasts do not necessarily make any more milk than smaller breasts. (Of course, there are extremes to the size and shape issue which affect a very minute population, and they would need specialised assistance.)

Each breast has an areola (pronounced either "ah-ree'-o-lah" or "air'-ee-ola". Both are correct). The areola is the smooth, differently coloured skin that encircles the nipple. Its colour can be pale, pink, rosy, brown, black, blush, or skin-coloured. It can cover 1/3 of the exterior of your breast, or it can barely trace the shape of your nipple. Neither the babe or milk production has a need to rely on the size of a mother's areola. The mammary gland is basically the same size regardless of the areola's size or colour.

Each areola has a nipple. This is the portion of the areola that contains the vast majority of milk duct openings from the mammary gland to the exterior of your breast. When stimulated, your nipple may protrude (become firm and stick out from your breast) or it may simply form a firm ring to indicate its presence, or it may invert (pull inside itself ~ like pulling your lips in between your teeth). The mammary gland is basically the same size regardless of the nipple's size, shape, or directional characteristics when stimulated.

If your nipple protrudes with stimulation, you have perfect breasts for breastfeeding! If your nipple forms a firm ring to indicate its presence, you have perfect breasts for breastfeeding! If your nipple inverts, you have perfect breasts for breastfeeding! And you need to seek knowledgeable support before the birth. (Seeking support after the birth is OK, too, but before is less stressful for you as your baby is not yet in-arms. If there's nipple protrusion or a ring, then the portion of the nipple that extends from the areola to the edge of the firm ring is called the neck. If there's nipple inversion, then the would-be neck is extended along the interior. When everted, the neck would be identifiable. No worries.

The very front, flat portion of the nipple is what I call the face of the nipple. This front, flat portion contains almost all of the milk duct openings from the mammary gland to the exterior of your breast. There may be one or two wild ducts that open on the neck or areola, but that's OK. They usually don't interfere with feedings.

The breast, the areola, the neck and the face can all be further defined by locating any point on any of the areas in terms of a clock face. For instance, if I had a lump on my right breast, I could describe the position of the lump to you by saying, "It's located in the 9 o'clock position on my right breast." And you'd know that I was meaning a lump in the breast tissue of my right breast on the side closest to my armpit. Or if I had an open wound on the face of my nipple, I could describe it as, "a blister in the 10 to 2 o'clock position on the face only of my left nipple." And you'd know that I was meaning a blister that almost covered the top half of the part of my nipple that is flat.

When we use the same language to discuss breasts and breastfeeding, everything is better understood.

Lesson Two: know what breastfeeding looks like. If you've never seen another mother nurse her baby, then you're already at a disadvantage when it comes to nursing your own. Breastfeeding is learned, not from books or articles or teachers, but from each other. We used to be able to watch our mother nurse our siblings, our aunts nurse our cousins, and our neighbour mothers sit with our own mothers while they all nursed their babies on and off, and enjoyed each other's company. As young wombyn, we could watch our friends nurse their first babies while we excitedly awaited our first babies. In the back of the church, where all the mothers of young children and babies sat, we could sit with other mothers and observe their responses to their babies' silent nursing cues.

By being around other nursing women, common knowledge is exchanged. For instance, to be talking to a mother when her babe in-arms begins to root for the breast, and she almost absent-mindedly slips him on to the breast without stopping her conversation, is to learn about 'rooting' being a feeding cue, and latch-on need not be an all-consuming endeavour. To be present when a new mother winces in pain at latch-on, disconnects the latch and replaces the baby on the nipple, is to learn that a comfortable attachment to the breast can be achieved. To be shown myriad feeding positions that a baby can lie or sit in to nurse, is to learn that one, restrictive, way of holding your baby is not mandatory. And, to be close enough to a nursing mother that you can see the child's lips flanged over her nipple, his little tongue curled around the underside of her breast, thereby providing a cushion between teeth and breast, and observe his eyes gently shut to the rhythm of his suckle, is to learn that nursing is not nipple feeding, but breastfeeding (much breast tissue goes into a nursling's mouth: not just a nipple), and that breastfeeding is pleasurable and soothing to the babe, and comfortable to the mother.

La Leche League understands that new mothers need to see this and much more. If a group meets near you, go! Begin attending during your pregnancy, and continue long after the birth. You'll never regret seeing the nursing mother or being the nursing mother.

Lesson Three: know the most common breast ailments of breastfeeding. In that realm, mother is the most knowledgeable professional of us all. With just a little factual information, you can diagnose and treat yourself, thereby avoiding even the first step, "terrible nipple damage". If you have in mind what might go wrong and how those conditions happen, then you're already 95% closer to avoiding it. If you know what the symptoms are of the most common nursing pitfalls, then you're 100% closer to diagnosing and beginning the "treatment" yourself. Should any of the following fail to relieve your immediate discomfort, please call a lactation supporter for early assistance.

Nipple pain ~ pinching: This occurs with latch-on. The squeezing sensation makes your toes curl, and causes you to inhale sharply.

Cause: Your baby is squishing your nipple between his gums. The nipple is not located properly in the back of his throat, and not enough breast is in his mouth. When just the nipple is offered and taken, then the baby must clench his jaws to hold on to the nipple. When just holding on is the focus, the baby is unable to place his tongue between the breast and his lower gum, cushioning his powerful lower jaw and the underside of your breast.

Correction: Gently un-latch your infant. With your fingers and thumb well away from the nipple and areola, cup your breast, and stroke your infant's mouth with the face of your nipple. When he opens his mouth like a yawn, pull him onto the breast. Keep bringing him toward you until he closes his mouth on the breast. (If the fingers of your hand holding the breast are too close to the nipple, and he touches these first, he'll be triggered to shut his mouth at that point. Be sure to place your fingers well away from the nipple and areola.)

You should feel an immediate difference, as your baby is now breastfeeding, and your nipple is encased safely away from his jaws, in the smooth back regions of his throat.

If left untreated: The pain will escalate, and nipple damage is likely to occur. A bad latch left uncorrected will eventually cause the skin of the nipple to blister or crack, and the neck of the nipple to become sore and severely cracked ~ most often due to the tongue rubbing the skin off the face of the nipple, or the gums gripping the neck. You'll become engorged. In addition, an infant latched onto the breast in this manner isn't transferring milk in the quantities that he needs to grow: he may be fussy, gassy, "always hungry". His wet nappies will be OK, but he'll have little to no dirty nappies. His weight gain will be poor or absent.

If you've practised the latch-on, and believe it to be correct and the pain continues, or if damage occurs, please seek a lactation supporter for assistance. In addition, be sure the consultant evaluates your infant's tongue for a condition commonly referred to as "tongue-tied" ~ the frenulum, which attaches the tongue to the floor of the mouth, may be restricting the tongue's natural movement for breastfeeding. This can be corrected quickly and easily, and with very little pain to the infant.

Nipple pain ~ burning and itching: This is most likely caused by a thrush infection.

A yeast, or thrush infection commonly occurs in any dark or clothed area of the body that remains moist with sweet biological fluids: mouths, vaginas, nipples and diaper areas. Itching when dry, and burning when wet, are the identifiable symptoms of a yeast infection. If located in or on the nipples, the pain usually lasts throughout the feeding, and is unresolved by correcting the latch. If you had previously damaged nipples as described above, and they won't heal after correcting the latch-on process, please consider a secondary thrush infection as the culprit preventing the healing process.

Causes: if you or your baby has taken antibiotics recently, you're prone to a yeast infection ~ usually a vaginal yeast infection. If you're also nursing, the sweet milk left on the breast and areola, or in your baby's mouth, is a growing bed for thrush. If you suffer from frequent yeast infections even when you're not nursing, the susceptibility continues, and you're at risk of a thrush infection of the breasts when you are nursing. If you're diabetic, deficient in essential vitamins or iron, or use asthma medications (corticosteroids), you're also at increased risk. Nursing pads that stay moist can be culprits in creating an environment that breeds yeast growth.

Editors' note: *olive leaf extract and/or Propolis will get rid of candida/thrush.*

Correction: unfortunately, there are no tests to confirm a thrush infection, and other infections of the skin should be considered also (eczema, psoriasis, etc.). The diagnosis should be based on your description of the sensations. While your baby should be examined by a knowledgeable practitioner, it's entirely possible that he'll be "free of signs and symptoms" of thrush. Regardless, if thrush is the final conclusion, both of you need to be treated at the same time.

There are myriad treatment regimes! Some are medical, some are home-remedies, and some are over-the-counter concoctions. If you have Internet access, type "breastfeeding thrush" into any search engine, and enjoy the response. The amount of curative information is so broad and readily available that no mother should suffer one day longer than necessary with this annoying infection. If you're happily computer-free, most reputable books on breastfeeding will cover a few of the treatment options, and La Leche League is just a phone call away!

If left untreated: good luck. Thrush shall not be ignored! Nipple tenderness and pain will increase until the nipples are barely touchable. As the yeast moves up the ducts through the nipple, you'll begin to feel sharp, shooting pains in the breast from the nipple to the chest wall. Damaged nipples ~ cracks, blisters, open sores ~ will not heal.

Your baby will become fussy with the same itchy, burning pain in his mouth. He'll want to nurse for comfort, then pop off because it causes that little burning sensation, then cry because he wants to nurse. He'll get a diaper rash as the yeast moves from his mouth through his gastrointestinal system and out his bottom.

Engorgement: the misunderstanding is that these are BREASTS, not bowling balls. Engorgement is the condition of overly full milk ducts in combination with swollen, hard breast tissue. It's not, as some mothers like to announce, that "your milk is in!" Well, it is "in". But, the true problem is "It's not getting OUT!"

Causes: engorgement is a painful and unnecessary condition that makes nursing mothers cry in pain and frustration. Common causes are situations that create separation for you and your baby; delayed breastfeeding due to attempting to schedule infant feedings; incorrect latch-on for excellent milk removal, being instructed not to express any milk; breast infection; and unlatching a nursing baby because you think they must only nurse for certain lengths of time.

Correction: PREVENTION!

But, if it does happen, treat the swelling with cold. Treat the immobility of milk and blood flow with heat. REMOVE THE MILK. Discover and correct the cause.

If separation of you and your nursling must occur, hand-express or request/bring a dependable breast pump. Express milk from each breast every two to three hours even if you "don't feel full". "Not feeling full" is the hallmark of successful breastfeeding! Your body makes milk regularly in anticipation of frequent removals ~ so, remove it. Don't attempt to put your nursling on a schedule. This frustrates your baby and causes a backlog of milk in your breasts. Sit back, relax and let your body and your baby make and remove milk in tandem. Offer the fullest side first for effective milk removal.

If both sides are equal, then it really doesn't matter which side is nursed first; just don't delay a "full" side because it's "the other side's turn" to go first.

Likewise, artificially deciding how long your baby should nurse on one breast, and then switching him to the other for an equal amount of time, is confusing to the baby, and chaos to your milk production. Foremilk and hindmilk are produced in the mammary gland at different rates and amounts throughout the day. At a single nursing, the foremilk is available first, then the hindmilk is made and served. If you pop your babe off one breast to switch him to the other just because the clock says "ding", you may be depriving him of the fresh, rich hindmilk the first side was ready to serve. This could leave an unknown amount of milk in the breasts after each feeding, causing an engorgement to build over time. (These mothers often complain of recurrent plugged ducts, as well.)

Latch your baby comfortably to one breast. Let him nurse unfettered. When he's done, he'll let go. Offer the other side. If he's not interested, and you're uncomfortably full, express. Free milk! You'll make plenty more. I promise.

If you've had nipple pain or damage that hasn't been evaluated and corrected, it is likely that your infant latched incorrectly and has now caused an engorgement situation. If he's using his gums to grip the nipple, his tongue can't be placed under the nipple and areola to stroke the flowing milk out of the breast in efficient quantity. So, while he's capable of stimulating a grand milk production by nuzzling at the areola and creating a let-down, he's incapable of removing the majority of the milk mechanically with the proper action of his mouth ~ and engorgement occurs.

If you're one of those lucky mothers who produces enough milk for her own babe, and still has enough to feed two or three more, you too are at risk of engorgement. Don't listen to the nay-sayers! Express that extra milk. Pumping your breasts to remove excess milk doesn't increase your production. If you express each side until the streaming from let-down stops, you're likely to produce exactly the same amount as you just removed. However, if you express only enough milk to relieve the uncomfortable fullness and leave the rest in the breast, you've assisted your body in decreasing the overall production rate (because you left some milk in the ducts) without damaging your ducts and mammary gland by engorgement.

An infection of any type will usually have engorgement as a by-product illness simply because the milk removal may be delayed or ineffectual due to pain. The important thing to remember is that the engorgement is not part of the infectious disease; it's a secondary, opportunistic condition that can be easily resolved. Use whatever you can find (frozen bags of peas, heated rice socks, cabbage leaves, etc.) to relieve some of the pain so that you can either nurse the baby or so that you can express your breasts.

Seek assistance for the infection, and continue to provide for regular milk removals while the infection resolves.

If left untreated: engorgement will resolve itself ~ but, not in the manner in which the breastfeeding-public-at-large believes. "They" instruct to "just leave it alone; you'll be fine in a few days". Or, if they believe engorgement to be a sign of "finally, your milk has come in!", they'll say things like, "Oh good! I'm glad you had those free samples of formula to feed the baby while you didn't have any milk!" If you're actively weaning, they'll say things like, "Yep. That's what it's supposed to do. If you don't like it, don't breastfeed next time."

That's not how it works. First, you have the perfect amount of milk the day you give birth, and it grows proportionately with your baby. Second, engorgement is not a sign of anything good. In fact, it's a hugely indicative sign that a number of things are wrong. And, third, forcing oneself into engorgement in an effort to wean is ridiculously painful and cruel, and totally unnecessary.

If left untreated, engorgement will cause the destruction of milk-producing cells from the inside-out ~ cells that will not be regenerated for the duration of this baby's nursing span and perhaps beyond. A supreme loss of cells during the engorgement period could affect the amount of milk a mother is capable of producing after the engorgement has resolved. In the short term, the milk supply will most definitely be affected, simply due to the sitting milk triggering the mammary gland to produce less because no one is removing what it has already made.

The swelling in the tissues of your breast surrounding the mammary gland (similar to the swelling surrounding a sprained ankle) creates an external pressure on blood vessels supplying the mammary gland with fluids, nutrients, antibodies and oxygen, and delays or prevents their flow capabilities. Without this exquisite exchange from the outside, and in addition to the incredible pooling of milk on the inside, the entire system is set to grow the most fabulous bacterial infection a nursing mother can imagine! Not to mention, plugged ducts, abscesses, and all the symptoms of having the flu: fever, pain, chills, lethargy.

So, yes. The engorgement will resolve on its own (sic), but in this case, the resolution can be worse than the illness.

End of Primer

Unlike birth, which demands your attention, knowledgeable support, and physical effort to accomplish, breastfeeding is not a rite of passage. Nursing peacefully in your arms is your baby's gift: their hostess gift, if you will, to you. Embrace and accept this gift as you would any other, pain-free, with grace and gratitude.

My breastfeeding career:
feeding a baby with Down's Syndrome
by Jemima Hoadley

My baby boy was born at home in Penzance, Cornwall, 24th January, 2003, after a long but peaceful labour and a wonderful healthy pregnancy. He was born two weeks before his 'due' date, so about four weeks before we were expecting him to arrive. I hadn't done any research into breastfeeding as I presumed that apart from getting sore, cracked nipples it was going to be a natural process.

The joyful moment my beautiful boy was born into the world was truly awe inspiring, the most profound relief and elation at meeting in the flesh this gentle being I had connected with so deeply throughout the months he danced around in my womb. I had immediate skin-to-skin contact with him, and the midwives left me to bond and establish breastfeeding with my little baby, after cajoling me into pushing out the placenta 10 minutes after he was born. I felt our bonding time was not respected completely as it seemed like no time at all before the midwives returned to clean up and weigh my fresh new babe, who I'd waited so long to meet. I'd asked if they could wait until the next day before weighing my baby, as I wasn't interested in statistics and wanted unbroken skin-to-skin with him. They had initially agreed. It was an anxious moment for me, when they took him from me and I quickly asked Gilly, my partner, to keep physical contact with him as I seemed too heavy to move from the mattress I'd given birth on.

Our little babe didn't show an immediate interest in the breast, but Janet Balaskas (Active Birth Pioneer) had warned us of this on an Active Birth workshop we did with her. I just thought that he would in his own time, but I feared that if I'd left him to find his own time, he may have been taken from me.

As we settled into our freshly made family bed upstairs, the midwives and Leif, our birth partner, joined us for cooing and pats on the back. One of the midwives tried to take my nipple to baby's mouth (without asking me first), and when he showed no interest she said it didn't matter in the first 24 hours. So, after they all left, we didn't think too much of it until the next day, when our baby still hadn't fed.

I started to worry, as he was sleeping so much: much more than I had expected. I thought he must be getting dehydrated and was getting low blood sugar, which made him sleep so much, so I gave him a drop of fruit sugar in boiled water to drink from a syringe. Although it really saddens me to think that the first thing that entered my baby's body was not his own Mummy's milk, but sugar and water, it did seem to wake him up a little, so I could attempt to feed him myself. After many, mostly unsuccessful, times over the next day of trying to help him onto the breast, I started to get very panicky. He was ALWAYS sleeping.

Another midwife brought us a breast pump, which meant I could express milk and feed it to him, again through a syringe or with a cup. I found this desperately upsetting and clinical, so Gilly took over, while I struggled on with trying to get breastfeeding established. I consulted a breastfeeding book, which thankfully happened to be lying around our house (left by the homebirth midwife landlady), and I also called the NCT helpline for some guidance and encouragement.

My partner Gilly was so completely supportive during these emotionally agonising first days and weeks, always commenting when we were getting it, and bringing me a supply of food and drinks. He complimented us on how good we were looking, even though my shoulders were attached to my ears with tension!

I received quite a lot of conflicting advice from different sources on how often to feed; and so we woke up every two hours, often more, to attempt a feed. Baby and I were really struggling with latching on, and so a feed would often take up to two hours to complete. I felt like such a failure and was terrified and appalled at the suggestions by professionals that I may need to top up with formula. "No WAY!" I said.

Eventually, four days after our beautiful, perfect and very sleepy baby boy had arrived into the air-breathing world, our midwife asked us to go in to hospital to check out a couple of her concerns about a dimple in the base of his spine, his small mouth, and feeding problems. What the hell was anyone going to do about a small mouth, I thought?! And anyway, I hadn't noticed him having a small mouth. No mention had been made of these things so far, and a terrible dark feeling loomed over me. We didn't want to interrupt our Babymoon, but with a chill down my spine, I agreed to take our tiny baby out of the house for the first time, to the bright lights of the frightening hospital.

The paediatrician told us that although he wasn't concerned

about his lumbar dimple, he believed that our baby had Down's syndrome, and did a blood test, which even though he performed very sensitively, tore my heart apart. I felt a wave of shock engulf me, and I heard myself saying "Really, it's obviously meant to be then", but the bottom dropped out of my world, and I clutched my baby and Gilly to me, suddenly feeling so uncertain about our future. The midwife cried with me when I confirmed her suspicions. She helped us choose a name, as she knew its meaning. Nathan ~ meaning Gift. It felt right to honour with special attention his presence in this world and our lives, in his naming.

The next two weeks were exhausting, as I continued the challenge of breastfeeding my little babe, who lacked the coordination to suck, swallow and breathe at the same time (a common problem for babies with DS, I found out). The Down's Syndrome Association was supportive, and a feeding advisor gave me some excellent tips on stimulating Nathan in his waking time, so that he became more alert and ready to feed. After the third week, Nathan was feeding much better, although his weight had dropped so much (from 6lb3 to 5lb10) that I had to feed him very often, and Gilly continued to top him up with breast milk from a syringe.

My terror of Nathan being taken into hospital to be monitored or tube fed drove me on through this tense time. He was born at home for a reason, and formula feeding never crossed my mind as an option. With the knowledge that my baby had DS, I felt that we needed, more than ever, to have a bonding and fulfilling breastfeeding career.

Looking back to that difficult time often brings up anger, frustration and sadness that I wasn't given the expert guidance I needed at the time, and that proper action was not taken by the professionals involved.

After Nathan and I had established breastfeeding well, my dad, who lives in Australia, came across a booklet on breastfeeding babies with DS which was very informative and gave excellent advice on waking up sleepy babies, positions to try, stimulation tips, and, most importantly, encouragement that what I was experiencing was not uncommon and could be overcome in a short time. Why wasn't this kind of information handed to me the day I found out about Nathan's condition? Why, when I reached out for help from my 'professional support' team, was I not guided to a relevant source of information? I gave the little booklet to my local Breast-is-Best (or just 'normal' as

Michael Odent puts it) group so that they could photocopy it and pass it on immediately to anyone needing guidance. After all, two babies are born with Down's syndrome every day in the UK.

Today, fifteen months after Nathan came into my arms and our lives, we're joyfully breastfeeding through the day and also at night (not always SO joyfully!). And, needless to say, after the initial trauma of discovering that my baby has a condition I was not prepared for, he's our constant joy and love. I felt so proud of myself and Nathan on his first birthday for being so good at breastfeeding together. WE ARE EXPERTS! It was so healing for me to hold him to my breast to nurse on the hour he had been born a year before, for a long loving feed. Incidentally, people with DS are meant to have more vulnerable immune systems and be prone to infections and illness. Nathan is totally unvaccinated and enjoys excellent health, never having had any infections, etc. I've found that his immune system is actually more robust than many other babies (particularly those who've been vaccinated, and often filled with antibiotics). Nathan has a very good friend, Mary B, a cranial osteopath, who has treated him for free since he was just two weeks old, and my homeopath aunt regularly suggests remedies for any of his ailments.

I would be really interested to know of any other readers who attachment parent a baby or child with Down's syndrome.

Is Baby Bottle Tooth Decay relevant to breastfeeding?
by Veronika Sophia Robinson

When my youngest daughter, Eliza, had her first pearly whites coming through, I was as excited as most other parents are at this milestone. The excitement, however, soon turned to upset and despair as her precious, beautiful teeth turned brown, then black. Over the space of the next five years they crumbled and eroded right down to the gum line. The roots came out when her second teeth emerged.

I received the standard dental advice: "They need to be extracted, and you really must stop breastfeeding." I've heard this advice countless times, through other dentists perpetuating the same misinformation to parents who've had a similar experience with their own children.

The positive side of going through such an experience is that it really does make you stop and pull your socks up. It makes you question everything about your lifestyle, especially diet, nutrition, and yes, the relevance of breastfeeding.

One of the downsides to editing The Mother magazine is hearing how many parents have been persuaded by 'well-meaning' dentists to have their child's teeth extracted, and to stop breastfeeding.

My own journey to discovering the truth ~ that breastfeeding does NOT cause tooth decay ~ started by listening to my intuition. I knew that dental work has a deleterious effect on the cranial rhythm, and given that the child is constantly growing, I was very wary of any work that would impact on that. Such a belief became even more heightened when discovering that the dentists in question didn't even know about the cranial rhythm.

As a mother, I always look to my intuition, and to Mother Nature, long before looking at medical and scientific studies. It seemed wrong to me that Nature would provide mammals with the perfect infant food, but would also damage the milk teeth. Where's the common sense in that? I wondered how humanity's teeth had survived all these generations if breast milk really was that damaging. It all started to seem rather stupid. And so, my investigation began. Firstly, I found that there's not a single published study to show any evidence that full-term, on-cue breastfeeding causes Baby Bottle Tooth Decay (BBTD). This disease is native to the realm of artificial infant feeding. What has been found is that there is a reduced risk of decay in the teeth of breastfed children. Family dentist Dr. Brian Palmer does not see a connection between cavities and breastfeeding, and says that studies which have suggested a link were population-based studies, not studies where breast milk was used as the control. He calls this 'guilt by association', rather than a true study.

Dr. Pamela Erickson published an article which showed that breast milk is not cariogenic, unlike some infant formulas, which dissolve tooth enamel (causing decay).

Baby teeth are formed long before they pop through the gums. There are various reasons for imperfect enamel on a child's first teeth, but one thing is clear: the health of our children's milk teeth begins at conception, not when we first see teeth rise above the gums.

Pregnancy
Studies show us that if a pregnant woman experiences grief, trauma, major nutritional deficiencies (such as insufficient calcium), illness or antibiotic use, these can contribute to tooth decay by damaging enamel in-utero.

Dealing with grief in pregnancy
The events of our life aren't predictable. We don't know when we'll be facing situations of grief. Regardless of what comes our way, there are practices to help ourselves and our gestating baby.

[] accepting rather than suppressing the emotions/talk to baby about what you're experiencing
[] Bach flower remedies, such as Rescue Remedy
[] deep breathing
[] massage
[] meditation/yoga
[] rest and relaxation
[] drinking plenty of water

Night-time nursing
Breastfeeding is the best health care a mother can ever give her child. She should be wary of any health practitioner ~ doctor, dentist, health visitor (even alternative ones, such as homeopaths), if they encourage her to wean the child from night-time or full-term feeding. If a mother isn't breastfeeding, she'll be using formula: research shows it can be very cariogenic.

Our prehistoric breastfed babies

Research into prehistoric human skulls provides evidence that breastfeeding does not cause tooth decay. Children from 1,000 years ago were breastfed full-term. Evidence has shown that mammals have been around for up to four millions years. The modern version of a human mammal ~ Homo Sapiens ~ has been on Earth for up to 35,000 years. Anthropologists have found that dental decay didn't become an issue till about 10,000 years ago: at the very time humans started cultivating their own crops, rather than eating 'wild foods'.

Our prehistoric babies were almost certainly breastfed throughout the night, and well into toddlerhood and older. If breastfeeding were a factor in tooth decay, this would be evident in the skulls which predate agriculture.

The physiology of breastfeeding

When a child breastfeeds, the milk doesn't pool around the teeth as milk or juice from a bottle does. The breast milk enters the baby's mouth from behind the front teeth, and is then swallowed. The mechanics of breastfeeding makes it unlikely for human milk to stay in the baby's mouth for long.

During the act of breastfeeding, the mother's nipple is drawn deep inside the baby's mouth, and milk is taken directly into the back of the mouth. Before the child can take in more milk, s/he must swallow. When a baby drinks from a bottle, the milk still drips in even when there's no active sucking. This is where 'pooling' of milk occurs. Unlike the human nipple, the teat on a bottle is short, so the liquid almost certainly has to pass over the teeth before the child can swallow.

A child who is breastfed on cue is unlikely to experience a dry mouth, a common factor in Early Childhood Caries (ECC). A breastfeeding child (even one who nurses at night) produces enough saliva to maintain normal pH in the mouth.

Breast milk as a tooth protector

Breast milk contains a substance called lactoferrin, which kills the bacteria (Strep Mutans) that cause tooth decay. It was found in a study by Dr. Torney that early dental caries were not caused by feeding a child to sleep, frequently feeding at night, or longer-term breastfeeding. He did find that if there were defects in the enamel, the protective effects of breast milk were not necessarily enough to protect the teeth from this bacteria. He has based his work on an extensive study of long-term breastfed children with or without caries. His advice is that if there is soft, or no, enamel on the teeth, weaning a child off breast milk may speed up the decay, due to the lack of lactoferrin.

Dr. Erickson's 1999 study found that teeth become stronger when covered in breast milk, and that it was virtually identical to water in terms of how teeth reacted to the liquid.

Causes of tooth decay
[] although sugar is not recommended for humans, it's actually the frequency of contact with the teeth by sugars and carbohydrates which is a key factor in the development of decay.
[] lack of saliva flowing in the mouth (caused by dehydration ~ very common in babies who are fed to schedule).
[] foetal stress.
[] poor dietary and oral hygiene habits.
[] genetics (minor factor).

Breastfeeding studies show how important the act of breastfeeding is for oral and dental development, such as reduced risk of: malocclusion; snoring; obstructive sleep apnoea; and poor facial development. Breastfeeding is always going to be humanity's best form of health insurance.

Preventing Caries While Pregnant
[] Eat well, and include adequate calcium in your diet (raw green leafy vegetables, parsley, watercress, tofu, tahini, broccoli, Brazil nuts, almonds, figs, sesame seeds, swedes).
[] Reduce stress levels, through meditation, deep breathing, etc.
[] Avoid antibiotics. If you feel that you MUST have them, make sure you take a good probiotic, such as Nature's Living Superfood.

Preventing Caries in Infants
[] Delay solids until nearer to nine months, rather than the standard advice of 4 to 6 months.
[] Avoid your baby using artificial nipples ~ e.g. bottles, dummies. If they 'must' use them, ensure no-one else (adult or child) sucks on them, as they can pass on bacteria.
[] Ensure the family diet is rich in wholefoods; raw, fresh leafy greens; and only natural sugars.

[] Breastfeed on cue, rather than demand, to ensure your child doesn't get a dry mouth.

So, the four main triggers of BBTD are:
[] Enamel defects in-utero
[] An infant diet high in carbohydrates
[] Poor oral hygiene of the mother and child
[] Pooling of milk in the baby's mouth from a dripping bottle

Early Childhood Caries
The following factors have been found as significant factors in ECC:
[] Complications in pregnancy
[] A traumatic birth
[] Caesarean section
[] Gestational diabetes
[] Disease of the kidney
[] Maternal viral or bacterial infection (e.g. herpes)

High risk factors for babies:
[] Prematurity
[] Allergies
[] Malnutrition
[] Rh incompatibility
[] Infectious diseases
[] Gastroenteritis
[] Severe diarrhoea

The following factors are also implicated:
[] Sucking on a dummy
[] Iron deficiency (weaning off the breast, partially or fully, before seven months)

Remineralisation and natural healing remedies for tooth decay
Soft teeth can be treated through natural means, such as increasing exposure to sunlight (vitamin D). Our Sun-fearing culture encourages us to hide from the Sun, or lather ourselves with sunblock. We need exposure to this vital nutrient every day, for good health. Even in grim climates like Britain's, we can still obtain vitamin D from the Sun, provided we get outside even on the cloudiest days, and in

Winter. One of the reasons that saliva is so important in the mouth is because it allows teeth to remineralise from the calcium in it. Most people are severely dehydrated and have dry mouths.

It's a rare dentist who doesn't religiously advocate fluoride; however, this toxic ingredient inhibits the body's ability to absorb calcium.

To remineralise teeth:
[] The homeopathic remedy of Calcarea phos. is recommended on a daily basis
[] Avoid sugary foods and drinks (fresh home made juices are fine)
The good news is that the health of the first teeth does not affect second teeth, and those pearly whites which come through second time around are just as precious!

Resources
*Liquid vitamin D
*Orthobone
*Nature's Living Superfood

References
Population-based studies do not support a definitive link between prolonged breastfeeding and caries (Slavkin 1999).
Prolonged demand breastfeeding does not lead to higher caries prevalence (Weerheijm 1998).
Breastfeeding may act preventively and inhibit the development of nursing caries in children (Oulis 1999).

*There are various reasons for
imperfect enamel on a child's first teeth,
but one thing is clear:
the health of our children's milk teeth
begins at conception,
not when we first see teeth
rise above the gums.*

Health, well-being, natural immunity

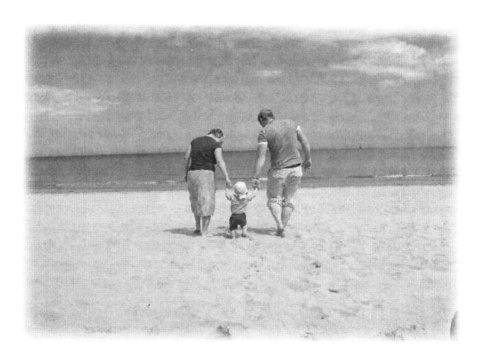

Anna, Leon and Joss enjoy a walk on the beach.

Matridonal Remedies
by Harriet Wood

Harriet is a qualified, registered homeopath. She specialises in working with women before, during and after pregnancy, and working with families to create and maintain better health. Harriet practises from The Brunswick Clinic, Penrith, Cumbria, and can be contacted on 01768 890800

Matridonal means gifts of the mother, and these are a collection of remedies made from the gifts of breast milk (Lac Humanum), oestrogen (Folliculinum), placenta, the cheesy varnish that babies are born with (Vernix), amniotic fluid, and umbilical cord. Surprisingly, these remedies are relatively recent in being developed, despite their obvious importance in our lives. The key theme in all of these remedies is 'finding ourselves'. It's these things that bring us into being when we're being created, but it can be so easy to lose ourselves on the rest of our journey. These remedies help bring us back to that which is truly our self. I've actually only used these remedies on adults, but as with any remedy, they can be for anyone. In Melissa Assilem's (one of the homeopaths instrumental in the making of these remedies) book, Matridonal Remedies of the Humanum Family, she writes a beautiful description of the journey from when we're conceived, to when we're born; and I would recommend finding and reading this part of the book. It's aimed at homeopaths, but the beginning would sing to all. This journey, of coming into being ~ and what happens when that is interrupted or lost ~ can be seen throughout the remedies.

Lac Humanum
This is probably the best known of the matridonal remedies. By looking at the symptoms that it helps with, you can see the potential effects of not breastfeeding. Although someone who has been breastfed might need this remedy at some point in their lives, it's often seen in those who missed out on that crucial experience. Lac Humanum grounds ~ bringing us into our bodies. The need for this can be seen in disconnectedness, detachment, and indifference. How many children (and adults) do you see like this?

Breast milk is the substance that teaches us about desire. In health, when a desire is met, we're satisfied. However, desire can become about experiencing lack, not enough, when nothing can satiate that desire, and this can lead to addictions. Lac Humanum is a great remedy for this, for all sorts of addictions. The scope and depth of Lac Humanum is vast, and this is just the tip of the iceberg. Its key is nurturing and grounding.

Folliculinum

This remedy is made from human oestrogen. We're surrounded by a huge surge of this at birth. Esoterically, this is about forgetting where we came from, which is necessary to make it easier to be on the Earth plane. And homeopathically, it starts the journey back to remembering, and to our true selves. This remedy allows you to see that there is a self and identity to reclaim. It can be seen in people who lose their sense of self in relationships, and are very much full of self-denial. It's a big remedy for depression, especially post-natally. On a physical level, it's great for the after-effects of using synthetic hormones, such as the Pill, or HRT.

Placenta

This is a lovely remedy. You can have your baby's placenta made into a remedy that is uniquely yours. This will hold the same themes as the remedy here, and is a wonderful gift to give. The placenta is made from cells from both mum and baby, and provides nutrition for the growing foetus. It also absorbs and takes away any waste products. You can see this in the remedy, as it can really clear out things that aren't needed, both physical and emotional: from synthetic hormones to no longer needed emotional issues. It can help with mother-daughter relationships, and gives new energy to discover who we really are.

Vernix

You can see the potential problems created when this important substance is washed or rubbed off a new baby. Vernix contains Vitamin K, which will be absorbed by the skin if left on, which leads to the question: why is the heel prick needed?

Vernix, as Melissa Assilem describes it, is the 'shell within a shell within a shell'. It's the final layer around a baby ~ after the amniotic fluid, and the womb itself. People who need this remedy need protection, from the surrounding world, as this is what it provides. They're very sensitive to environmental pollution and chronic disease. I've used this with a woman who was sensitive to everything, and it brought peace. These people can be disconnected from their feelings; because they are so sensitive it's too painful to feel them. The remedy enables us to be open, but protected, like a mirror, not a sponge. Physically, as you might expect, it's an excellent skin remedy, for eczema, dermatitis etc., where the other issues can be seen too.

Amniotic Fluid

I've not used these last two remedies, so I only know of them intellectually, rather than from experience. This remedy is deeper, and very spiritual. It has a connection to the ancestors and past life experiences. People who need it can have heightened senses, and issues around water. It's about how we live our lives, and makes it safe to explore our issues and our selves. It helps us to really find our identity, and brings calm and tranquillity. It's also a remedy for grief; and can be used if a twin dies in-utero.

Umbilical Cord

This is the final remedy in the matridonal remedy journey. It's the deepest of them, going into the heart of who we are. People who need this have deep identity issues, really not knowing who they are, even to the extent of not recognising themselves in a mirror. It's also about feeling excluded, not part of the group, or of humanity. This remedy will help to feel part of a group, but retain your own identity. There are also a lot of dreams of children in the remedy picture, children who need protecting, or who have been abandoned. It's the deepest, most connecting remedy in the group.

So that's a little about each of the remedies. There's so much more that could be said about each one, and I would really recommend Melissa Assilem's book for those who want to find out more. These remedies deal with very deep issues, and so are best used under the guidance of a practitioner who can help support you through the journey. For some people, all of the remedies are needed, and can be given in sequence over months or even years. They are great tools in helping with fertility, as so many of the issues that are in them can be found in women (and men) having problems conceiving. They're a wonderfully powerful group of remedies, and really do show the importance of our time in gestation.

Chiropractic
by Dr. Christophe Vever

Chiropractors can remove interference from your nervous system, so that information can flow freely and fully to all parts of your body, allowing full health.

Your brain co-ordinates and regulates every single cell in every part of your body and mind. It does this by sending and receiving messages via the nerves.

Everyday life stresses and tension interfere with this nerve flow ~ a condition called subluxation (a bit like plaque build-up on your teeth). This lessens the connection between all the parts of the body, resulting in decreased function and decreased health. Subluxations lessen our performance.

Chiropractors perform adjustments to release the interference caused by subluxations. This restores the nerve connection to all parts of your body and mind, so that every single cell, in every part of your body, can perform at its best.

The body has an in-built programme for health and balance, called the innate intelligence. Problems only arise when the communication and delivery of this intelligence are compromised. Subluxation represents one of the major interferences to the normal expression of our innate intelligence.

[] Health and healing come from within us, not from some treatment given to us from the outside. So we just need to be free of interference, in order for our innate intelligence to manifest its plan.

[] Adjustments don't fix or heal anything. They just reconnect us so that we can heal from within.

[] The spine is the most common area of the body to be subluxated, so this is where chiropractors tend to concentrate most of their efforts.

[] Interferences in nerve function (subluxations) don't always cause pain. Chiropractic care is recommended for those who feel fine, as well as those who don't. For this reason, people bring their children for regular care. This keeps their spines free of interference as they grow and develop, allowing them to reach their full potential.

[] Chiropractic is not a treatment for bad backs or headaches. It's a healthy lifestyle activity which promotes optimal health. Hence why so many people with bad backs notice an improvement with chiropractic. Feeling better is just a pleasant side effect of being fully connected.

What exactly is innate intelligence?

This is not an easy thing to explain. Modern humans love concrete things, and tend to only accept that which they can see, hear or feel. Innate intelligence is a concept which explains the perfection of living systems. We can't see, hear or feel it, yet we know that it's there because we can see what it does.

The easiest way to explain it is with examples. Each cell in your body will have millions of chemical reactions going on inside at any one time, yet none of them is random. Modern mechanistic science would have us believe that the chemicals just whiz around in our cells, and randomly come into contact with one another, thus creating the activities of the living cell. But on closer inspection, we see that, in fact, nothing is random. The activities of all of these chemicals are beautifully coordinated and orchestrated in a purposeful way, even if we can't see the control mechanisms through a microscope.

It's this innate intelligence that gives us living things our defining characteristic-adaptation. A living being can adapt to the circumstances around it, whereas a non-living thing cannot. For example, if we step out of a warm house into the cold Winter air, the body temperature remains constant. We don't just randomly become cold, nor do we randomly create warmth. Rather, we increase our metabolism in a specific way to suit those particular temperature conditions. This isn't something which we need to do consciously; it's all taken care of at a subconscious level. Likewise, when cells choose to take up passing nutrients from the nearby bloodstream, they don't do so randomly ~ there's a specific innate plan which decides which ones are needed, and which ones are not.

It would be tempting to say that this is just a function of the nervous system, but then how do we explain the continued co-ordination of metabolic processes in paraplegics, whose nerves are severed? The innate intelligence therefore exists at a deeper level than just our organs and systems. It exists inside every cell, and uses the nervous system (and other systems) to communicate the plan with all the other parts of the body.

How is it that a sperm and an ovum can unite, and create a perfect little human being within nine months? How is it that we can go to work, and yet our digestive system takes care of breakfast without us having to spare a thought? When was the last time that you had to give specific instructions to your worn-out cells to replace themselves while you got some sleep? These are all examples of what it is that our innate intelligence does for us. "It needs no help – just no interference". (B.J. Palmer)

What about our genes? It's been tempting in the last 50 years to assume that our genes, in fact, represent our innate intelligence, but they don't. Remember, as soon as you die, your body ceases to adapt to and interact with the world around, yet your genes are all still there and intact. You see, the genes are not intelligent. They're just inanimate tools which the innate intelligence uses to get things done. Genes don't switch themselves on randomly, they get activated by the innate intelligence. That includes genes which create diseases. So when our body creates a disease, it's not the fault of the gene. It's the innate that chose to create that disease in response to an environmental stressor.

Innate can't be very intelligent then if it creates disease, you might be thinking. This is where understanding genes gets complicated. In order to explain how the creation of a disease can be considered an intelligent response, we would need a lot more space than is available here. In simple terms though, think of it this way: if we're subjected to a stressor which has the potential to kill us, such as metabolic acidity, it's far more intelligent for the innate to channel that acidic stress into a chronic disease like cancer, which will take 20 years to kill us, rather than to let us die immediately of acute acidosis.

The best doctor in the world is already inside you. It's called your innate intelligence, and it's this magnificent life-force that chiropractors aim to unleash, in order to allow people to express their full life potential as healthy, happy, purposeful beings.

My journey into Lemonhood:
escaping 'product' on half a lemon
by Anton Saxton

I never thought I would fall in love with a lemon. I am, of course, making reference to the yellow citrus fruit.

My journey into Lemonhood was the next logical step in my quest to wean myself off commercial body products, having already given up using moisturisers. A homeopath friend of mine explained that using moisturisers is, from the skin's point of view, akin to using hard drugs. As fast as you moisturise, your skin is trying to do the opposite, in order to achieve perfect balance. Soon after giving up moisturisers, the inevitable happened: I stopped needing to use moisturisers!

It was now time to take a serious look at shampoo. To others, the Lemon may appear to be nothing more than a little, yellow, rugby ball shape that's hardly worth getting out of bed for ~ yet, get out of bed for it, I do. Most mornings, I venture into the shower, cradling my half lemon (which lasts about three or four washes) as I ceremoniously anoint my head with a squeeze of lemon drizzle. My humble lemon now takes pride of place where once the bottle of shampoo used to sit drooling and slobbering gunk all over itself.

A short time into my Lemon honeymoon, I've already noticed a shift in my well-being. I can allow myself a couple of drops of smug satisfaction that I'm saving: money (compared to the price of organic shampoo); water (LJ washes out of hair more quickly than shampoo); conditioner (though distilled vinegar is a good conditioner); and the environment (no manufacturing of product or packaging). All I need to do to complete my eco credentials/smugness, is to learn how to grow my own lemons, or switch to using locally-produced cider vinegar. I think I'll stick with lemons for now.

But the greatest joy is from not having to make decisions on which darn shampoo to buy. The plethora of choices of whether it's organic, locally produced, paraben-free, SLS-free, parfum-free…the list goes on! This is even before choosing which flavour and which hair type. This cultural pre-occupation for making a different product for each hair type is a marketeer's dream, and a consumer's nightmare.

In my mind, the road to happiness starts by simplifying everything to its essence, and just enjoying simple pleasures. I now have only two choices to make: use lemon juice or don't use lemon juice. Now that I have so much more free time available, I've come up with some alternative marketing hype for Nature's own product:

Wash your hair in new improved LEMON JUICE ™. Suitable for ALL hair types (even combination problem types). Comes in ONE zingy fresh flavour (yep, Lemon flavour). Packaging for LEMON JUICE ™ is TOTALLY BIO-DEGRADABLE, and is even EDIBLE (when grated up and used in cooking). Please note, terms and conditions apply. Lemons can be fatal if used incorrectly. Always read the small print.

I've even started using Lemon Juice on my children's hair. My five year old, Hugo, used to hate having shampoo on his head, for fear of getting it in his eyes. Now I squeeze a lemon on his head, and the only thing he complains about are the pips which he finds in his hair a day or so later!

When I share my enthusiastic discovery with others, I either get a blank stare (it's ok, I'm used to this: being a tee-total vegan brings about this kind of response), or I get asked if I'm trying to get my hair to go blonde. "Ha," I say. "I couldn't give two oranges about what colour my hair is. Just so long as I don't ever have to buy another bottle of shampoo."

So now I wake up fresh and lemon-headed, ready for the day. My hair feels clean, and I no longer get dry skin. I had thought this was due to the hard water in our area, but actually it was due to the natural shampoos stripping the oils out of my skin. Today the Lemon ~ next stop ~ making my own toothpaste!

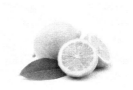

Growing Pains
by Dr. Christophe Vever

We've all heard of growing pains, either in others, or more unfortunately, from personal experience; but what exactly are they? In common parlance, growing pains seems to be a term that we throw at any little niggles that afflict children which we can't seem to explain any other way ~ the idea being that as kids grow, certain tissues are being stretched and enlarged at such a rate that they become uncomfortable, or that some bits grow too fast relative to other bits, and that things get out of balance, putting more pressure in certain areas, thus causing pain. On a simplistic level this seems plausible, until we ask one fundamental question: should it really hurt to grow up?

This was the question put to us many years ago by one our university lecturers, and it has always stayed with me. It's easy for us to equate growth with pain, not only because so many of us will have experienced growing pains at some time or another, but also because it's common nowadays when we have an unpleasant experience, to realise that we can learn from it and create a silver lining. We, therefore, find it easy to link emotional pain with emotional growth. But does this need to be the case physically?

Before we deal with this question further, let's clear up one issue which might potentially confuse things.

We've all heard athletes cry "no pain-no gain", meaning that when they train they're pushing themselves to the point of pain, and from this is stimulated muscle growth. Certainly this seems true, given our current understanding of physiology. Essentially, what we understand currently is that when a physical force is put on a tissue, it distorts the shape of the cell, which opens up channels which release electrolytes (charged particles), thus creating an electrical current known as the Piezo-electric effect. This electrical current is then thought to stimulate the cell to make new components to increase the strength and/or size of the various intra and extra cellular tissues ~ but this is adaptive growth, which the innate intelligence uses to make sure that the body is strong enough to deal with the environmental stresses to which it subjected. This isn't the same type of growth as seen in childhood. The innate genetic growth in children will happen anyway, whether there's an outside force applied or not. Outside pressures will certainly affect the extent to which growth occurs in children, but once again, that's just adaptive growth combining with innate genetic growth. So the "no pain-no gain" idea doesn't apply to children.

Getting back to the idea that we're all familiar with growing pains because we have probably all experienced them at some stage, leads nicely into what is likely to be the real reason for growing pains: toxicity and deficiency. The familiarity of growing pains is dangerous, because it fools us into thinking that this situation is normal, just the same as we accept menstrual pain as though it were normal for women, or like we accept degeneration of the spine as being a normal process of aging. "Oh well, it's just growing pains, everybody gets them. It's normal." These things are only normal in toxic, industrialised humans living in the captivity which we call modern civilisation. This means that we accept and soothe growing pains, rather than trying to understand and avoid them.

In order to get somewhere with this we have to make one fundamental admission. Sickness and disease are not normal or random. There's always a cause. The innate intelligence doesn't make mistakes, it simply adapts to whatever its environment throws at it. Therefore, if the body ever experiences a pain or a sickness, then it's been created by the innate intelligence in order to overcome an overwhelming stressor. From this, we have to then admit to ourselves that all disease is environmentally-caused by some form of toxicity (too much bad stuff), or deficiency (not enough good stuff). Once we can accept this, we can then learn to improve our bodies' environment (lifestyle), and hence regain control of our health/ disease profile. This will apply equally to children and growing pains.

The first likely problem is that of subluxation. A subluxation is an interference to the transmission of nerve signals, meaning that the connection between the brain and the body tissues is decreased. In the growing child, this means that certain tissues may grow and develop without proper guidance from the central nervous system, meaning that they may in fact grow out of proportion to surrounding tissues, thus causing a problem. The child therefore grows in a distorted way, which shows up as postural imbalances and loss of normal spinal curves and motion. Next time you're helping your child to get dressed, ask them to stand up straight, and look at the level of their shoulders and hips. If they're not level, then chances are your child is subluxated and needs an adjustment (same applies to grown-ups too, by the way). All modern humans develop subluxations, due to the physical, chemical and emotional stresses of modern industrial living.[1] This includes children. Probably the biggest single cause is prolonged sitting, which most children do ~ it's called school. The reason that most people don't know about their subluxation problems is that the subluxations themselves don't cause pain.

The pain that eventually comes is from tissues which have been degenerating instead of regenerating, due to a decreased nerve supply. Modern stress increases our levels of circulating stress hormones ~ which heighten our sensitivity to pain. So a child need only have a minor trauma ~ a slight slip or fall will do it: or how about jumping up and down on the settee, or collapsing into an armchair, or horsing around with a mate, etc.? This will be enough to create a slight tissue tear in the degenerated area, and instead of healing quickly, the stress hormones flare it up, and it becomes pain.

Compounding this is the fact that most modern humans are deficient in omega 3 essential fatty acids. This deficiency not only hyper-sensitises our nervous systems so that we feel every little pain more acutely, but it also creates a pro-inflammatory state. When our body needs to heal something that's damaged, it uses inflammation to do the healing. A group of hormones switches on this swelling, and then a slightly different set switches it off. In simple terms, omega 6 based hormones switch on the inflammation, and omega 3 based hormones switch them off again. So, as we predominately have an excess of omega 6, and a deficiency of omega 3, this creates the pro-inflammatory state. This pro-inflammatory state means that healing processes start, but then don't appropriately finish, leading to swelling, and therefore pain. Apart from the fact that modern foods are virtually devoid of omega 3 fatty acids[2], our modern diet is grain-based, and grains raise our omega 6 levels, so that instead of having a healthy ratio of omega 3 to 6 of about 1 to 1, our ratio is more like a very unbalanced 1 to 20. Way too much omega 6 means pain and inflammation. In children, this means growing pains, and then as we progress to adulthood it slowly worsens into arthritis and the like.

The simple fact is that growing pains aren't a condition on their own, but rather, modern children suffer needlessly because of a toxic lifestyle; but with a better approach to everyday life there's no reason for our kids to go on suffering with these growing pains.

Especially if we think that raising them as healthier kids will give them a better chance of being happy, healthy, well-adjusted adults. Imagine a society with healthy, natural children, rather than toxic ones.

***

(1) Think of subluxations like you would plaque on your teeth. Plaque is a build-up on your teeth caused by the unhealthy (stressful) nature of modern eating. This plaque doesn't cause pain in the short term, but if it's not dealt with it leads to decay, and eventually pain. Subluxations, then, are like a plaque build-up in the joints of the body, especially the spine.

(2) Don't be fooled by modern marketing promising that foods have been fortified by added omega 3. Omega 3 and 6 essential fatty acids are very delicate substances which are easily damaged by heat, light and oxygen. By damaged, I mean that they change shape and become no longer useful to our physiology ~ in fact, they become toxic. Some of the terms used to describe this damage include trans, hydrogenated and rancid fatty acids. So that means that omegas have to be raw, or uncooked. Heating these omegas over body temperature (37 degrees C) will rapidly damage them. So, for instance, cooking with olive oil is no good, because you damage the mono-unsaturated omega 6s in them. If you don't believe me, cook some olive oil, then let it cool, and notice how much thicker and gluggier it is. This is because the molecules have been heat-damaged and have changed shape, making them stick together, which is how they would behave if they were saturated. This is also why an egg yolk hardens when it's cooked. The fats in egg yolks are healthier when they're raw, or runny at the very least (assuming you're eating organic, free range eggs in the first place): likewise if you cook seeds. For example, in bread, you damage the omega essential fatty acids in them. So, these processed foods which promise omegas are usually a joke, because they have all invariably been exposed to heat, light or oxygen. Manufacturers can get away with this because technically they're still omegas, even if they've been damaged by the time they get to your mouth! You notice that they don't guarantee that these omegas are still in their healthy "cys" form.

Amber:
an ancient, holistic remedy for teething pain
by Mary Marks

Your baby is in pain, cheeks are flushed and new teeth are coming through. What can you do to ease the discomfort? There are many over the counter treatment gels and products containing paracetamol, but what about a gentle and side-effect-free remedy? Amber teething necklaces are a natural solution, providing a holistic choice, and are easily available on the Internet.

Amber is an organic and ancient remedy. Organic, as it's not a chemical, stone or mineral, but comes from the fossil resin of extinct conifer trees, buried in the Earth for 30-90 million years. Many of us recognise amber as jewellery, but its medicinal properties pre-date its decorative uses.

Introducing our babies to the ancient beauty of amber gives them gentle, non-invasive pain-relief, while fostering a deep connection with the Earth. Amber has been known to us since prehistoric times, and has been used continuously for the past 7,000 years to treat a variety of illnesses, both mental and physical. Hippocrates described medicinal properties and applications of amber that were used through to the middle-ages. Amber beads were also worn in the middle-ages for treatment of jaundice, while Romans used it to heal swollen glands and to ward off madness.

Mothers in the Baltic region, Germany and Austria recognised amber's benefits for teething pain, placing the beads around their babies' necks, a common practice through the beginning of the last century. Women in Lithuania today wear amber beads to help with goitre. Since amber is a natural analgaesic, it will help to calm a baby, without any known side-effects or use of drugs. It's not surprising then, that in places like Germany, teething necklaces are now sold in local pharmacies.

Amber is also currently used in Chinese and Homeopathic medicine. In the homeopathic Materia Medica, by Dr. William Boerke, amber, listed by its Latin name, 'succinum', is a treatment of nervous symptoms, asthma, headache and migraine. In the Oriental Materia Medica, by Hsu Hy, et al., amber's listed with the 'heavy and settling' sedatives, and is frequently used to treat epilepsy in children. It's also used for treatment of rheumatism, due to its warmth.

The Baltic region has been the source of most of the world's amber for 5,000 years. Baltic amber contains a substance called succinic acid, also referred to as Succinite. When rubbed against the skin, the amber beads collect an electrostatic charge, with the surface containing the highest amount of succinic acid. This is a bio-stimulant, which has a positive influence on the body. When it comes into contact with our skin, negative ionisation occurs on the skin surface, which is believed to benefit our nervous system, kidneys and heart. It's also said to neutralise negative moods, and stimulate healing processes. With such a long history of use, mothers in Britain and America are turning to amber and discovering what many Baltic mothers have long known ~ that amber eases teething pain.

The idea of a teething necklace can sound confusing at first, since we normally think teething = mouth. But the relief comes from amber's contact with the skin. It's not for chewing on.

Amber necklaces that are designed specifically for babies and children have individually knotted beads for safety (in case of breakage), a plastic screw clasp, and are generally 12-14" in length. They can be worn by babies and children of both sexes, and many sellers are offering various darker bead styles in an attempt to provide more appeal for boys. The necklaces are available in a variety of different bead shapes, including oval, round, and 'chips'. Quality varies as well, and many on-line sellers are offering certification and money-back guarantees.

We began using an amber necklace on our daughter when she was five months old. She was showing classic teething signs, and appeared calmer once the necklace was on, particularly at nap time (it's generally recommended to remove the necklace before sleeping). At ten months now, she's grown used to wearing the necklace. She's now more curious about it, and has sucked on it, and given it a few good tugs. I'm pleased to say that it appears well-made, and has survived so far without breaking.

These simple beads around my daughter's neck have a continuous history with the planet. Primeval sunlight and energy are contained in every bead, capturing the past, while illuminating the present, a true gift from Nature.

References:

Gintaro Galerija Muziejus
www.ambergallery.It/english/muziejus.htm
Andzia's Amber Jewelry and Beads, "Amber Reading Room"
www.AmberJewelry.com/amber_reading_roomp1.htm

Emporia State University "World of Amber"
www.Emporia.edu/Earthsci/amber/amber.htm
www.itmonline.org/arts/amber.htm "*Succinum (Amber) Use in Chinese Medicine*" by
Subhuti Dharmananda, Ph.D, director, Institute for Traditional Medicine, Portland,
Oregon. May 2006. — Oriental Materia Medica: A Concise Guide by Hsu Hy, et al.,
1986 Oriental Healing Arts Institute, Long Beach, Ca.
Homeopathic Materia Medica by Dr. William Boericke
www.homeoint.org/books/boericmm/s/succ.htm
www.ambermines.co.uk.
Healing Crystals and Gemstones, by Dr. Flora Peschek-Bohmer and Gisela Schreiber.
Konecky & Konecky, Old Saybrook, Ct. English translation copyright 2003.
Necklace purchasing info:
www.threesisterstoys.com US based, priced at $12.95
www.novanatural.com US based, priced at $15.90
www.teethingnecklace.com CDN $42.00. Canada based, ships to the US Claims that their
necklaces are Swiss lab certified.
www.Mamageo.com Ireland based also ships to the US
www.wondrousgems.com England based, also ships to the US. Offers a 30-day money
back guarantee. This is where we purchased our necklace.

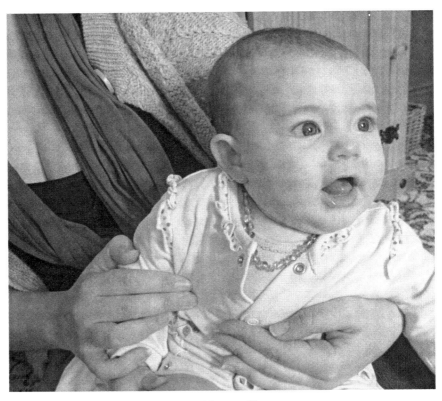

Elena Loulli wearing her amber teething necklace.

Vaccine Marketing Techniques
by Joanna Karpasea Jones

I'm often asked, "If vaccines are so bad, how come so many people choose to have them?" Let's look at the marketing techniques which have entranced whole nations to accept vaccination.

Reinventing History

This is the first technique used. Vaccination has been credited with the eradication of smallpox, which is the basis of the theory of inoculation. Many doctors will tell you that vaccination saved thousands of people from the scourge of smallpox, but they are relying on you to not actually pick up a history book. Anyone who researches this claim will realise that the opposite is true.

Vaccination was thought to be started by Edward Jenner, when he theorised that dairy maids didn't get smallpox because they worked around cattle with cowpox. He then suggested that if someone was infected with cowpox, they would be immune to smallpox. He first vaccinated his baby son in 1791 and again in 1798. The baby was never well after the first vaccination, and actually died at 21 from vaccine-induced TB. Jenner did the same with a boy named James Phipps, who also died at 21 from TB.

There was never a vaccine for smallpox, the human disease. What was used was an animal disease. The medical profession was fully aware that these two diseases bore no resemblance to each other, and it questioned how immunity could be obtained, even after years of vaccinating the general public. According to The British Medical Journal, January 17, 1880: "A little consideration will suffice to show that the vaccine disease is suigeneris. In no sense does it owe its origin to smallpox. There's no such relation between the two. The true attitude of cowpox towards smallpox is an attitude of antagonism."

The London Medical Observer (vol. VI, 1810) held an article, '535 cases of smallpox after vaccination' and 97 fatal cases of smallpox in the vaccinated.' It listed the names and addresses of those who had died.

There were many epidemics of vaccine-induced smallpox, and a particularly bad epidemic in 1838, where thousands died; and it was this event that caused the British government to BAN VACCINATION in 1840, under threat of imprisonment if the procedure was performed. It was not legalised again until 1853, and made mandatory in 1871. This caused the death rate from smallpox to skyrocket again.

According to Dr. William Farr, compiler of Statistics of the Registrar General, London: "smallpox attained its maximum mortality after vaccination was introduced. The mean annual (smallpox) mortality to 10,000 population from 1850 to 1869 was at the rate of (only) 2.04, whereas (after compulsory vaccination) in 1871 the death rate was 10.24, and in 1872 the death rate was 8.33; and this after the most laudable efforts to extend vaccination by legislative enactments."

Clearly, this shows that rather than saving us from smallpox, vaccination was causing the spread of the disease.

Supply and Demand

People never want a product unless they're convinced they need it; so firstly, the risk of diseases must be hyped-up in order to create fear, and the need for a vaccine. For instance, before the measles vaccine was invented in 1968, the disease was described as a mild illness which didn't require a doctor's treatment. After the vaccine was introduced, it became a killer disease. The same is now true of chickenpox. On the UK's NHS Direct website, they describe chickenpox as "a mild disease that most children catch at some point. It's most common in the Winter and Spring, and usually affects lots of children at the same time, around once every three years." However, on the CDC website in America, where the varicella vaccine is in use, they state: "chickenpox can be dangerous and even deadly. Before the introduction of the varicella vaccine in 1995, approximately four million cases of the disease were reported annually, including 4,000 to 9,000 hospitalisations and 100 deaths. While varicella is the greatest vaccine-preventable killer of children in the United States, only 26 percent of children ages 19 to 35 months old had received varicella vaccine by 1997." (Chickenpox: It's more serious than you think, article, CDC). You can see that once there's a vaccine, what was harmless becomes a killer, so parents demand a cure. This is the supply and demand technique.

Social Conditioning

In recent years, vaccinations have been referred to by the medical profession as immunisations. There's a specific reason for this, in that it implies that vaccines confer immunity, and, just by using this term, doctors can increase compliance rates. They also call the shots preventative medicine, to achieve this same affect. In reality, the only thing that truly immunises is breast milk, or having the disease itself, and numerous studies have shown epidemics occurring in vaccinated populations. Even minor side-effects, such as fever, occur in one in two vaccinated children, and considering most babies are in perfect health prior to having the jabs, this can hardly be called 'preventative medicine'.

Withholding Information

In the UK, doctors are not required to give full information on safety studies and side-effects in their parental information leaflets. The limited side-effects they do mention, as well as the proposed benefits, are usually not referenced. Any epidemics mentioned are suggested to result from low compliance rates, and never referenced. When I've attempted to get information on the vaccination status of subjects, I was told that, due to patient confidentiality, I wasn't permitted to have this information. This means a medical authority can make up any epidemic they want to, if they don't have to verify their claims.

Doctors don't inform parents of the manufacturer's data sheet, which comes with the vaccine, and contains fuller information on side-effects and contraindications. Health visitors don't inform parents that they, in fact, have a choice; and in my children's 'red book' health record, on the consent page for vaccination, it lists all the vaccines offered, and then, next to BCG vaccine, it states 'optional' in brackets. This implies that the other vaccines aren't optional, which is misleading. Even in countries such as the US, where jabs are mandated, there are exemption certificates.

Bullying

If parents question vaccination, they're told 'the benefits outweigh the risks' (a standard mantra), but when I asked what those risks were, no-one would elaborate. Parents who aren't reassured by this, are often told they're being selfish or irresponsible, or they're even threatened with child services. I was told my second daughter would die of whooping cough, by an irate GP who was standing behind his desk, literally yelling. I've received many tearful phone calls to the Vaccination Awareness Network UK helpline from new mothers subjected to this kind of treatment. One mum was so traumatised she sat in the surgery for half an hour, crying, before she could even walk home, and her breast milk temporarily dried up from the shock.

Other tactics include removing a non-compliant patient from the doctor's list. Doctors don't have to give a reason when striking someone off. This happened to me three times, and on one occasion I received a letter stating 'you repeatedly refuse to comply with our efforts for preventative health care'. Even the practice assigned to us by the local authority removed us after the obligatory three months. We had to take the case to a tribunal in order to have access to the National Health Service. Ours was by no means the only case. Many parents will crumble under the pressure, and submit to the vaccinations.

Word Games

Even when side-effects are admitted, words shift the blame from the vaccine. For instance, the DOH states on its website <u>www. immunisation.org.uk</u>, that 'very rarely (in less than 1 in 1,000 children), a day or two after they've received this vaccine, babies have been reported as suffering from febrile convulsions, that may be caused by a rise in body temperature'. So, rather than say the vaccine caused the fit, it's the temperature that caused the fit. But what caused the temperature? The vaccine! They're just mincing words.

It also states: 'Remember that young babies can have fits at any time ~ it may be that your child is suffering from an illness that is totally unrelated to the vaccine.'

Can babies have fits at any time? I'm sorry, but I don't think a baby having a fit is normal. Even as a first-time teenage mother, if someone had told me it was normal for babies to have fits, I'd have thought it ridiculous. This is called 'normalisation', where doctors will normalise side-effects to make it appear as if babies are like this anyway. They've clearly forgotten what health is.

The Guilt Trip

The argument about social responsibility is another commonly used technique: for instance, when medics inform us our children must be vaccinated with MMR to protect a pregnant mother from congenital rubella syndrome. As a parent, my responsibility is to <u>my</u> child, not a pregnant woman. If my child is one of the 11% of children to develop chronic arthritis after the rubella component of the vaccine, then it's only her and my family who have to deal with the consequences, not the pregnant woman whom we were trying to protect from congenital rubella syndrome. No-one should be coerced to submit to medical procedures for the benefit of someone else. If my neighbour needed a new kidney, would I be dragged off the street and forced to donate mine?

Another aspect of the guilt trip is the herd immunity argument, where apparently we all need to be vaccinated in order for it to work. That a lot of unvaccinated children will spread disease to the vaccinated is nonsensical. If vaccines truly worked, then vaccinated people would be protected, and only the unvaccinated would get the diseases.

The Big Brother Effect
If you're not the type to be swayed by the guilt trip, then the big brother technique will be used to try and force you. For instance, when people refused MMR, but opted for single vaccines, the government withdrew the licence for single vaccines on the NHS. Parents then travelled to France to obtain them, and shortly after, French hospitals were threatened with legal action if they continued to supply single vaccines. This left parents with no choice but to submit to MMR or pay hundreds of pounds at a private clinic. The DOH continues to say that single vaccines aren't licensed in the UK, but this isn't because they were withdrawn for safety reasons; the government didn't renew the licences because it wants everyone to have MMR.

Bribery
Offering free gifts to parents who vaccinate is another technique. For instance, last year, Third World mothers who accepted MMR vaccine were given a free mosquito net. In one tragic case, a mother presented her child twice so she could obtain a second mosquito net. The child died from MMR overdose later that day.

Skewing Statistics
Doctors will tell you that only one in a million children is ever damaged by vaccines, but the yellow card reporting system is voluntary, and most doctors will not report a vaccine reaction, so the damage statistics they have are only about 10% of the actual figure. An example of this is in the word games paragraph, where the DOH states: 'it may be that your child is suffering from an illness that is

totally unrelated to the vaccine'. The doctors and drug companies are protected from prosecution by a government-funded compensation programme which only pays out a maximum of £100,000; and even then, you have to prove your child is 80% disabled by the vaccine. Any lesser disabilities are excluded, and many families who try to take their cases to court have their legal-aid funding removed.

Herd Immunity: treating our children like cattle
by Joanna Karpasea Jones

When my oldest child was a baby, after telling the health visitor I didn't vaccinate, she promptly exclaimed, "Oh well, she's lucky, as she has herd immunity from the vaccinated children to protect her!" She then went on to say that not everyone had the luxury of my decision, because if less than 95% of children were vaccinated, then it wouldn't work any more. I thought this was a silly concept because if vaccination truly worked, then any child who was vaccinated would be protected from disease, no matter how many 'infectious' unvaccinated kids there were; and if the 95% herd immunity figure was a genuine argument, it only points to one thing: the medical profession doesn't really believe in the effectiveness of its own vaccines.

What Is The Herd Immunity Theory?
The herd immunity theory was originated in 1933 by a researcher called Hedrich. He had been studying measles patterns in the US between 1900 and 1931 (years before any vaccine was ever invented for measles), and he observed that epidemics of the illness only occurred when less than 68% of children had developed a natural immunity to it. This was based upon the principle that children build their own immunity after suffering with or being exposed to the disease. So the herd immunity theory was, in fact, about natural disease processes, and nothing to do with vaccination. If 68% of the population were allowed to build their own natural defences, there would be no raging epidemic.

Later on, vaccinologists adopted the phrase and increased the figure from 68% to 95% with no scientific justification as to why, and then stated that there had to be 95% vaccine coverage to achieve immunity. Essentially, they took Hedrich's study and manipulated it to promote their vaccination programmes. (You can read about this in Greg Beattie's book, 'Vaccination', by the Oracle Press, Australia, 1997).

Why Vaccine-Induced Herd Immunity is Flawed

If vaccination really immunises, then your vaccinated child will be immunised, and therefore protected against that disease if it occurs in an unvaccinated child. If he isn't, his shots didn't work.

We should also examine whether or not the vaccines actually do provide immunity, and in which populations epidemics occurred. Was it the unvaccinated children spreading disease, as they would have parents believe? Or were those epidemics already in previously vaccinated people?

To do this, I've listed several epidemics that have occurred in the last 100 years or so, including smallpox, which medics claim that vaccination eradicated.

There was a smallpox epidemic in Pittsburgh, USA, in 1924. This epidemic was started by a mandatory vaccination campaign in which people were imprisoned if they refused the shot. A health club then started a suit against Dr. Voux, who had headed the vaccination drive, for bringing disease upon the people. Legal counsel for the health club stated: 'There have been NO deaths from smallpox in Pittsburgh during the previous nine years from 1915 to 1924, including the years when there was no vaccination or re-vaccination, at all ~ and hence, no vaccine immunity.'

They pointed out that the vaccine campaign had caused 22 deaths and 112 cases of vaccine-induced smallpox. (You can read a detailed history of vaccination in Eleanor McBean's book, Vaccination Condemned, Better Life Research, 1981.)

In Germany between 1947-1974, there were ten outbreaks of smallpox, including 94 people who had been previously 'immunised', who then became ill with the disease. (The Vaccination Nonsense, 2004 lectures, Dr. Gerhard Buchwald.)

Here are some more recent epidemics in vaccinated populations:

In March, 2006, 245 cases of mumps were confirmed in Iowa, US, where the law requires vaccination for school entry. Eleven year-old Will Hean of Davenport was diagnosed with mumps, and his 21 year old sister Kate. Both of them had got the measles, mumps and rubella vaccine (or MMR). "He had all the shots and everything. You don't think you're going to get the mumps after you've been inoculated," said Will's father, Wayne Hean. (2006, The

Associated Press.) In 2002 an outbreak of Varicella (Chickenpox) occurred in a US day care centre for <u>fully vaccinated</u> children. Varicella developed in 25 of 88 children (28.4 percent) between December 1, 2000, and January 11, 2001. A case occurred in a healthy child who had been vaccinated three years previously, and who infected more than 50 percent of his classmates who had no history of varicella. The effectiveness of the vaccine was 44.0 percent against disease of any severity. Children who had been vaccinated three years or more before the outbreak were at greater risk for vaccine failure than those who had been vaccinated more recently. Conclusions: In this outbreak, vaccination provided poor protection against varicella. A longer interval since vaccination was associated with an increased risk of vaccine failure. Breakthrough infections in vaccinated, healthy persons can be as infectious as varicella in unvaccinated persons.

(Outbreak of Varicella at a Day-Care Centre despite Vaccination) 2002 Karin Galil, M.D., M.P.H., Brent Lee, M.D., M.P.H., Tara Strine, M.P.H., Claire Carraher, R.N., Andrew L. Baughman, Ph.D., M.P.H., Melinda Eaton, D.V.M., Jose Montero, M.D., and Jane Seward, M.B., B.S., M.P.H.).

And here are some vaccine failures for measles: five cases of measles secondary vaccine failure with confirmed seroconversion after live measles vaccination (Scandinavian Journal of Infectious Disease vol. 29, no. 2, 1997, pp.187-90); two, five, seven and twelve years after vaccination with further attenuated live measles vaccine, three of five patients experienced modified measles infection, and the remaining two had typical measles. "This may be the first SVF case report that confirms the existence of completely waning immunity in recipients of the further attenuated live measles vaccines."

And whooping cough: Journal of Infectious Diseases, vol. 179, April 1999; 915 − 923. Temporal trends in the population structure of bordetella pertussis during 1949-1996 in a highly vaccinated population "Despite the introduction of large-scale pertussis vaccination in 1953 and high vaccination coverage, pertussis is still an endemic disease in The Netherlands, with epidemic outbreaks occurring every three to five years." One factor that might contribute to this is the ability of pertussis strains to adapt to vaccine-induced immunity, causing new strains of pertussis to re-emerge in this well-vaccinated population.

So What Happens if People don't Vaccinate?
Are the unvaccinated really infectious?

According to Archives of Disease in Childhood, vol. 59, no. 2, February 1984, pp. 162 – 5): 'Severity of whooping cough in England before and after the decline in pertussis immunisation', "Since the decline of pertussis immunisation, hospital admission and death rates from whooping cough have fallen unexpectedly...The severity of attacks and the complication rates in children [who were] admitted to hospital were virtually unchanged. That is, hospital admissions and death rates reduced when people WEREN'T getting vaccinated, meaning that avoiding shots is actually good for your child's health and may save his life, and in those cases which were admitted to hospital there were no increased complications in the unvaccinated group. Basically, at best the shots don't make a difference, and at worst, they kill or disable.

But there has never been one double-blind controlled study of vaccinated vs. unvaccinated children. Why? The medical profession says it is unethical to withhold vaccination from children. Therefore they cannot gain an accurate indication of what health is, because everyone is getting the shots and suffering colds, ear infections, eczema, asthma, and there is nothing to compare it with. If they did do a study, they would undoubtedly find the unvaccinated are healthier, and maybe that is why they refuse.

Not one of my four daughters ever suffered from any of the common childhood ailments that so many of their friends did. Whilst all the babies in the nursery were catching colds every other week, my baby was happy and healthy. "She's got an excellent immune system even though she's never been vaccinated", remarked the health visitor at her check. "No," I corrected, "She has an excellent immune system BECAUSE she's never been vaccinated".

So the herd immunity theory was, in fact, about natural disease processes and nothing to do with vaccination.

...vaccinologists adopted the phrase
and increased the figure from
68% to 95%
with no scientific justification
as to why,
and then stated that there had to be
95% vaccine coverage
to achieve immunity.

Tetanus Vaccine
by Joanna Karpasea Jones

In my years running VAN UK, a persistent theme which reccurs again and again from worried parents, is 'okay, so I know vaccines harm, but what about tetanus?' Even some 'alternative' practitioners seem to be on the fence with this particular disease, but are their fears founded? Here, I will look at the facts about the disease and the vaccine.

Tetanus ~ The Disease

Tetanus, also known as lockjaw, causes stiff muscles, particularly in the neck and jaw. Other symptoms are a hard abdomen and painful spasms of the muscles and respiratory tract, which can cause breathing difficulties. The disease is serious, but it's extremely difficult to actually contract tetanus. It's primarily caused by the improper cleaning of wounds, where the wound has been bandaged up without being cleansed, or stitched using unsterile instruments, something which rarely occurs in developed countries. Even then, the clostridium tetani spore would also have to be present in the wound, and unlike what medics tell you, these spores aren't 'everywhere'.

During the Second World War, only five American soldiers died of tetanus, despite being up to their eyes in mud in the trenches. All five of these soldiers had been vaccinated against tetanus, one had received a full programme of shots, the others had been partially vaccinated.

The British Army had 22 cases of tetanus in which 11 people died. All of the deaths were in tetanus-vaccinated soldiers. The 11 survivors were unvaccinated. (Dittmann, S. Atypische Verläufe nach Schutzimpfungen. Johan Ambrosius Barth Leipzig, 1981; 156.)

Most tetanus cases occur in Third World countries, and many of these are caused by umbilical stump infections in newborns, where the cord has been tied off in unsanitary conditions.

In Western countries, tetanus is rare. For instance, Germany has only 17 cases a year. (Mass für Mass - Tetanus-Impfung (Tetanol u.a.). Arznei-Tel, 1994; 7:60.)

Isn't the low Tetanus Rate because of Vaccination?

Unlike childhood diseases, it isn't possible to gain natural immunity to tetanus. If you've had it once, you can have it again. The body doesn't produce antibodies to Clostridium Tetani. Vaccination is the act of injecting a viral or bacterial substance into the body to make it produce antibodies to that disease. However, since no natural antibodies can be made, then there's no possible way that artificial antibodies could be made either. If the disease cannot give you protection, then how can a vaccine? It's likely that any raised antibody level seen after vaccination is the result of adjuvants (toxic heavy metals which are added to increase the body's antibody response). In the case of tetanus vaccine, this substance is aluminium.

Antibodies themselves are not an indication of immunity ~ this is just one function, which is vastly different from whole body immunity.

According to Vieira et al: 'This minimal protective antibody level is an arbitrary one and is not a guarantee of security for the individual patient.' (Vieira, B.l.; Dunne, J.W.; Summers, Q.; Cephalic tetanus in an immunised patient. Med J Austr. 1986; 145: 156-7.)

It's widely known that even those antibodies caused by tetanus vaccine adjuvants will wane or disappear completely within five to 10 years. That is why children have a preschool 'booster' at four years old, despite being vaccinated three or more times as a baby, and why it's repeated again at 15, and in some countries, at 12. It's estimated that over 50% of the adult population is not up to date with their tetanus vaccination, and therefore, unvaccinated. If it was truly vaccination that was keeping tetanus rates low, then why are there not dozens more cases of tetanus with all these adults running around? It certainly isn't in line with their herd immunity theory, where they assert 95% of people have to be 'immunised', or it won't work.

Vaccination also mimics the way in which people get tetanus (the spore entering through a deep puncture wound) ~ exactly the same as with an injection, so it's possible to get tetanus from the vaccine.

Many diseases have declined rapidly in the last 100 years because of improved sanitation, hygiene, and diet, and those who recovered from disease appear to be the ones who didn't get their jabs.

The Vaccine

In the UK, single tetanus vaccine is no longer given. Children are given it in the combined five in one 'super jab', and if an adult attends an emergency department with an injury, they're given DT vaccine (Diphtheria and Tetanus). If a parent wishes to have only the tetanus vaccine, they'll have to pay a private clinic hundreds of pounds to secure the old vaccine. However, any vaccine containing tetanus toxoid can cause reactions, even the single one.

Reactions

There are four general reactions in every 500 vaccinations given, and one death in every 500. (Sisk, C.W., Lewis, C.E.; Arch Environm Health, 1965; 11:7,34).

Reactions include: swelling; redness and pain; headache; tiredness; muscle pain; high temperature; rashes; swollen glands; joint pain; numbness and tingling; nausea and vomiting; shock; paleness; breathing difficulties; collapse; allergic reactions; lymphadenopathy and peripheral neuropathy.

Tetanic spasms may develop, and rigour, after vaccination. (Stalikamp, B.; Hating, A.; Lung, L.C.; Dtsch med Wschr, 1974; 99:2579.)

Peripheral Neuropathy is a neurological disability which my children's father suffers from, and causes the myelin sheath on the nerves to degrade. This means messages from the nerves to the brain are 'scrambled', causing muscle wastage and bone deformities. My mother-in-law had elected to give him only DT, instead of DPT. Needless to say, he was shocked to read that his disability could be caused by tetanus-containing vaccines.

Shock reactions are also common after tetanus vaccine, and tend to become worse with each vaccine you have. For instance, a 24 year old woman, with a history of asthma and wheezing, died half an hour after receiving a tetanus vaccine. (Staak, M.; Wirth, E.; Zur Problematik anaphylaktischer Reaktionen nach aktiver Tetanus-immunisierung. Dtsch. Med. Wschr., 1973; 98:110-111.)

A 14 year old boy was bitten by a dog, and on receiving his vaccine, died five minutes later (Spann, W.; Medical Tribune, 1986; 19:10.)

Immune system damage is commonly written about with this vaccine, perhaps the most concerning is that research has indicated that tetanus toxoid causes a massive drop in T cells, comparable to that of an AIDS sufferer: 'Tests of T-lymphocyte subpopulations were done on 11 healthy adults before and after routine tetanus booster immunisations. Tests showed a significant, though temporary, drop in T-helper lymphocytes (a class of white blood cells which helps govern the immune system) in all of the subjects. Special concern rests in the fact that in four of the subjects the T-helper cells fell to levels found in active AIDS patients. If this was the result of a single vaccine in healthy adults, it's sobering to think of the consequences of the multiple vaccines (twenty one at last count) routinely given to infants, with their immature systems, during the first six months of life. However, we can only speculate as to the consequences, as this test has never been repeated' ~ Dr. Buttram (Abnormal T-lymphocyte subpopulations in healthy subjects after tetanus booster immunisation. N Engl J Med. 1984 Jan 19;310(3):198-9.)

Contraindications: (reasons people shouldn't have the vaccine)
Infections; asthma; hayfever; allergy to a previous vaccine; allergy to any of the vaccine components (tetanus toxoid, aluminium hydroxide, formaldehyde, thiomersal); liver and kidney conditions; hepatitis.

Natural Prevention of Tetanus
Proper hygiene! If cut, allow the wound to air first. Tetanus spores are killed before they enter the bloodstream if they come into contact with oxygen. In the case of more severe wounds, make sure it's cleaned out with water or saline before being stitched at hospital. Adequate cleaning is usually enough to deter tetanus.

In the case of newborns, any instruments used to sever the cord should be previously boiled thoroughly.

Homeopathic remedies Ledum and Hypericum have been successful in treating tetanus, and act preventatively for years. These are simple and effective measures, without a fraction of the risk.

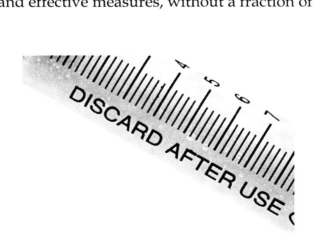

Holistic Living

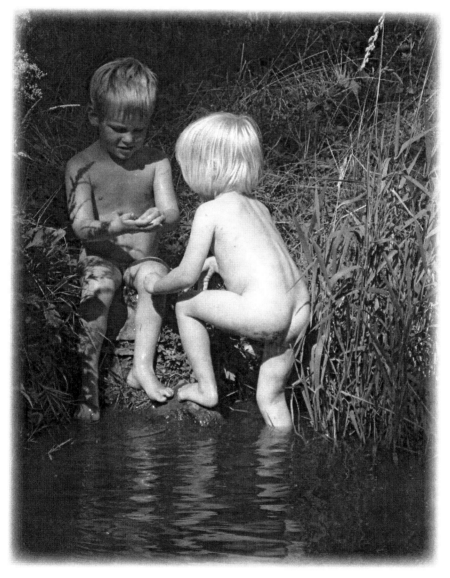

Aaron and Emily.

Beyond Attachment Parenting
by Jeannine Parvati Baker

Dear Jeannine,
There's a lot of writing and talking around about Attachment Parenting. When I read this, I'm confused: what else would one do? What are others doing if this feels like a new idea? What happened?
Jane, Midwife & Mother
Sydney, Australia

Dear Jane,
Indeed, what else would one do but continue the unity begun at conception throughout our children's lives? For that is the way Nature intended it, and doing so brings the fullness of joy to the entire family. Yet there are as many reasons for parents to separate themselves from babies and children as there are egos. Throw in the vested interests of a post-industrial society which benefits by selling the props needed when there's separation, and there we have it.

Look around ~ it's just about everywhere. Babies put in cribs, strollers, in high chairs, left with babysitters or nannies, in day care, preschool, and in front of televisions. There are monitors to check on the baby while the parents are in other rooms, and all sorts of substitutes for relationship in the form of baby bottles and pacifiers (also called "dummies" ~ aptly named, for indeed they dumb down dyadic communication). Parents who use these substitutes cannot hear the messages from their babies, so it's no wonder that when these babies grow into children and teenagers, they stop trying to communicate their real needs. Toys are sold to distract babies from their need for relationship with their families, and loads of toys fill family homes to placate parents who suffer the loss of unconditional love, yet know not why they feel so empty.

But, readers of The Mother are examples of another way. There is a multitude of babies who are carried on the parent's body. We continue to sleep and dream with our babies, so that they know the original lovers who called them from that place before here. Our babies are honoured, and even adored, for who they are. We have the courage to be loved so deeply by our children that our egos may disappear in precious moments when we surrender our selfish desires, and serve the needs of our new ones. I have pondered that one of the ways that separation between the generations is sustained is that to be so unconditionally loved by one's child is terrifying to the ego because it dissolves the illusion of separation. Thus, the rise of Attachment Parenting, which proposes to address the needs of new families in a holistic way. This is a noble intention. It identifies the malaise of our society; the estrangement of parents and children. It then prescribes a cure that begins from before conception, through childbirth, and beyond: So far, so good. Yet as the Greek Goddess of Healing Hygieia counsels, the wound reveals the cure. The wound upon which I focus is separation. What is wrong about this matter is the word "attachment", and all it implies, because the concept sabotages the ultimate goal of wholeness. To imply "wholeness" as a goal also undermines wholeness. Babies, if left to be with their mothers, are already whole. It takes about nine months to grow a baby on the inside of a mother's body, and similarly, nine months to continue to grow on the outside of mother's body.

Attaching a baby to the parents is like attaching a foot before walking. So, let us walk through the journey of how we abandoned ourselves ~ or, as you query, Jane: "What happened?"

We Westerners have a legacy of rebellion from the mother country. In America, we are prideful about being the "Land of the Free", and celebrate Independence Day as our national holiday. Yet, most parents view children as needy dependents, and urge separation (even from before conception vis-à-vis birth control ~ see my tome, Conscious Conception, for a fuller treatment of this theme). The estrangement is reinforced by viewing prenates (the unborn) as basically separate individuals. Perinatal medical management further deepens the split. (For example, we have obstetricians for mothers, and pediatricians for babies.) Toward healing the wound of separation, I first propose a new view of attachment parenting: interdependence. The mother, father, and baby are already one. In conscious conception and optimal birth, there's nothing broken, and nothing in need of re-attachment. The parents' genetics are present in every cell of the baby. The father's genetic material is found in the mother's brainstem and bloodstream. Therefore, the family genetically is an interdependent psycho-physiological system. In other words, the family is a unity of cellular consciousness. To reiterate: what is wrong with attachment parenting is the language. It presumes that the mother and father need to attach the baby, as if they're a separate appendage. This makes no physiological, much less psychological, sense. My perspective is that parents need the baby as much as the baby needs the parents. For example, a mother whose baby is taken away at birth is compromised in her postpartum, and can suffer for it through myriad gynaecological problems throughout her life.

As a midwife, I would often perceive a psychic hole in the mother's belly if the baby was taken from her after birth. The psychological and physiological need of the neonate is well documented. The baby's immunity, cardiovascular, pulmonary and neurological systems are all negatively affected by separation from the mother after birth. The way to sustain the unity of the new family is articulated through conscious conception, natural childbirth and breastfeeding, plus baby-wearing and co-sleeping: precisely what The Mother magazine is all about! If I were the Goddess of this planet, we would refrain from using the terms "bonding" and "attachment" as applied to infants and children, unless they've indeed been broken (traumatised) and need to be glued back together again. Rather, we would speak of the innate bliss of realising the wholeness of families when we keep our babies in our arms, next to the heart from whence they arise. There's a homely saying in America, "If it ain't broke, don't fix it." Let's focus on keeping intact the mother/baby/father unit rather than fixing the damage later. No wonder you're confused, gentle mother. In wisdom traditions, to be attached is to be bonded by illusion; and the separate pieces are put together without affection, but with fear. Indeed, the original meaning of the word family is a group of people sharing a house ~ not as bonded servants, but living together out of affection for one another: un-obligated, and free to love.

Let us language anew our experiences as parents who are free to love ~ rather than being attached to our children. We sustain the ecstasy of conception, birth, and breastfeeding long after our hearts have stopped melting into milk.

Rediscovering Elimination Communication
by Gina Sewell

'When you were a tiny baby, you were pure joy and love. You knew how important you were. You felt you were the centre of the Universe. You had such courage, you asked for what you wanted, and you expressed all your feelings openly. You loved yourself totally, every part of your body, including your faeces. You knew you were perfect. And that is the truth of your being. All the rest is learned nonsense and can be unlearned.'
~ Louise L Hay.

When we listen to our hearts, there is magic, and mystery, wonder and clarity. We cut right through the culturally acquired nonsense, and arrive at the truth of things, at the very core.

I've never felt comfortable using nappies on my babies. Even though we used soft cloth nappies, it felt wrong. Too bulky, too tight, that stiff, plastic wrap tight around their tiny bellies. But, I had no idea (well, my head had no idea, my heart was alert and still waiting for me to catch up, or more precisely, be still for long enough for its message to resonate). I thought babies had to wear nappies. I thought there was no other way...

Then a friend lent me a copy of Ingrid Bauer's book Diaper Free - The Gentle Wisdom of Natural Infant Hygiene. Its beautiful message spoke straight to my heart. Elimination Communication...Nappy Free...Natural Infant Hygiene...Of course, of course there's another way...Its story was the timeless song of the intuitive, innate mother and baby relationship. My baby would be birthed expecting all of her needs to be met. She would tell me when she needed to feed, just to be held, to be rocked, walked, when she was sleepy, alert, hungry, happy. So of course she would tell me when she needed to eliminate. Why would Nature have missed this out, made such a big mistake? How could our babies, who are born entirely vulnerable, and dependent upon us completely, not be capable of doing so?

'Stone-age babies don't know what century it is, or on which continent they are born, or anything about the cultural rituals and beliefs surrounding the beginnings of a new life. They hope their parents have the good sense to appreciate that they are born knowing everything about being babies and that they are master communicators.'
~ Jody Mclaughlin

That my baby could be, no, should be, nappy-free, was a joyful discovery for me. I was pregnant with our third baby, and our EC journey had begun. Last Summer, Willow was born peacefully at home, in water. For the first few days, we snuggled skin to skin, inside Ash's huge dressing gown! I kept a small, organic terry square nappy folded beneath her to catch the first wee and meconium (Note to self: do not use brand new, organic terries to catch meconium if you want to have any chance of ever being able to wash them clean enough to use again: cut up an old cotton sheet or similar, instead!).

It was a revelation to me that babies don't wee constantly! Willow would wee as soon as she awoke from a nap, and just before or after a feed. If she wriggled, as she surfaced from a nap, but wasn't fully awake, she would usually wee then, too. It was extremely rare for her to wee when she was in the sling; this only happened if she woke up and I didn't get her out in time.

When she was three days old, Ash caught the first wee (over the sink!); and from then on we held her either over the potty, sink or toilet when we thought she needed to go.

People often ask about the night time. In the beginning, we used a soft cloth nappy without a wrap, and an organic cotton waterproof pad where she slept between us in the bed. Or we lay her without a nappy, on a pre-fold, and kept a stack at the end of the bed so that we could change them easily if they got wet. It was easier than changing nappies at night, and kept everything much more peaceful and undisturbed.

As Willow grew, we were amazed how beautifully she responded to us responding to her needs. But, one morning, when she was about six months old, I realised that I'd fallen into the habit of putting a nappy (without wrap) onto Willow more and more often during the daytime, as things were hectic, with three children under five years old. We'd also bought one packet of 'Eco' disposable nappies for the night, as we were so tired, and thought it would help. It didn't, it felt wrong: deeply, irrevocably wrong. I went out for a walk with Willow in the sling, and thought about it all. And then I tried not thinking about it, and listening instead to the quiet, but insistent, voice of that primal cave mother within me. I'd chosen nappy-free because I didn't want my baby to wear nappies, and also because I knew in my heart that it was the only way. I went home, my heart filled with the words "If you're going to do it, do it bravely", and we stopped using nappies completely that day.

It's Willow's first birthday next week, and we don't have a single nappy in the house. We have the occasional pair of damp trousers, and sometimes even a poo on the floor! But most days we make it to the potty every time, and I can't remember when we last had to change Willow's trousers because we missed when we're out and about.

One of the most important aspects of Elimination Communication for us is our understanding that it's not a duty, or just an alternative to using nappies. It's a natural part of gentle, conscious attachment parenting. It's just one aspect of being fully in the present moment with your baby. It's cutting through the 'learned nonsense', and listening to the timeless voice of our primal mother instinct.

Our babies need us to reclaim this ancient, instinctive knowledge of their elimination needs. Just as we birth, breastfeed, co-sleep and carry our babies joyfully, we can listen to our hearts, and respond to their need to be nappy-free, bravely and lovingly. They deserve nothing less.

'We don't have to 'do' love, we just have to let go and find ourselves in it. That's how it is with becoming diaper-free, too…We try so hard to get it right. But everything we need to know is already there inside, simply waiting for a quiet moment to be recognised.' ~ Ingrid Bauer.

Useful bits and pieces for EC:
[] A small bowl to use as a potty while babe is tiny. Much easier to balance on your lap, and use at night!
[] Soft, flat terry nappies (or prefolds/cut up cotton sheet) ~ organic cotton is best.
[] A few soft cloth nappies, without wraps, as backup in the early days.
[] A soft waterproof pad (or two) for the family bed in the early weeks.
[] Not essential, but fun, and definitely useful as they get mobile: split-crotch trousers, baby size training pants and baby legs.
[] A sling. HUGELY essential. Being in constant contact with your baby is an essential part of Elimination Communication.
[] Most importantly, a willingness to let go and just be with your baby. Shrug off the expectations of the world outside, and spend as much time as you need Babymooning with your baby.

50 TV-free things to do with your family in Winter
by Veronika Robinson

Make a seasons table, gathering goodies from Nature to display, such as acorns, holly berries. Light a candle, and give thanks for all the beauty around you.

Make a Winter ring (wreath) to hang on your door, or above your fireplace, using ivy, holly and pine.

Try making your own candles using plant wax, essential oils and dried flowers.

Craft your own soap, and share your scented delights with friends.

Sew lavender bags.

Celebrate the Solstice with mindfulness and joy.

On New Year's Eve, write three wishes on paper, then bury it into the soil before the clock strikes midnight. Mother Earth will hold your prayers in her bosom as you walk forward into the New Year.

Bake sourdough rye bread with caraway seeds, and share the 'starter' with friends.

Invite friends for a themed pot luck dinner.

Join (or start) a local storytelling group.

Take a Moon bath by walking under the full Moon.

Build a bonfire beneath starlight.

Collect conkers, then string them together to make figures or dolls.

Join a local knitting café, and enjoy this traditional craft. You can also use hemp, rami and other plant-based yarns.

Go sledging!

Build a snowman.

Write a poem, song, play, novel.

Bake stöllen (German Christmas bread with layers of marzipan throughout), then wrap in lovely paper and ribbon, and give as a gift to friends.

Make a yule log.

Perform a Phoenix ceremony for New Year's Eve. Write down things you'd like to release from your life. Burn the pieces of paper in a fire, and imagine them being replaced by good and wonderful people and experiences.

Make lanterns for an evening starlight walk.

Snuggle up on the sofa, and read to your family ~ no matter what their ages.

Nature rubbings: colour crayons over leaves, bark, and make pieces of artwork.

Write to your grandmother.

Learn about healing herbs, and how they can benefit your family.

Make spicy warm fruit punch when visitors come.

Compile a list of goals and dreams for the new year.

Create a dreamcatcher from shells, ribbons, feathers and beads. Hang it in your window.

Start a gratitude journal. Write five things each day for which you're grateful, and watch your life change.

Feed the birds! They're hungry.

Discover flower essences, and how they can soothe the soul.

Learn the Japanese art of origami, and include pieces as delightful surprises when you post a hand-written letter.

Make a friendship bracelet for your best friend.

Learn a new recipe ~ be adventurous.

Create your own paper, and use pressed flowers in your design.

Learn yoga asanas for health, peace and vitality.

Treat every day as a miracle.

Go walking each day for vitamin D, exercise, fresh air and inspiration; and to reconnect with Mother Nature.

Collect sticks, moss, pine cones and berries, and craft a mobile to hang from your window.

Massage your family with essential oils blended with almond oil.

Discover five new ways to become more eco-friendly towards Mother Earth, and commit to these changes.

Prepare a salsa salad rich with herbs such as flat leaf parsley, coriander, mint and basil.

Contribute to your community through volunteer work or by starting a group based on your interest/hobby.

Commit to creating DIY holistic beauty products.

Play Scrabble.

Make chunky root vegetable soup. Invite friends to share in the feast.

Redesign clothes found in charity shops.

Give ten things away on Freecycle/Freegle.

Learn salsa, belly dancing, circle dancing for peace.

Make a superfood smoothie and a vegetable juice every day, for vibrant vitality.

The Birth of a Mother
by Liz Pilley

How often have you heard people talking negatively about the changes motherhood has brought? Or wondered yourself where 'you' went after the baby arrived. In our society, the transformation from maiden to mother is generally seen as a negative one ~ involving limitation, self-sacrifice, a loss of the woman as an individual, and often, isolation and depression. I would argue that this huge upheaval is actually a positive one, if only we're prepared and helped to view it in its correct context.

In modern Western society we're severely lacking in rites of passage, so much so, that teenagers have been forced to invent their own ~ first cigarette, first car, first drink. And life is generally so safe that adrenalin sports have been introduced to give people that rush of danger and brush with mortality that they crave. But women don't need either of these things, as we're lucky to have a natural alternative far more powerful than any teenage initiation or bungee jump could be: motherhood.

Pregnancy, birth and the first year of motherhood, together form a long process of change and reinvention, which, if supported, can be an intense and exhilarating journey of self-discovery; and yet, sadly, too few of us are able to take advantage of this opportunity, due to lack of support, exhaustion and sheer shock. We don't realise in advance how it's going to be, and afterwards the general cry is 'why didn't someone tell me?' The answer to that is partly because it's different for everyone, and it's very hard to articulate to someone who hasn't yet experienced it, exactly how big an upheaval ~ physically, emotionally, spiritually and socially ~ having a baby represents.

But another part of the answer lies in how little our society values mothers and their experiences. Motherhood, particularly early motherhood, is hidden from view, deemed as rather distasteful or a bit boring. Women are only allowed to speak again once they've 'got back to normal'. Heaven preserve us from being 'baby bores'.

ı go to great lengths to not allow their babies to change
ıs life, including the use of 'cry it out' methods of
, early day care, and actively discouraging a too close
ın the part of the child. But this is missing the point.
ѕ many women a long time to realise is what Naomi

Stadlen quoted a mother as saying, in her book 'What Mothers I 'normal has changed'.

And this is the whole point of a rite of passage ~ it's an intense experience, one which breaks down your barriers, and tests you to the limit, and yet gives you enormous insights. You'll be a different person when you come out of it, and this is a positive change, a welcome one. In the weeks running up to the birth, women in our society are encouraged to work as long as they can; check they have all the baby equipment they 'need'; go to birthing classes; and yet none of these things attend to a vital need on the part of the woman: to prepare for a dissolution of who she has been up until now, and the long process of learning who the new person who has emerged is.

This is not the work of one night, though one night is often the first time many women realise what's ahead of them. When the first pangs of labour kick in, the enormity of the enterprise also kicks in, along with panic. From now on, you'll be a mother. Who will that mother be?

Labour is the entrance to this transformation, a real baptism of fire, a test of character. But, as is typical in the West, when we hear the word 'test', we immediately think we can 'fail'. You cannot fail at labour, although many women, me included, have felt that we have failed if we didn't live up to our expectations of ourselves during this time, or if we didn't 'manage' the kind of birth we'd planned. It's taken me five years, and another birth, to understand the lessons of my first labour. The test was not a pass or fail scenario, but one which uniquely allowed me to see myself clearly.

How did I react under pressure? How did I deal with fear? With pain? With the unexpected? With things not going as planned? Not too well, as it happened. It took a second birth, two years later, to properly learn the lessons of the first ~ to surrender to the experience, to open up, and to face the unknown with courage. And also to realise the strengths of character I had shown in the face of difficulties the first time around: that I hadn't failed at all.

Many people assume that once the birth is over, the rite of passage has ended and you'll 'go back to normal'. And it's a terrible shock to the system to discover that you're not the same person as before, that you don't even know who you are any longer, that there's no 'normal', that your whole viewpoint has changed. Birth may be the crucible, but you have only just begun your transformation. Like a ding its armour, you're now soft-bodied and vulnerable, grow a new shell. The whole world feels dangerous, big as you venture out clutching your precious newborn. the news makes you cry; you can't bear to read about children being hurt. You're tired and hormonal, and that's all it is, right? Wrong.

You have changed, and the process is still ongoing whether you embrace it or fight it.

It's terrifying, you think your self is 'lost' and you'll be in some kind of limbo for evermore. But, this is a mother's 'dark night of the soul', and it lasts for the first nine months to a year of her baby's life. You're in the process of being reborn as a mother, and this is your gestation period.

Naomi Wolf, in her book, Misconceptions, quotes one new mother as saying: "I wish someone could have let me know I would lose my self in the process of becoming a mother ~ and that I would need to mourn that self."

It's entirely natural to grieve for parts of yourself which have gone, but you're not lost as an individual, merely changed. As Joanna Macy, author and Buddhist scholar has said: "What disintegrates in times of transformation is not the self, but its defences and assumptions." Preparing for this feeling, and discussing what you think might happen and how you will cope, can take away the panic and isolation this can cause, and make it easier to see from the outset that it's a temporary, natural and positive journey. If you're awake to the process, prepared and supported, you can take an active part in it ~ rediscovering yourself, re-making yourself, you may discover strengths you never knew you possessed, ways of coping with the weaknesses, and a much more thorough self-knowledge.

Wolf also comments, "Many women I spoke to learned with surprise that new mothers are not born, but, through a great effort, made." And this is a great truth which is rarely covered in antenatal classes or mainstream pregnancy and birth magazines. It's a source of great distress for many women, as they feel they 'failed' at labour and are now 'failing' again at motherhood. Why isn't it coming naturally? Why don't they know immediately how to breastfeed, what their baby's cries mean, how to dress and undress that tiny body? The reason is that motherhood is learnt, literally through blood, sweat and tears. For many, love, or at least a truly primordial sense of protectiveness, comes naturally (though not for everyone), but most of the other skills of motherhood are grasped over the days and weeks that pass. And the new sense of ⌐ with that as we meditate on things during the night, when with a tiny alien creature in the dark and silence.

Old pursuits which we used to define ourselves are not possible, or changed, with a newborn ~ career, creative outlets, hobbies, likes and dislikes, socialising, the kind of person we used to think of ourselves as. We're used to defining ourselves by outside activities, by social status, by society's view of us. When that's stripped away, we can feel there's nothing left. But there is, there is our inner self ~ what we are like, the characteristics we show, our fundamental beliefs and values. Some of these, even, may have changed. But many people have never learned to define themselves by these core inner values, and once the external has disappeared, they feel their self has gone with it.

This is often experienced as depression, a kind of terrified floundering around, loss of status, and utter shock. But it needn't be like that. The pressure of the constant needs and constant change in the first year of a baby's life can be, as described by one mother to Naomi Stadlen, "relentless", but also, "pushes me forward". Like birth, it has to be surrendered to, to truly be able to appreciate it and use it as a personal transformative tool.

That first year requires skills you never knew you had. Just when you think you've got to the end of your tether, you find more tether. Again and again. You redefine the meaning of patience and love. You also redefine the meaning of tired. Your focus in life changes, you reassess everything, and come out with new priorities, new ideas, and hopefully, a new confidence.

Wolf comments in an incredulous aside, that motherhood requires "even a kind of warrior spirit", but this should not be a casual comment, it's central to the whole rite of passage. It, as they say, separates the women from the girls. It's a final growing-up in a society which currently tries to put that off indefinitely. It does take a warrior spirit to get on with it, get through it and come out the other side, battered, bruised, but with new experience, knowledge, self-knowledge and a whole new sense of self.

It's a shame that we don't seem to have the time and support required to get through our rites of passage joyfully, and with conscious preparation, in our current society. All it really requires is an acknowledgement of the change about to take place, some ebriefing with experienced and sensitive mothers to make sense of the birth experience, and then the social and emotional support after the birth to integrate those new experiences into our new sense of self, gradually, and at a pace which suits us and the baby. Yet we're ignored and rushed. How often have you heard someone speak admiringly of a woman who is up and about within a week or even a day of giving birth? This is clearly what our culture finds admirable: someone who can brush off the physical and emotional maelstrom, and carry on, 'business as usual'. If that's what feels right to you, then good luck, but many women find they wish to hibernate after the birth, bed down for a Babymoon, find their feet in their new role, and make some mental readjustments. Most women feel the need to talk about their birth experience, to make sense of it and understand its significance, despite this often being frowned on.

We also need to acknowledge the changes that motherhood brings for individuals, but in a balanced way; and to encourage realistic discussions of the positive and negative, so that women aren't so stunned at the strength of their feelings and the intensity of the experience ~ so that mothers are allowed to step outside the normal bustle of life, and enjoy the rite of passage they're participating in, to learn their lessons, and glory in the wisdom they've gained.

Further reading:
Misconceptions, by Naomi Wolf
What Mothers Do, by Naomi Stadlen
A Path for Parents, by Sara Burns

Babies don't need to cry
by Emma Lewis

I'm writing this in dismay, having recently read a number of articles in various magazines which usually support meeting the basic needs and rights of babies and children, and more often advocate 'attachment parenting'. The articles I refer to regard some new theories that imply an aware parent would let their babies cry; moreover, that it's OK, even desirable, for them to do so as long as they're being held.

Firstly, I'd like to make a comment about the term 'attachment parenting'. For me, it's a bit like the terms 'demand feeding', 'breast is best' and 'extended breastfeeding'. Sometimes we do ourselves, and others, a disservice with the language we use.

Replace 'demand feeding' with 'feeding on cue', and not only does it become accurate, it feels better. Rather than say breast is best, we should say breast is normal. The devastating physiological and biological (not to mention emotional) fact is that babies deprived of, or unable to have, the breast will be compromised and never reach their full potential. Mothers who breastfeed their children as long as needed don't extend breastfeeding, they breastfeed 'full-term' ~ in our culture, breastfeeding is generally severely limited.

Hence, parents who 'attachment parent' do not, in effect, attach their child, and 'attachment parent', they simply don't create a detachment, and, in a culture where children are generally parented in a detached way, instead parent 'fully'.

It appears to me that we now have a bit of a wave of articles, offering repackaged advice regarding babies and crying, that are playing on the vulnerability of 'attachment parents' whose resources are being challenged; and these articles are creating some fear around 'attachment parenting'.

It's suggested that parents dealing with feelings of resentment, and issues around angry toddlers, are somehow linked to babies not having support to cry. I would like to suggest that these phenomena are very normal reactions to being a family in a modern, Western setting. We're absolutely not meant to parent in isolation.

Even if we parents do manage quite a full social life, the reality is that, as a parent in our culture, we're excluded from many social settings. And, even if we do manage to find truly supportive peers, for most of us the everyday living ~ the heart of our lives ~ tied up with essential work like food preparation and other domestic chores, is carried out in isolation. We're not honoured, respected, revered or supported by our culture as we should be for doing the most important work of all.

No wonder we feel resentful.

As for angry toddlers, I believe that, due to the everyday social isolation, often their world becomes quite child-centred. As attachment parents we can fully include them in OUR world and lives, but it's difficult to fully include them in life in a wider context. They innately expect a tribe, and most of the time, most of us cannot provide that.

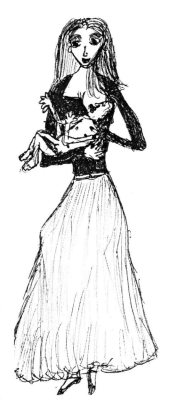

Instead of having the arms of many adults and children of all ages to snuggle and learn in, many of our babies and toddlers have one or two parents, and occasionally the availability of extended family, and maybe a playgroup or activity group for a few hours a week with similarly aged children. They have no tribe, and little acceptance in their wider community, as they expect and deserve. No wonder some toddlers react in an angry and frustrated way!

It's very important not to confuse the needs of a toddler with those of a baby. Toddlers are in a very different space and stage of growing and learning, and maybe do occasionally need to scream out their frustrations in a safe, loving space, as they start to negotiate their way in the world, and begin separating themselves from their 'oneness' with their mother. This absolutely does not mean that babies should cry!

Yes, parenting can be tough and wildly challenging, particularly in our unsupportive culture, and especially in the everyday isolation most of us parent in. Often the issue is whether or not the parents have the support, energy or resources to be able to respond fully to their baby's needs. I mean this as no criticism of those who are unable to, for all the reasons mentioned. We are doing it tough. And alone.

But, please, as aware adults, let's OWN this. Let's work on changing the isolation and lack of support, understanding and reverence of parenting. And, in the meantime, let's own our shortcomings.

Let's acknowledge that, in an ideal situation, we would all respond fully and wholly to our children's needs without needing to compromise ourselves.

Let's not undermine the messages from, and dismiss the needs of, our babies by having them cry in our belief that somehow they need to!

Babies whose needs are being heard and met, and who are involved in life, passively from loving arms or a sling, absolutely do not (need to) cry. They don't generally get stressed, bored or overstimulated. At least, if/when they do, they can easily resolve it themselves by 'letting off' stress through the movements of their carer, snuggling at the breast or wriggling close to 'opt out' with a snooze. They receive all the love, nutrition, hormones, quiet, stimulation etc., they need. They're in a state of bliss. Where's the stress?

Apologies to those who are parenting a baby who is crying because they have special needs as yet unidentified. I certainly don't wish to undermine your difficult experience. It can be so hard. Keep plodding at finding the solution. It's not uncommon in today's world where so many babies experience traumatic births, early separation, or reactions to the artificial environment or some food sources. I hope that you're able to find all the extra strength needed for such difficult times. Be comforted by the knowledge that your baby really needs you, even when you feel that you can do nothing right. Babies crying in-arms (who are seemingly not comforted) still cry for significantly less, overall, than those left in isolation. They also fare better emotionally in the long-term. I absolutely believe that all parents KNOW with their whole being exactly how to respond to a baby crying, and will react appropriately wherever possible.

So, instead of regurgitating old and devastating trends about babies needing to cry, please let's support parents to confidently hear the needs of their babies, and listen to the truth of the consistently reliable, age-old, worldwide messages that are held in their HEART.

Let's not undermine the messages from, and dismiss the needs of, our babies by having them cry in the belief that somehow they need to!

Crying and Babies
by Veronika Sophia Robinson

With respect to the new fad of following the Aware Parenting technique of allowing babies to cry, The Mother magazine presents the following facts:

It used to be that when babies were born, they were hung upside down and their bottoms were smacked. The idea behind this barbaric thinking was to open their lungs and get circulation going. A gentle and conscious parent would, instead, massage the baby's skin to stimulate the nerves.

It has been proven (as if an intuitive parent needs proof) that it's physiologically harmful for an infant to cry. This happens on many levels. Firstly, it can cause hoarseness. It reduces blood oxygen levels, dramatically increases the heart rate, disturbs digestion, and can lead to fainting. Crying drains a baby's energy.

The hormone cortisol floods the bloodstream. This negatively impacts on the developing brain. Other negative risks include distress on the respiratory system, breathing troubles, puncturing of the lungs, and intraventricular haemorrhage.

When we allow our baby to cry unnecessarily, we're teaching it negative socialisation skills. It's here that our infant learns that its caregiver doesn't in actual fact 'care'. As a parent, when we allow our child to cry without attending to its needs, we become detached emotionally. All the traumatic states listed above in turn lead to our child having a delayed (psychosocial) adaptation to life after birth.

Our baby, when left to cry, will make poor eye contact after such distress, and may not breastfeed as effectively. He is, in essence, shutting down to the relationship with the caregiver.

Hard crying leads to poor learning, and affects sleep patterns. If you view a good cry as positive for your infant, then you're not realising that the sleep induced state it brought on is, in fact, a response to stress. This is NOT healthy or safe. Be aware that this negatively affects your baby's organs and internal systems.

The purpose of a baby's cry is to alert its mother, and ideally, if she's in tune with her baby, for her to feel upset, and attend to her baby. This is a NORMAL, natural and biologically designed response. It should make the mother's heart rate and blood pressure increase. Her nipples should become erect, and milk let down will occur.

Crying is designed to alert a baby's mother to danger. In our culture there's far too much crying. An in-tune mother will not need her baby to cry. She will see and hear her baby cue her for food, nappy, sleep. And she'll respond by cuddling; or by changing the baby's position; feeding; or getting him to sleep.

At one extreme of parenting, we have the barbaric Gina Ford style, which encourages complete distancing between parent and child. And then we have the Aletha Solter style, promoted to attachment parents, ironically. Her style states that if you love your child and stay near her, she can cry all she likes. Both are completely ignorant and out of touch with an infant's needs. Both are based on utter selfishness.

While crying may be healing for adults, this does not mean it's the same for infants. Infants are non-verbal, and have not developed their other systems: adults have.

The Aware Parenting approach is a short cut to eliminating the intuitive tie between mother and child. It leads to separation, and does nothing to maintain bonding between mother and child. The practice suggested by Aletha Solter is passive, detached and creates emotional separation. As mammals, this is completely contrary to our biological evolution and needs.

Many studies have shown that this very act of emotional separation and detachment can lead to violence later on in life. It's emotional neglect. When we do this to our children, we're teaching them, in a non-verbal way, that it's 'normal' and therefore 'right' to not feel the pain and hurt of other human beings.

We fool ourselves if we believe that not attending to the needs of a crying baby is any different than if we were to leave them crying in a room alone. Babies who are denied comfort through the breast will be deficient in tryptophan.

An infant doesn't WANT to cry. It cries so that its mother will come and stop the crying. It's a late call to needs. Whatever the needs: comfort; heat; breastmilk; suckling for comfort, the baby is calling you to relieve its problems. It <u>relies</u> on you.

By forcing a baby to self-soothe, we're inadvertently interfering with their development skills. They're compromised.

Our culture has a high rate of thumb sucking and the need for dummies and pacifiers. Cultures which allow babies to nurse on cue have no incidence of thumb sucking. When we meet the needs of our infants, they'll have no need to suck fingers, thumbs, artificial objects, or even more sadly, to bang their heads, self rock, body rock or head roll. Most humans would be horrified to see these actions occurring in animals kept in captivity. Yet we don't notice it in our own children?

It's so easy to recognise when our baby needs attention. We don't need to wait for her to cry. Look and listen to her fidgets, grimaces, fussing and agitation. This is her way of COMMUNICATING. Some babies never need to cry. When we truly care for our baby, nurse on cue (not on demand), and carry the baby so they have sensory stimulation, they have very little reason to cry.

It can take just over a minute for the unmet needs of a baby to go from a small cry to a crying scream of pain. Quick and intuitive responses by a mother lead to happy, contented babies.

Many studies have shown that this very act of emotional separation and detachment can lead to violence later on in life. When we do this to our children, we're teaching them, in a non-verbal way, that it's 'normal' and therefore 'right' to not feel the pain and hurt of other human beings.

When we allow our baby to cry unnecessarily, we are teaching it negative socialisation skills.

Further reading:

Anderson, G.C., *Crying in transitional newborn infants: Physiology and developmental implications.*

Dinwiddie, R. Patel, B.D., Kumar, S.P. Fox, W.W. *The effects of crying on Arterial Oxygen tension in infants recovering from respiratory distress.*

Drane, D., *The effects of dummies and teats of oro-facial development.*

Fagen, J.W. *The effect of crying on long-term memory in infancy.*

Ko, M., *Crying is not good for babies.*

Prescott, J. W., *Essential Brain Nutrients; Breastfeeding for the development of human peace and love.*

Deprivation of physical attention as a primary process in the development of physical violence.

Woolridge, M. W., *Baby controlled breastfeeding; Biological implications*

Too young to be a mum?
by Amelia Loulli

When Veronika asked me to write about life as a young mum in our culture, I wasn't sure where to start, and what follows are some of my thoughts on the ways our society treats its young women, and whether age is what makes a capable mother.

"In 2004, there were 45,094 births to women under the age of 20 in England and Wales" (www.brook.org) ~ my beautiful daughter, Sophia, was one of them. As an unmarried mother in her teens, without a 'completed education', I was, for the British government, a statistical nightmare. It's no secret that Britain has the 'worst rate of teenage pregnancy in the world', and there's much written by the government and corresponding organisations about how they intend to reduce these numbers as dramatically as possible. Whatever the causes of this high rate, or circumstances of individual women, it's undoubtedly tough to be a younger (than average) mother in this country. Stereotypes abound regarding the abilities and circumstances of teenage mothers, and it's often assumed that we all fit into one neat, little, uneducated box, taking advantage of copious benefits, and lacking true competence to be mothers, as we are "only children" ourselves.

And it's amazing how I was often treated like a child during my pregnancy and early days of new motherhood. One of the midwives who looked after me through the course of my pregnancy, did little to hide the rolling of her eyes and judgmental sigh. She wrongly presumed I was living at home with my mum, unaware of the loving fiancé and family home I was lucky to have. Back on the ward, after my wonderful, natural birth, it was simply presumed that I would be bottle-feeding my gorgeous new bundle, with artificial milk. They were unaware of the beautiful ease with which my new daughter had latched-on minutes after birth, and that there was nothing else I would rather be giving her than my own precious milk.

My negative experiences with health professionals didn't stop when I left the hospital, and I was often told at various check-ups that breastfeeding was "unnecessary", and that at my age, motherhood would be tough enough! This terrible advice only increased once Sophia passed six months; and what little encouragement there had been for breastfeeding on-cue and co-sleeping, completely stopped. (Luckily for me, my daughter knew [almost better than her mother!]

what was best, and would not have stopped breastfeeding at six months for anybody.) I know of many mothers, though, who after giving birth in their teens, have had their lives irreversibly damaged by such ignorant guidance. One mother spoke to me about how she gave birth, at 17, to her son, and began to breastfeed. She was later advised that she "wouldn't be able to keep that up", because she "would be up all night, and nobody would be able to help her". This is a betrayal of a vulnerable new mother at its worst, and I wonder how often it happens. Younger mothers, and indeed, mothers of all ages, are so often bullied into making choices 'for their own good', at the cost of their mothering experience. Our culture so often likes to know best! And consciously or not, we sow seeds of fear and doubt when we label women as too young and immature, and suggest that they can't possibly know how to be mothers yet.

Often I hear that women of 17 or 18 haven't had enough time to "find themselves", and lack the life experiences necessary to mother effectively. This puzzles me somewhat. Regardless of what you've discovered before children, motherhood is a massive, irreversible shift of self for all women. It's a stop on our journey to self-discovery, not the destination. So it's short-sighted to believe that anyone has truly learnt who they are before having children, because motherhood changes us on every level. I've seen shocking decisions made by mothers of all ages ~ what distinguishes them is not their age, but their inability or unwillingness to truly open themselves up to the mother/child relationship, and to fully embrace their new role. Just as birth is often made easier when a woman opens her mind, and visualises an open body ~ and milk let-down is facilitated by relaxation, belief and visualisation of 'open' breasts pouring with milk ~ so motherhood is easier if we can imagine our arms and hearts open to our children, and agree to let them in. Whilst it is without doubt that all the experiences we have culminate in the person we are, and so have a bearing on our responses in parenting, it's surely naïve to believe that they alone determine our ability to mother.

It's beyond the scope of this article to discuss all the possible reasons behind England's high rate of teenage pregnancy, but I would like to briefly address one issue which is very close to my heart ~ that is, the way in which we're treating our daughters as they become women, and the way we're failing to teach so many of them about the wonder and wisdom of their own bodies. Little girls like dolls ~ they mother them and pretend to feed them. Little girls are often maternal and caring, and whilst I don't wish to spark a debate about how real the gender differences between boys and girls really are, there's no denying that most little girls are programmed with the 'mothering gene'. This is surely as Nature intended it. How I wish we could all start embracing and honouring the changes their bodies will go through, and actively encourage our young women to prepare for the roads their journey will lead them down. Motherhood will more than likely be one of them, and so it should be: the human race depends on it. We're so often forgetting to marvel at the special magic of a woman's body and role ~ a giver of life, maker of milk. This is the knowledge we should be openly gifting to our daughters, because we can teach them the ins and outs of sex education all we like, but until we respect, and, in turn, allow them to respect their own bodies for what they are ~ a place to grow and nurture their future babies ~ until we honour their deep, inner desire for children, and allow them to understand where this comes from, and delight in what it means, we will change nothing. We have to start putting the wonder back into women and motherhood. Once we start reinstating and revering motherhood as a highly honourable, life-altering, spiritual experience that young women can look forward to, but not rush in to, perhaps our daughters will be able to benefit from the full knowledge and appreciation of all the paths open to them, and then feminine power will be able to truly take hold.

Yet, so often, we seem frightened of this reality in our young women. We tend to push education and success in other areas, and encourage them not to waste the gifts they have, which we feel can only be best used at University or in a 'successful' career. This was certainly my experience of becoming a young woman in our culture. The beginning of my menstrual cycle was far from celebrated, and whilst my parents were always supportive and loving of all that I was, I never felt as though becoming a woman, and eventually, one day, a mother, was something to be proud of. I'm sure that the message my family and society gave me was the same as it is for most young women today: "We must not waste our intelligence on babies and domestic life, because we could do so much better than that". I was on the right track to being someone, you see. I did very well academically, and was bound for a first degree, and a successful career. It was inevitable that with so much expectation put into this side of my life, my impending motherhood would carry a sense of disappointment for most people who knew and loved me. Despite the immense joy and support, it was impossible for people not to feel like I had wasted so much of what I could have been. Now I would just be a mother.

I can only hope to give my daughter a very different experience. I know I'll never be afraid of, or try and deny her, her desire to have children. In fact, at 3½, she talks about it often enough already (her father, however, is terrified!). Instead, I will marvel with her at the wonder of her body, be excited, and celebrate when her period comes, and she turns from girl into woman. Because, how marvellous it will be. It fills my heart with joy when Sophia tells her baby brother, "Sorry, Nico, I haven't got any milk in my booboos, yet!" I think it's vital to her growing sense of self and self-respect, that she understands (in age-appropriate language) what her body is capable of, and how wonderful that is. I don't want these things to be mysteries to her, encouraging a lack of respect for her own body, born out of a lack of knowledge. I think it's hugely important to introduce my daughter to the concept of conscious conception, something I don't think they include on the National Curriculum just yet, and which I'd never even heard or thought of, until I opened my first copy of The Mother magazine.

I want her to know that she can take control of her own body in many ways, choosing to take the next step only when she's ready physically and mentally. Because surely this is where our power lies as women. To be given all the information and support for all the options open to us. Not all 18 year old girls may want to become mothers yet, or indeed ever, but we should be no more proud of those at University, than those nurturing the future generation, for theirs is surely a most precious job.

And for those women for whom the issue of motherhood in their teens is a reality, I wish them strength to find and follow their own path, despite the negativity of our society. I envision that we'll be able to start honouring and caring for these women with hope and admiration, rather than isolating them in the group of 'teenage mums', and labelling them as a problem. Because, we mustn't forget that it's certainly irrelevant to their babies how many years their mothers have lived. Their needs remain the same as all babies, and they expect their mothers to be free to bless them with the same loving experiences as any other mother. So if we could just stop interfering in the beautiful hormonal dance between new mother and baby, if our culture could just quieten down and let each mother do

her own footwork, then I'm certain each mother-child relation
would be filled with beautiful music, regardless of age. The natur
hormonal responses to birth give <u>all</u> mothers the power and instincts
to nurture their babies, but when we undermine or underestimate a
young mother's ability (or any mother's ability), we're jeopardising
these responses.

We must remember that motherhood transcends all issues such
as age, race and location. It is a universal experience, which connects
all mothers. We are, ultimately, all the same, with the same instincts.
No matter what age we are when we give birth, whether society
judges us as a child or an old woman, we are reborn ~ as mothers.
With this rebirth should come celebration, joy and a view for our
future journey.

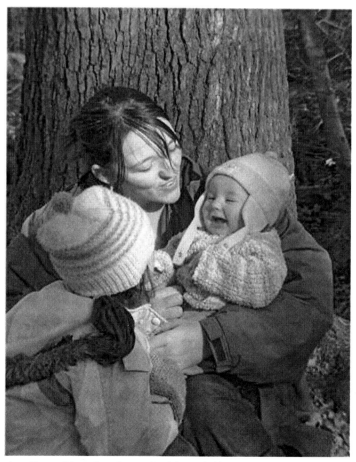

Amelia and her daughters Sophia and Elena.

The Highly Sensitive Family
by Liz Pilley

ou've never heard the term Highly Sensitive before, the chances are that you know a child who fits the profile: they have a very sensitive nervous system, are aware of the subtleties in an environment, and are easily overwhelmed in stimulating surroundings. They're often labelled fussy, shy, spirited, spoilt, ADHD, inflexible, explosive, or even Autism Spectrum; but none of these labels quite fits. They take things very much to heart, they're fussy about food, temperature, texture and many other things. They often hate group settings, and have many fears, but they're also creative, curious, loving and empathetic.

Bringing up a Highly Sensitive child can be a challenge; but that's just half the story, because the Highly Sensitive Trait is genetic. So, if you have a Highly Sensitive child, the chances are high that at least one parent will be so, too.

I'm a Highly Sensitive mother, and this has heavily coloured my parenting style in every possible way. Before I had any children, I had fantasies of a big, happy, noisy family living in loving chaos. It was only after the arrival of my first child that I realised this wouldn't be possible. My baby daughter was a huge challenge, but what was the problem exactly? I wasn't sure. She didn't have colic, but she also didn't sleep ~ the slightest thing woke her, and it took literally hours to lull her off. Gradually, I realised how sensitive she was to noise, temperature, texture, colour and the number of people around her. Shopping trips were hell, and any kind of playgroup was completely out of the question.

In desperation, I started researching what might be 'wrong' with her, came across Elaine Aron's ground-breaking work on Highly Sensitive Trait, and had a major epiphany. Not only was this what was 'wrong' with my daughter, it was also what was wrong with me. I'd thought I was going crazy ~ other people seemed to manage perfectly well, why did I find the demands of early motherhood so tricky? The health visitor kept testing me for post-natal depression, but I wasn't depressed, I was just way too stimulated. The intensity of the connection with my baby freaked me out, and when she cried, I cried ~ for months. I felt like my skin had been ripped off, and my nerves were in shreds. Other mothers only seemed to understand up to a point; they didn't seem to feel the soul-ripping agony that I did every time my daughter cried. They didn't seem able to feel their baby's anguish at being abandoned every time they left the room, as I did. It took me months to get my feelings ~ or rather, my reaction to them ~ under control.

By this time, I'd read and absorbed a lot of information about the trait, and realised that I could never have this huge family I dreamt of. Just having one or two children was going to be a challenge for me. I grieved, and still grieve, over this loss; and also felt inadequate that I couldn't cope with perfectly normal things that other people could. It took me a long time to realise that there were also positive points, such as my increased empathy to my children's feelings, and my heightened instincts about their welfare.

While my daughter and son were small, I soon realised that the world of modern parenting is not set up for Highly Sensitive children and parents. The noisy, crowded playgroups and sing-a-long groups made the children cry, and I wasn't far off either. Children's attractions and events were always crowded, full of music, singing, bright colours, flashing lights ~ and were a total nightmare. Children's food in cafés and attractions was often unacceptable to my children ~ mixed flavours and textures. We'd dash out first thing in the morning to go to a Children's Farm before anyone else got there, and then scuttle off as soon as any other children arrived.

In the library, my daughter would announce loudly that she hated songs in Storytime ~ it was Storytime, and there shouldn't be songs in it. A well-meaning friend prompted a huge tantrum by offering us a lift home in the car when we'd told my daughter we'd be going back on the train. Any slight change to the expected programme of events would cause huge problems and upset. Guiltily, I realised that I tend to be somewhat lacking in spontaneity myself.

Once, my daughter fell over in the playground, and there was blood on her knees, and she was so distraught ~ more at the thought that she was hurt than at the actual pain itself ~ that she screamed for a good 30 minutes. Several well-meaning strangers came running to help ~ did we need an ambulance, a first-aider? I knew we just needed to get home so that she'd feel safe after her shock, but I could feel the eyes on me, and hear the comments about what a fuss my daughter was making over a relatively minor trip. They should see her when she has a paper cut! By the time we struggled home, I was absolutely spent with nervous exhaustion, and burst into tears myself. My husband had to put me to bed with a cup of tea and a book, to calm me down. My son's sensitivity takes a different form. He's very funny about colours and textures, and he's so imaginative that he actually enters the pretend world of play that he creates, and terrifies himself on occasion with baddies that he's made up himself. He has dreams and nightmares, and won't wear corduroy, and thinks he owns the colour blue. I find him easier to deal with, as we don't find the same things stressful, so I can stay calm when he's over-stimulated.

I soon learned that the best way to deal with problems was to remain utterly calm and soothing at all times. If only I could have done that. Sadly, my daughter and I are too similar for our own good. The things which over-stimulate her have the same effect on me. So, I'd be completely rattled by a certain environment, and not at my best when she would throw a major wobbly, and I'd be unable to keep calm and deal with her, as I was already at breaking point myself.

You're probably reading this and thinking I'm exaggerating. After all, no-one likes children throwing tantrums, and everyone thinks soft-play centres are actually the seventh ring of hell. But this is more than just a normal reaction ~ this is fingernails-down-a-blackboard style lack of tolerance, for both me and the children.

Over the years, we've worked out how to adjust the environment for both me and my daughter so that we can cope, on the whole, without major meltdowns, but it's often entailed detailed explanations to friends and acquaintances ~ why we can't stay for lunch, why the children can only cope with one outing a day, why they need a quiet day to recover from some minor excitement ~ why quite routine events, such as visits to the doctor, dentist or even a party, have been awful challenges.

The first party my daughter went to, she took one look inside when the door was opened to her, and then shut her eyes and went rigid. We had to lead her inside into a quiet room ~ eyes still closed ~ and let her acclimatise. It took about an hour before she opened her eyes. And even then, she refused to join the actual party, and just sat in a room, mainly by herself, as it was all too much. To get her to the dentist was a major feat of planning that I can't even think about without a shudder of horror. And, as for the time she was supposed to be a bridesmaid, words fail to describe the sheer awfulness. It took me about a week to recover from that experience myself. Seriously!

But it isn't all doom and gloom. My Highly Sensitive children are also amazing. They're intuitive and highly imaginative. They're nurturing towards each other, animals, and other children. They cuddle easily, and are hugely affected by the natural world. They notice tiny details which other people miss, and they're full of love. As much as I feel drained by their constant chatter, by the stress of taking them on a day out, I also feel recharged by their sleepy, cuddly bodies next to me in bed, their sticky kisses, and curiously wise insights.

So they get carsick and loathe busy theme parks ~ so do I. We can just be one big Highly Sensitive family together.

Common HSP Dislikes
Big groups of people.
Noisy places or things, such as washing machines, aeroplanes.
Rough textures, such as towelling, corduroy, clothing labels.
Strongly flavoured food, or foods mixed together.
Being put on the spot and having to think quickly.
Plans being changed.
Strong odours.
Even the slightest amount of pain.
Surprises.
Dealing with stressful situations in public.
They get very upset if someone else is upset or in pain.
They get very distressed if they're told off or feel they've done something wrong.

Ways To Help A HSP
Let them know what to expect, and don't change plans once they've been made.
Don't plan too many activities on one day, balance stimulation with calm time.
Make sure they get enough sleep ~ give them plenty of time to wind down before bedtime.
Don't try and force them to join in, they need plenty of solitary time.
Listen very carefully to them ~ even if it seems to be said quite casually, it might be incredibly important to them.
Deal very quickly with emotional upset or physical pain.
Don't let people 'test' them.

Go with preferences about food, clothing textures, colours, smells. Soothing physical therapies such as massage, reflexology and reiki can be very helpful.

Positive HSP Attributes

Very intuitive, and they notice every subtle undercurrent.

Deep thinkers, very curious, and tend to remember lots of odd facts. Wide vocabulary, and very articulate.

Very empathetic and nurturing, especially good with younger children and animals.

Very open to plants, animals and Nature.

Feel everything deeply, and tend to be tactile and loving with those they know well, but reserved and apparently shy with those they don't.

Very creative ~ often artistic, and good with language

What the weeds have taught me
by April Coburn

Weeds inspire me. How many gardeners make a claim such as this? Yet for this gardener, it's true. I welcome the weeds as they appear among their tame and pampered cousins. Some are old, familiar friends who I greet fondly. Others are newcomers to my Earth space, that I welcome with joy. All have come for a reason. All have gifts to share and lessons to teach. We have only to watch, listen, and open our hearts and minds to the voice of Nature as she speaks through her emissaries, the wild plants.

Yes, I'm speaking here of the same plants much cursed by farmers, gardeners and lawn cultivators ~ the thistles, ragweeds, and pigweeds, the lamb's quarters, dandelion, chickweed, and the like. They are trodden, ploughed, sprayed and pulled, accused of crowding out flowers, robbing crops of water and nutrients, and disrupting the lawn. We speak of them as stubborn, tough and tenacious because they're not easily removed, and ever persistent on returning.

But look…growing through cracks, pushing up the asphalt, persisting in life in vacant lots where the ground lays wasted: what strength of life force allows a mere plant to be so strong? It begs a closer look, this force of Nature that comes back and back each time we rip, tear, pave, pollute or wash away our Mother's life-giving surface skin. We curse them when we should be thanking them ~ really down on our knees and thanking them from the bottom of our hearts for their silent work. You see, they're always there to make things right. Like wild mothers, they do their nurturing work with or without our appreciation. And they've become my teachers.

The weeds reach down with strong roots to break up the hardpan. They make tracks in the earth for other roots to follow, and for water to rise up. The weeds call forth the pollinators, and pull up the trace minerals from the depths of the earth, and share them with their neighbours. They offer us food and medicine, for our own needs often mirror those of the land. Their song is that of wisdom and strength. It's the feminine song that is not written in books, but carried on the wind for those willing to be still long enough to hear.

Can I emulate the weeds in my mothering practice? Can I take into my heart these lessons of strength and wisdom from the silent Earth healers? Can I allow their roots to reach into the soil of my heart, to mend its parched and barren places? There are times when I need

...nis primal teaching/healing: when my confidence falters, and the questions of society ring in my ears ~ when the culture that doesn't value weeds asks... "Don't you think it's dangerous not to vaccinate? To co-sleep? To birth at home? Are you sure a vegan diet is healthy for children? Shouldn't they be in school? Why can't they have a lollypop at the bank?"

"Lighten up," the voices say, "but be firm, you don't discipline enough. Do you want them to be spoiled? They should have chores by this age! They need to learn responsibility. Aren't they reading yet?"

The culture that hates weeds can't see the silent work, the work of love, the work of roots that go deep, reaching into the heart of things. The lessons learned in long hours of play, or silent moments of quiet reflection, aren't easily measured and tested for. The wisdom gained from immersion in Nature is unquantifiable. This culture says that the heart knowledge of a mother birthing at home, sleeping with her children, and nursing them for years must be verified by supporting data.

To mother from our hearts is to move into wilderness. These paths are overgrown, not much used since generations past when our great-grandmothers last walked them, following the footsteps of their mothers. Now they're thick with weeds, and where they lead exactly, we can no longer see. And yet we know this way. It's in our blood, and the weeds have kept the ground fertile, and kept the wisdom of our great-grandmothers for the day of our return.

And so, I invite the wild weeds into my garden.

I invite them for their many and varied gifts for the Earth, my garden and myself. I invite the wild weeds into my garden because they're part of the natural order of things, like the wind, the rain, the bees, and the snakes...like mothers and babies. But more than anything, I invite the wild weeds because they've become my teachers. They remind me to be strong, to send my roots deep, stand my ground, do my Earth work with grace and beauty (even though it may never be valued), and to always be ready to offer my gifts, even after having been trampled and cut down countless times.

I take these lessons into my mothering. The wild weeds in me whisper, "You're here to do this work. Stand up tall and let your wild mother nature flow through you." They are there to remind me to be the rooted and strong foundation my children can rely on. They remind me to shrug off the criticisms of others, who may not understand the wild, instinctive ways of my mothering. They remind me that I have gifts to offer to my children and the world, and even though they may be devalued now, I must be ready to offer those gifts when they're needed. They remind me that I have work to do now. It's work I may not be paid for, thanked for, or even accepted for: but it's my work; and I'm inspired to perform it with grace and beauty, like the weeds.

The culture that hates weeds
can't see the silent work,
the work of love,
the work of roots that go deep,
reaching into the heart of things.

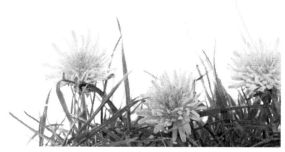

Stretch Marks

Countering televisual assault
by Dr. Richard House

'The senses become disordered when too much of a simulated world is inserted between our body and the surrounding world.'
Robert Sardello Ph.D. and Cheryl Sanders M.S.

I can just about remember being in my rural English primary school in the late 1950s and early 1960s, when television was first introduced. As I remember it, there were very clear rules that went with its introduction into our classroom: we had to sit, strictly, at a certain distance from it, and we could only watch it for a certain (limited) length of time each day.

In retrospect, over 40 years on, it's as if there was an intuitive understanding that this technology needed to be treated with great care, respect and judiciousness ~ as excess might well prove to be harmful, and that it was a technology possessing the potential for great harm as well as educational good ~ or, as Martin Large puts it in his important book Set Free Childhood (see The Mother, issue 5, p. 48), this technology can be an excellent servant, but also a very bad master indeed.

A Kaleidoscope of Damning Research Findings...

'...the potential loss of imagination, the inability to maintain a long attention span, the tendency to confuse fact with knowledge, and a homogenisation of an entire generation of minds.... These risks could even actually change the physical workings of the brain.'
Prof. Susan Greenfield on the dangers of IT

There's a whole host of research evidence ~ ably and comprehensively summarised by Martin Large ~ which convincingly exposes the damage done by TV watching, in terms of both the content of what is watched and also the developmental effects of the medium itself upon the growing child. For example, Large devotes over 80 pages to the physical and social hazards of TV watching. We have recently seen Britain's Chief Inspector of Schools, David Bell, bemoaning today's preschool children's lack of language skills compared with previous generations ~ and television is top of the list of culprits (cf. 'Should the tots be tuning-in? ~ The Independent newspaper, EDUCATION Suppl., 11 March 2004).

The present article was prompted by a recent high-profile media report that reached the world's newspaper stands, citing a research paper authored by Dr Dimitri A. Christakis and colleagues, of the Department of Pediatrics, University of Washington at Seattle, from the prestigious journal Pediatrics (Vol. 113 (4), April 2004, pp. 708-713) ~ 'Early Television Exposure and Subsequent Attentional Problems in Children'. This article's highly disturbing (but entirely predictable) findings are worth recounting here in some detail.

The research objective was to test the hypothesis that early television exposure (at ages one and three) is associated with attentional problems at age seven. Using the National Longitudinal Survey of Youth representative longitudinal data set, data were available for 1,278 children at age one and 1,345 children at age three.

The authors found that 10 per cent of children had attentional problems at age seven. Moreover, hours of television viewed per day at both ages one and three was found to be associated with attentional problems at age seven. The authors concluded that: 'Early television exposure is associated with attentional problems at age seven. Efforts to limit television viewing in early childhood may be warranted, and additional research is needed.'

These findings merely add to the existing kaleidoscope of research findings pointing to very similar conclusions. It may be instructive to offer an explanatory framework that helps us to understand just why it is that television-viewing is so harmful to young children.

Sensory Nourishment instead of Sensory Overload and Assault

'In the first part of his life, before the change of teeth, the child is... altogether a sense organ. This we have to take very literally... He is the sense organ reacting to everything to which he is exposed'.
~ Rudolf Steiner

Within Steiner education, we place great emphasis on the central importance of the senses and their early healthy development. Steiner actually referred to twelve senses (rather than the more conventional five or seven), and Steiner-inspired researchers have developed Steiner's insights on the senses in great depth.

In early life, then, the environment we create for our children is at least as important as what we say to them. We 'intellectually dominated' adults have commonly long since forgotten what it's like to be a young child; and we wrongly assume that it's quite appropriate to treat children like 'mini-adults'. But children are not 'adults in miniature'; and Steiner implores us to try to understand as far as possible the world of the child, and then meet her in that world, rather than imposing ~ often unwittingly ~ premature adult-centric ways of being and relating upon them.

The increasingly pervasive incursion of tele-visual culture into children's lives is a classic example of the adult world brutally intruding into that of the child.

For Steiner, what infants imbibe in the way of impressions influences their life forces, and therefore the actual ways in which their physical bodies develop, and also the capacity of their organs to function in a rhythmical way. Norbert Glas agreed: the awakening of the sense organs in the young child should, he writes, be 'gentle and gradual…, because the meeting with the outer world brings about a certain damping down of the forces of growth'. Thus, the sense impressions to which young children are exposed constitute a crucial influence upon healthy physical child development.

Martin Rawson emphasises how the sensory organs are not fully developed at birth, and how they first have to be 'fine-tuned, mastered and developed'. However, if they're overloaded before they're fully developed, their potential is enormously curtailed, and 'we impoverish the picture of the world that we're able to construct in our minds, as well as our understanding of it'. Rawson cautions against young children's exposure to 'random, rapidly appearing and disappearing sensory impressions that have no context [and] provide no meaning' ~ for such assaults on the senses can only lead to alienation and anxiety. In sum, young children need, first and foremost, 'to experience the world in concrete, tangible terms'.

IT technology, including TV, is entering the lives of the youngest of infants; and, perversely, sometimes this intrusion is even given a pedagogical rationale! ~ as any casual glance at the adverts in early years magazines indicates.

In the 1950s, Norbert Glas, M.D. was stressing the harmful effects of cinema and (the then new) tele-visual technology ~ for, he wrote, they 'bring about a disharmony in the activity of the sense organs…, disturb[ing] the formation of the right relationship between eyes, ears and the senses for the perceptions of thoughts, speech and the other ego'. He argued that TV 'is responsible for preventing at least five of the senses from working together in their natural relationship'. And we should rejoice that modern empirical research is, at last, increasingly confirming Glas's prophetic observations.

The self-protective 'buffer' which we adults have progressively built up between ourselves and the world is developed through a maturing understanding of that world, but the small child has not yet had the life experience which will enable it to do this. Up to about the third year, the child identifies in a very natural way with the environment in which it finds itself, and all the impressions are assimilated in an uninhibited way, and (sub)consciously assimilated. As Steiner argued, these sense impressions are combined with the other physical processes, and a kind of 'print' is made, with the child's being modelling these manifold environmental influences.

The Steiner (Waldorf) early childhood approach therefore takes great care with both the quality, and, increasingly, the quantity of sense impressions to which children are exposed. Not least, with the sensual bombardment that typifies modernist culture, young children are in mounting danger of losing the capacity to discriminate subtle sense experience ~ with quite unknown and unpredictable 'knock-on' effects into adulthood. Subtlety in the Waldorf Kindergarten is seen as a crucial developmental experience for the child ~ not least because of its healing, therapeutic role as a haven from an increasingly hyperactive technological culture.

We find great attention paid to the sensory environment: in the words of Kindergarten trainer Lynne Oldfield, 'soft pastel walls, the absence of... "untrue" plastic food and plastic tools; the use of watercolours and beeswax crayons; the care of the environment'. The integrity and qualities of the materials are paramount; for positive, constructive impressions are those impressions in which the natural origin of materials, sounds etc. can be perceived by the child. For hearing, these are the sounds of real people and real animals, and natural sounds such as the rustling of wind and tree; for seeing, they are natural colours; and for the sense of touch, they are materials such as wool, cotton, wood, sand and water. How much more nourishing these experiences are for the young child, in contrast to the crude sensory assaults of tele-visual culture. Moreover, these same precepts can seamlessly transfer into the home environment, as many a family of Waldorf-educated children will testify.

Spiritual psychologist Robert Sardello, and Cheryl Sanders, have written at length about what they call 'the care of the senses', as being a neglected dimension in education. Their little known paper is by far the most comprehensive writing I've found on the senses

~ and their systematic bludgeoning within modern materialistic culture. We currently live in a world of sensory chaos, they argue ~ and we therefore live lives which are increasingly sensorily disordered. 'Without a capacity to recognise the sensory world in which we are cast, we have no proper medium to develop thinking in healthy directions, because the body is always disturbed...'. They write, further, that 'Our senses are very disordered in the present because the surrounding world has been largely replaced by a simulated world, a world of humanly constructed objects of every type imaginable, which changes our experience from that of sensing the fullness of the world, to being overwhelmed by sensory objects which capture our awareness.' And if our senses don't give us access to the true, authentic qualities of the world, then we merely become surrounded by artificial, materialised representations. The authors refer to the harmful effects of TV on five of the senses ~ those of movement, vision, hearing, thought, and the 'I'-sense. In the case of movement ~ an absolutely crucial one for young children ~ they write that 'if all we hear all day from birth are the mechanical, electronic sounds of television and stereo, this will inflict a certain character on the way we move'. A healthy sense of movement leads to a bodily sense of being free, but in modern materialistic culture, the sense of movement is 'either too cramped or it becomes too muscle-bound. We replace the inner movement of imagination and wonder with empty entertainment and stimulation to "hold" [children's] attention.' Moreover, its disruption is most dramatic in young children, and commonly leads to serious misunderstandings of behaviour. Thus, for example, 'Psychological reasons are sought for hyperactivity and a host of other "learning difficulties", while the basis for such disorders goes unrecognised.' (Cf. my article in issues 4-6 of The Mother.)

Visually, moreover, there is a world of qualitative difference between technicolour films and colour television, on the one hand, and 'the red and orange glow at dawn, the purple of the clouds at sunset, the play of light and shadow in the forest or of plants', on the other. And with the sense of 'I', the world of mass communications, television and films is very different from the actual, lived experience of perceiving what is unique about an individual, in real, authentic face-to-face contact. 'If the senses are effectively cut off from consideration as important to education,' they write, then 'there is no possibility of educating toward a harmonious relation between the individual and the wider world'... this is supported by research findings on the long-term effects of early TV exposure. For example, 'If the corporeal senses are disordered, then the relational senses cannot develop'.

Towards Empowering Remedial Action...

'Trying to assure a balance in the sensory world... is an education of the whole human being toward freedom... Knowing that the senses, and therefore the perceptions and experiences,... are going to continue to be disrupted by the simulated world of technology... must be attended to with conscious, fully awakened attention.'
~ Sardello and Sanders

For Sardello and Sanders, then, the proper response to the sensory malaise of modern culture is what they call education towards balance. It's easy to feel relatively powerless in the face of a soulless globally ubiquitous tele-visual technology, but there's one simple action that you, the reader, can take, right now, to challenge televisual culture.

If many or most readers were to summarise the main points from this article, or the disturbing findings from the recent Paediatrics research study, and communicate this information to all of your friends and contacts, urging them to do the same, before long this information would be cascading around the globe into literally millions of inboxes and letter-boxes!...and which the commercial vested technological interests can do absolutely nothing to stop! So I invite you to 'take the moment' and to responsibly exercise this power...knowing that you'll be contributing towards an act that will do untold good, restoring as it will at least some balance to a chronically unbalanced technological culture. Such action will be entirely in line with the admirable ethos of The Mother magazine: collective empowerment towards a better world for all of the world's children.

TV-free ideas
by Veronika Robinson

Play scrabble, dominoes, puzzles or other board games
Walk through woodlands, a park, by the river, near a marshland, in a wildflower meadow, rainforest, swamp...
Bake date and banana muffins
Sew a themed, family patchwork quilt as an heirloom
Paint a picture
Make your own gift cards
Learn an instrument ~ flute, mandolin, clarinet, saxophone, piano, banjo, violin, trumpet and so on
Ice skate
Belly dancing, salsa, line dancing, waltzing
Grow organic vegetables
Grow a vertical garden ~ strawberries in connected hanging baskets
Keep a journal of your family life
Make a family tree
Adopt a pet from an animal rescue centre
Volunteer at an animal refuge; meals on wheels; riding for the disabled; a hospice; a soup kitchen
Go for a lantern walk in the starlight. Sleep under the stars
Camping ~ try camping without relying on processed foods
Make a huge pot of vegetable soup and invite friends for lunch
Sing in the bathroom
Read a novel together each evening
Visit a museum
Swimming
Learn life drawing
Celebrate the seasons with a Seasons Table ~ collecting items from Nature
Join LETS ~ local exchange trade system. Share your talents
Save fruit and vegetable seeds to grow next season
Join a choir, singing or amateur theatre group
Hand write letters to friends near and far
Bike riding ~ discover your local cycle routes
Create spiritual nourishment through meditation, and time in Nature
Study the Moon's phases
Create a full and new Moon ritual
Learn massage; treat each other to the bliss of aromatherapy massage

Write short stories
Visit botanical gardens
Go for a picnic
Visit an astronomy centre
Find out which groups exist in your local community ~ LETS, National Childbirth Trust, La Leche League, Writers' group, Sustainability network, Allotment holders group, Friends of the Earth, etc.
Play rounders, hockey, hopscotch, skipping or volleyball
Make a family joke book
Keep mealtimes sacred ~ eat together, at a table, without a TV or radio on

If you choose to have a TV, limit its use. Keep it hidden under a cloth so it's not the focus of attention. Have it in the family room, not in the bedroom. Research all the effects of tele-visual technology so that you know, without doubt, that you've made an informed decision. Recommended reading: Set Free Childhood, by Martin Large (Hawthorn Press).

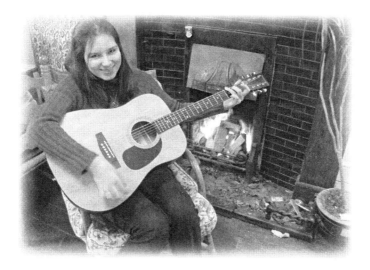

Bethany teaching herself guitar.

The ecology of attachment parenting
by Gina Sewell

I live with my lovely midwife partner, Ash, and unschooled children, Mia, Tarka, and Willow. We're nurturing our dream of finding a patch of Earth on which to walk barefoot with love, and live joyfully ever after. www. ourunschooledfamily.blogspot.com

Attachment parenting is the name we give to this: the awakening of deeply rooted awareness, an innate knowledge of mothering, which has always lived (maybe slumbered, but still lived) within the quiet truth of our hearts. I believe that when we practise gentle, conscious, attachment parenting, this is what we do. We strive to conceive and birth our babies gently and joyfully.

We hold a space for our babies' journeys Earthside with the fathomless depths of our love. We meet them skin to skin, heart to heart.

We nurture them with our amazing and magical breast milk.

We hold our babies *all the time*.

We carry them wrapped closely to us in beautiful soft cloth slings and pouches. We hold them while they feed and while they sleep, and we don't apologise, for it's as natural as night following day, and Winter giving way to the gentle strength and joy of Spring.

We have a family bed where we're all nurtured and held with love.

We respond to our babies' elimination needs respectfully and lovingly, choosing to be nappy-free, or to use soft cloth nappies against our babies' delicate skins.

As they grow, we nourish them with organic whole and living foods. And we nurture their innate need to bond with the natural world.

Put simply, we're humbled to have been chosen to grow with this beautiful little soul, and therefore we choose to parent with awareness of the sacredness of this gift every day.

Green Parenting is the name we give to living a life which celebrates the awesome interconnectedness of all living things. Everything around us is an embodiment of pure universal energy. If we be still, hold the silence, really be present with this energy, we can feel it absolutely. We can feel it in every blade of grass, every leaf, every weed, every pebble, every star, the trees which reach skyward above us, the Earth beneath our feet, and the ocean, whose energy dances with the Moon. All of these things are vibrant with joyful energy.

Our babies are this energy. How then could we choose to nurture one and destroy the other?

Choosing attachment parenting is choosing green parenting because it's about letting go of all that we're 'supposed' to want or need. We don't need to buy vast amounts of overpriced, environmentally damaging baby 'stuff'. When you're attachment parenting you are green parenting in a very concrete sense, because you don't need to be a mindless consumer. A sling, some organic terry cloths and some pre-loved baby clothes are the only things you and your baby actually need. When our first daughter, Mia, was born, almost five years ago, we'd never heard of attachment parenting, and had allowed the incessant mindless chatter of living in this crazy, consumerist society to drown out the quiet, but insistent, truthful whispers from our hearts. We bought a cot, a pram, bibs, a Moses basket, bedding, bouncy chair, highchair, musical baby night light (even now that memory jolts me... really, did we really do that?). I'm so grateful that the quiet truths of our heart don't give up and fade away when we seem deaf to their murmurs...

When Tarka was born, 22 months later, we had freecycled the cot, the bouncy chair, the cot bedding, the pram. We bought a beautiful pre-loved sling, some organic baby clothes and towels, muslin squares. And when Willow was born, almost 22 months after that, our only purchases were pre-loved baby clothes, organic terry squares and (another!) preloved sling.

Best of all, as we begin to awaken to the comforting heartbeat of our own innate maternal instinct, we discover just how wonderful it is to offer ourselves to our babies bravely, with joyful abandon. We realise, maybe for the first time, that we don't have to be a part of that huge illusion out there, where multinationals, advertising agencies, shopping centres and fast food chains reign supreme.

All of these things are exposed for the cold, fake, insignificant mistakes that they are, the first time that you hold your baby ~ your embodiment of pure loving energy ~ close to your heart, and really feel the quiet truth of it all.

Attachment parenting is green parenting because learning to listen to your inner wisdom liberates from the chains this consumer-driven society would like to bind around you. As attachment parents, we don't buy into the 'need' for fake follow-on milks, toxic plastic dummies (which first pollute our babies' bodies, and then spend centuries polluting landfill sites), cots which take our babies far away from our arms ~ arms which should be open to hold them close to our hearts for at least the whole of the first nine months of their precious lives after birth. Attachment parents don't make great consumers, so it's easy to understand why our path is belittled, scorned or viewed as plain scary. We're entering unknown (by our generation at least) territory here; this is the path which leads to the wilderness. The wild woman carrying her children at the park, breastfeeding her three year old, letting her children splash naked in the sea, run barefoot in the park, buying every item of clothing for the whole family second-hand ~ it all hints at something way too primal, it makes people uncomfortable; they stare, whisper, turn away, are compelled to look again.

Is it because they too can feel the surge, the connection to Earth that I feel when I bend down and hold my baby when she needs to eliminate, with the grass beneath her, and the wind gently caressing her soft, soft skin, or lift her to my breast, and even on the busiest, noisiest park day, get lost in the truth and beauty of her soulful blue eyes as she feeds. Attachment parenting is green parenting because how can we strive to raise strong, healthy children if the Earth, beneath our feet, is dying? All of life is part of a delicate interconnected whole, our children are themselves, they are of us and they are of the Earth. Loving and nurturing one, means loving and nurturing the other. We just need to be still, be present enough for long enough to hear the timeless, constant message of the Earth and of all the mothers who have trodden the path before us, leaving nothing but footprints. It's true that it's not the easiest path, but some things are worth fighting for.

"Look at a tree, a flower, a plant. Let your awareness rest upon it. How still they are, how deeply rooted in being. Allow Nature to teach you stillness. When you look at a tree and perceive its stillness, you become still yourself. You connect with it at a very deep level. You feel a oneness with whatever you perceive, in and through stillness. Feeling the oneness of yourself with all things is true love." ~ Eckhart Tolle (Eckhart Tolle, 'Stillness Speaks', Hodder & Stoughton 2003)

The Parenting Taboo
by Michael Mendizza

Michael Mendizza is an educational and documentary filmmaker, writer, photographer and founder of Touch the Future. www.ttfuture.org www.nurturing.us

Parenting is transient. Pregnancy morphs into birth. One transforms into two. Each age and stage opens a new threshold to something unknown and unexpected for the child, and for the parent. The skills used to meet the needs of a three year old are completely different at five. The environment is also changing, as dramatically as our children. This demands that parents reinvent themselves, in different ways, right along with their children. But they don't.

Parenting today is more challenging than ever before. Changing lifestyles, new information, fragmented families, economic challenges, more to do, less time, all confront traditional parenting models. Developing the right skills quickly, hopefully ahead of schedule, is best. Books and DVDs can help. Wisdom, however, demands experience. Today's parents must be explosive, agile learners, just like their children. But they're not.

Behind our future-shocked excuses lies an invisible force which prevents many, if not most, from mastering the art of parenting as one might master a sport or craft. There is a Parenting Taboo, and it must be broken.

Years ago, my grandfather cautioned against speaking openly about three topics: religion, politics, and how to raise kids. Core issues have their own immune system. The more entrenched the topic, the stronger the social pressure not to look or openly question, to stay away and keep quiet. When a foreign view comes close, the shields go up. The challenging idea is defended against, killed or absorbed, preserving the prevailing belief or behaviour. So strong is this taboo, that many patterns persist, more or less unchanged, for generations.

In the past, when the dynamic of cultural change was slow, when most people lived in closely-knit villages, and were bound by common stories, myths, beliefs and behaviours, this cultural immune system preserved and carried forward patterns generation after generation. There was an assumption that conforming to accepted norms was good and that deviating was bad, not only as parents, but in all aspects of communal life. Tribal, extended familial bonds are disappearing like the steam drifting off Sunday morning tea. The parent taboo remains, as strong as ever.

For a child, belonging, feeling safe and accepted are a matter of life or death. The driving force for an infant is to maintain the bond at all costs. This expresses as a deep need for physical closeness, touch, body contact, movement, audio-visual communication and gentle, affectionate play. Not being part of the group is devastating. The greatest punishment anyone, and especially a young child, can feel is rejection, abandonment. Sensory deprivation is more traumatic than physical punishment. Much of the rage we see in the world emanates from this rejection ~ religious wars, rape, domestic violence and endless cycles of child abuse.

Culture, the conservative body of accepted beliefs and behaviours, is keenly aware of rejection's primal force, and uses it daily. Everyone is caught in the net: gang members, church-goers, parents, teachers, employees and heads of state. Those in power use shame and rejection to control those who are not. There exists a global behaviour modification machine. Rejection is its currency.

Parenting is a communal, public event. Children are kin, part of the tribe or kingdom, not private property. Everyone is watching. A child's behaviour represents a daily display of our competence as an adult, not just as a parent, but as a respected member of the clan.

We think we're free, but we're not. Babies are baptised into the larger social web of believers. This, and a thousand other rituals, place the authority of the group, church, club or culture above and beyond the individual. Governments, political parties, social classes, corporations and gangs use shame and rejection to control parents; and parents use shame and rejection to control children. It's the same game everywhere you look. Misbehave, fail to conform to this rule or that, and the punishment is the same: go to your room, rejection.

As a force, built up for tens of thousands of years, the primal need to belong, and its shadow ~ rejection-induced behaviour ~ became an unspoken taboo, one that prevents many, if not most, from mastering the art of parenting as one might master a sport or craft.

In his most recent book, The Death of Religion and the Rebirth of Spirit, Joseph Chilton Pearce argues that culture operates as an invisible field. The brain translates the patterns or implicit meaning of these fields into information. Pearce began a previous book, Evolution's End, by describing how savants access vast bodies of information they have never experienced or learned. Entire populations are influenced profoundly by fields that operate beneath the level of their awareness. New human beings are imprinted by culture in the same way they are by language. The parenting taboo operates the same way ~ similar to an invisible virus; it affects almost everyone, without any being aware of the influence.

The classic tool for mass behaviour control is to invent an outside threat. It works every time. Culture tells us, it's a jungle out there. The world is full of terrorists, predators. Children must be conditioned for their own good, and it's our job to do so. There's a difference between modelling adaptive intelligence, and domestication. Chris Mercogliano argues in his book, In Defense of Childhood, that nearly all children are domesticated, fenced in like pets or livestock, and so are we. Domesticated children become domesticated adults.

Taboo means forbidden. Its opposite is freedom. Which invites more wisdom and adaptive intelligence: freedom or prohibition? Children are told 'no' eleven times to each encouraging 'yes'. No! Don't touch. Keep your hands to yourself. You'll poke your eye out. No. No. No. Do that again and it's time-out for you, Buster. Go to your room.

We're conditioned from early childhood to obey, to do as we're told, colour between the lines, always looking over our shoulder, knowing that someone will tell us to stop, do it this way, not that. We're compared, graded, judged, sometimes praised (a shadow form of punishment), labelled, pigeon-holed, categorised and certified. Yes, this child toes the line, behaves in predictable ways, can be trusted not to deviate from accepted norms.

Parenting is a communal, public event. Children are kin, part of the tribe or kingdom, not private property. Everyone is watching.

A child's behaviour represents a daily display of our competence as an adult, not just as a parent, but as a respected member of the clan.

We're led to believe that inner and outer anarchy will spread widely, without constraint. Taboos prevent us from even questioning this assumption. J. Krishnamurti insisted that intelligence is innate, not learned or accumulated; it's orderly, co-operative, kind and compassionate. All the so-called higher spiritual qualities, as the wise have said for ages, are innate. Only in freedom can these most valued qualities express. Maher Baba said it wonderfully. "Love must spring spontaneously from within, and is in no way amenable to any form of force or coercion." Inward, psychological freedom is our birthright. But we're not free ~ and that's exactly what taboos are designed to do.

To this we must add the weight of habituation. New perceptions, skills and capacities open and develop in a heightened state of energy and attention. Children call this heightened state play. As the new becomes familiar, through a well defined 'cycle of competence' (novel discovery, repetition, variation), the heightened energy and attention found in authentic play diminishes. Habits set in. Full spectrum intelligence is replaced with predictable reflexes. Physicist David Bohm insists that there's no real intelligence in a reflex. The more reflexive, mechanical and predictable our behaviour, the less intelligence we're expressing. All of these forces contribute to the parenting taboo.

Bev Bos, a most respected early parent-child educator, describes how parents are under a spell, caught in a trance. We, more or less, blindly do unto others what others have done to us. And we identify with these habits. When someone challenges our reflexive behaviour, we feel attacked personally, and react defensively. Fearing too much public attention, we impose strict boundaries on our children, for their own good of course, to cover our ass. We might be sent to our room, not belong, and our children pay the price.

Compare this to the attitude of a committed athlete or a sincere apprentice. The road to mastery is vast, always extending. We reach one level only to find another, unexpected and richer, opening before us. Lifelong learning and practice is the key to mastery, regardless of skill or craft, including parenting. We hit the ball and watch it fly. Learning takes place on the instant, as we watch with wonder. If the results match our intent, we stay the course. If not, we adapt and hit the ball again. The art of parenting is a skill anyone can master. But we don't.

If we're wise (or lucky), we seek the guidance of a trusted friend, a mentor, who whispers, only on occasion, 'that was as nice a shot as it gets', or, 'close your eyes and hit it again, softer'. We seek, even pay, coaches and guides for their counsel. We may confuse performance with our personal identity, but we don't relate defensively to the advice of our mentors. That would defeat the purpose. Defensive learning strengthens only our defence. Imagine what the world would look like if today's parents approached their ever-changing challenges with the same lifelong learning attitude as elite athletes, a master craftsman or artist. For this to begin, each must face and break the parenting taboo.

Rather than repeating the same stale pattern day-in and day-out, adults would approach each parent-child encounter as a learning opportunity. While the outer game might be exploring frogs or building a tree house, the inner game is all about relationship, how to be more present, attentive, listening, imaginative, responsive and empathic. The parenting taboo develops none of these. Rather, it prevents and corrupts them all.

Which will serve our children, us and the planet more fully: living under the spell, or creatively reincarnating every day? There's no choice. Adaptive learning grows more and more necessary as the world changes faster and faster. The question is, how?

To begin, we must understand the simple fact that child development is dependent on adult development. Nature invests in adult development, and upon that, the child climbs to the next evolutionary step. Personal and global transformation are model-dependent. Forget institutionalised (conditioned, behaviour modification-based) schooling. The latent potential of every child is activated and developed by interacting with the model-environment. Monkey see, monkey do. This principle is woven into our nature, and has been for millions of years. Information is great, but we, you and I, the adult culture, must become the change we wish to see in the world. The next frontier in education is addressing, head on, this urgent evolutionary challenge.

We must overcome the cultural tipping point that occurred at the end of World War II. Prior to the war, parent development took place (never perfect, of course) in the intimate human experiences we call the extended family, village or tribe. Parent mentors and coaches (grandparents, aunts and uncles), lived in the house, or next door. This was true for 80% of American households. After the war, 80% of those families did not have a grandparent living in the home. Sprawling suburbs, mothers entering the workforce, TV and institutionalised childcare replaced having morning tea with granny.

Working mothers, day care and TV crippled experiential-based parent development. Parents lost their mentors. They lost community, real family, and all the learning that takes place in these intimate relationships. Parents and children were the big losers.

Every intimate relationship represents the potential for explosive learning. This is how wisdom is born, how real development unfolds, in relationship. How can a mother or father master the art of parenting when commuting on the freeway or answering the phone in a corporate cubicle? Great musicians play music. Great athletes practise. Scientists wonder. Chefs taste, and they do so in the company of experienced mentors. The same is true for great parents.

Realising that we, not our children, are the next frontier in education, parents will naturally seek out and immerse themselves in dynamic, co-learning relationships with other adults and mentors facing similar challenges. Like the extended family of days gone by, this parent development community will gather on a regular basis, not just on birthdays and Easter, at least once a month, to experience and practise real acceptance and belonging, trust, respect, curiosity, deep listening and empathy, to be inspired by the best science and age-appropriate child development practices in the world, and to share with others what is working in their lives and what is not. They'll come together to practise the skills that need more attention, just like dancers and world class athletes. The goal will not be to fix the child. Kids aren't broken. The goal will be continuing adult development that mirrors in the adult's life the explosive learning and growth modelled by children, as Nature designed. And this adult development will take place neighbourhood by neighbourhood, in every city, region and country throughout the world.

This will take place when there's a place, a safe, sacred playground where parents gather, learn, practise and master the art of joyful, playful parenting. It will be close, convenient, cost little or nothing, be filled with up-to-date information, mentors and lots of hands-on experiences. Parents need playgrounds to practise and master new skills. But they don't have any.

There are safe, mentored playgrounds for just about anything you want to be or become, except being a parent. Martial artists have dojos. Basketball players have courts, balls and hoops. Dancers have studios and partners. Chefs have gardens and kitchens. Parents have books, DVDs, and a few mandated classes which are about as experiential as traffic school.

Don't be confused. Information is not experience. We don't eat the menu when we're hungry. Our bodies need whole, nutritious food, enriched, life-changing experience, and we need it every day. The parent taboo prevents this continued adult development. Now is the time to break the spell, and replace data with inspired, mentored, neighbourhood-based experience.

One final courageous act is necessary to break the spell. Early childcare providers, practitioners and educators must reinvent themselves. They are, by default, today's parenting mentors. They have the playground and the kids, everything adults need, to master the art of parenting.

What's missing is a broader vision, one that reunites adult development with child development. They go hand in hand.

The instant the early childcare and education network grasps this simple fact, the paradigm changes. The focus of attention broadens. Childcare providers will see immediately that they face two equal challenges: to provide optimal, play-based learning experiences for children; and simultaneously provide the same mentored play-based experience for parents.

The parent taboo falsely separated adult development from child development. Providers are well-trained to meet the needs of kids, but have little or no training, skills, resources or funding to meet the continuing education needs of parents. Providers need support, just like parents, and that support must come from the local community. The local community doesn't know what to do, how to get involved, so nothing happens.

There is a spell breaker. It's called The Nurturing Project. It holds a broader, balanced view of adult-child development. It makes available inspired tools and resources to help providers respond to the needs of today's parents with the same training and skill they now use to meet the needs of children.

The Nurturing Project creates the network, the local, non-profit funding and the open channels of communication necessary to engage the extended community in support of today's parents and providers, neighbourhood by neighbourhood, in every city, region and country throughout the world.

The spell has already been broken. One by one, like Sleeping Beauty, we're waking up, opening our eyes and seeing a new world, our children's world, blossoming like flowers in Spring. To find out how to be a spell breaker in your community, visit www.nurturing. us. Then stand back and watch what happens.

Skin care in the Sun
by Star Khechara

Star Khechara is a naturopathic nutritionist, holistic beauty advisor, workshop leader and writer.

The sky is blue, the Sun is shining, and finally we can start leaving the house without a million layers plus hat, scarf and umbrella just in case. However, a new concern now grips us: the fear of the Sun! With all the media hype surrounding Sun and skin cancer, what loving parent wouldn't be smothering their precious ones in layers of gloop, which promise to protect with an army of SPF artillery against the evil menace which is skin cancer? While it's true that cancer can be a deadly disease, there are certain facts that just don't add up in the 'sunscreen use = protection from skin cancer' formula.

The burning issue

To put it another way, sunscreens are meant to help protect the skin from burning, by preventing most of the UV rays accessing the skin, provided they're used in the manner intended by the manufacturer.

The issues are how many of us do reapply these lotions thickly every two hours, or after sweating? How many of us believe that the sole cause of skin cancer is Sun exposure? And how many of us believe that sunscreen is the only way we can protect our skin from burning? We're all the targets of outrageous marketing and media hype. A quick glance at official statistics will show that skin cancer rates are steadily rising, as are the sales of sunscreen (does that not seem odd?). In fact, in 2005 there were almost 2,000 deaths from malignant melanoma (the fatal form of skin cancer), and yet, in that same year, sales of sun-protection in Britain were up by 17%.

One of the most important issues is the chemicals present in sunscreen, and their toxic effect on the body and planet, and also that the sunscreen itself plays a part in the overall cancer picture. This isn't necessarily as a direct causation; but the fact that people believe themselves to be protected may mean they spend more time exposed to the stronger Sun rays, and therefore still burn, suffering skin damage, potentially leading to cancer.

Of the two types of sun-protection (chemical and physical), the chemical ones are worse. The UV-absorbing ingredients are known to be toxic to many forms of life, and many have hormone mimicking properties ~ not really the sort of thing you want on your brand new babe! The other types use minerals, such as zinc oxide, which work as a physical barrier, reflecting the Sun. These are more 'natural', however a lot of companies have come under fire (yes, even 'green' ones) for their use of nano-particles in these products. Nano-technology is one of the newest threats to human and planetary health, as the particles are so small they can enter the body through the skin, and even cross the blood/brain barrier. Shocking stuff! They're also now ever-present in our environment, and, like GM plants, once they're there, they're always there.

It's a topic of which I've only scratched the surface. As to what we can do for ourselves in the holistic sun-protection sense, there isn't really any potion to make that will count as a proper SPF. However, it's important to use common sense:

[] The skin needs Sun exposure for health, and to form vitamin D
[] Over-exposure and burning will damage the skin (whether it causes cancer or not)
[] The Sun is hottest between 11am and 4pm
[] Clothes, a hat, and sitting in the shade are the only truly healthy options for protection from the Sun
[] A healthy lifestyle and an excellent (high in raw plant foods) diet will create healthy, resilient skin, which burns less

If you've been over-zealous with your Sun exposure, then these will help:

[] Keep a bottle of witch-hazel in the fridge, and splash onto sore areas liberally
[] Cold tea, cold yoghurt and cold water all help, too
[] Keep in the shade after being burnt, to let the skin recover
[] When the redness/hotness has gone, use a really good plant butter (e.g. shea butter), to nourish the parched skin
[] Drink plenty of water, to hydrate from within
[] Have cool baths, with drops of lavender oil added, to speed up the healing process
Have a wonderful Summer, and love your skin.

Nourishing The Mother
by Tish Clifford

Nourishing the mother is the way back home to the return of biological and spiritual sanity here on this awesome planet we share.

For over six years I've been closely involved with the work of radical plant bio-chemist and independent researcher, Tony Wright, on his astonishing model of consciousness restoration from the unusual and unprecedented mechanical angle that is presented in his book, Left In The Dark. It would appear that it's taken me almost as long to fully understand the implications of such research, and then to fully update my reality to encompass such a multifaceted piece of scholarship. Ultimately, what I'm realising most is that this work only continues to awaken the truth that I've felt for a long time in my own life. Nourishing the mother is so profound a truth, that it can almost be overlooked as some fluffy crap! And yet, if we take a logical look at this statement, we can begin to understand how radical and crucial this is.

As mothers, we're the 'biological factories' for our children. If we choose the role of staying at home, and providing the foundational sustenance for our children, we're their 'biological factories' for 18 years or more. The chemicals which flood our children's and our own brains have a key effect on how we think and how we behave, and I'm not just talking about food here. Our neuro-endocrine system, in effect, governs our behaviour, and everything affects our neuro-endocrine system (either positively or negatively) ~ how each of us behaves, then, ultimately, collectively creates what we as humans experience; how we treat each other; and how we treat the Earth, our home. There are so many loops to how we can, and need, to create restoration on planet Earth; and having pondered and explored these issues for over seventeen years, I continue to return to the mother... of course.

Nourishing the mother is the most crucial element because it's the mother who biologically creates the child's brain during pregnancy and breastfeeding. The brain, and what happens bio-chemically within it, somehow generates our sense of self: our consciousness. I believe that natural, child-led breastfeeding should be practised until around seven years of age, but irrespective of when this process ends, the mother needs to be held in the highest possible esteem.

A question that I continually ask myself is "how do we inspire the human race to ponder this truth and then act upon it?" How can we get our men to turn back towards us, nourishing their family through nourishing us in the multitude of ways that are needed? And how can we get society to turn back to our men, and nourish them, so they can nourish us? We're all part of this one, vast, continually-connected hub of Universal Life. It needs to start within our own self.

As women, mothers, we've come through a collective thought pattern that for hundreds of years has been dominated by a system that no longer reveres us: no longer holds us where we belong. We need to unravel and heal this thought patterning so that we can truly allow ourselves to be nourished and supported. Nourishment is needed in many different ways to heal, and to create a positive and healthy uterine environment that is optimal for growing life; and then beyond, through the breastfeeding years; then still, whilst our children are growing into puberty; and then adulthood. I envisage a time when, as a species, we start to really create nurturing, holistic environments for this sacred time, culturally, as well as individually.

Mothers, when they're supported thoroughly and naturally, yearn to give themselves 100% to their children; this is a biologically spiritual truth, hidden, or not so hidden, within each mother. Personally, I've never felt thoroughly supported. When we choose to bring our children up in radically different ways to the norm, it would appear to be even more difficult to get the support and nourishment we need. Yet, I know that inherited beliefs have also hindered my ability to create situations and relationships that fully nurture and support me through the journey of being a mother. Over the last few years, I've dedicated my life to a more reclusive path, meditating daily ~ sometimes for four hours or more, to try and gain some access to inner truth and energetic experience. This time out (or in!) has strengthened my connection to my feminine essence. It's allowed me to feel the truth that to manifest spiritual paradise on Earth, we need to turn to the mother in awe-inspired respect.

As women, we can recognise the current reality of a patriarchal dominated system, and still open ourselves up in trust. Not a naive trust, but a trust in a Higher Force that can guide our lives and enrich us. For many of us, even those who have supportive partners, financially, experience some strife. Those of us who yearn for a more simple life find the hectic world of creating an abundant income, so that we can buy somewhere to live our simple lives, challenging. There are now many more parents who are struggling to cope alone, having to do the job that was meant to be fulfilled by a tribe.

My meditative couple of years has left me feeling more nourished. I feel I've given my soul space and time to be. This, in turn, has allowed me a regeneration that has cleansed my home. It's allowed me time to create an even more beautiful environment to bring forth what I need in order to continue to relax and surrender into my feminine power, and creative force, as a mother and living-breathing woman. In my deeper spaces, I've been affirming choices that guide my life in the direction of nourishment and support. I yearn to give myself fully to my children, and yet, I also know that this can't happen without me being nourished too. I'd like to share with you some of the things that have come out of my meditations:

Appreciation of the masculine

It's very easy, when I'm frustrated with life, and in particular the men in my life, to become dismissive of masculine energy. Yet I've also discovered how important it is to really appreciate the masculine. In my own life, this has completely changed my relationship with my father. I can now appreciate the many masculine gifts he brought to my childhood. I feel more confident in my femininity when I'm appreciative of the men in my life. I now actively appreciate any acts of masculinity that aim at protecting, loving and caring for my family, or me, as a woman and mother.

Gratitude for life

Sometimes when I'm feeling really stressed with my circumstances, especially the financial and practical side of my life, I start feeling ungrateful. In my meditations, I can come across deeper spaces of gratitude for the many gifts I do have, and my life is always transformed in these moments. Even just sitting next to my children can fill my being with bliss.

Biological reverence

The utter awesomeness of Nature really rocks my soul. A way that I choose to nourish myself is by being in Nature. I never feel such divine power, energy and connection, as when I'm immersed in Nature, and all its beauty and majesty.

Simplicity

The more I meditate, the more I desire simplicity in my life, on every level.

Beingness

We're human beings, and although it's obvious we do need to *do*, I've also found that it's in my beingness where I feel most at home, alive and energised. As women, especially, I feel we need to spend much time surrendered to our beingness. When I'm filled up with beingness, I find it naturally spills over into my daily activities, such as food preparation, cleaning, and caring for the children. Being a Leo, and having a strong connection to my own masculine energy, I've realised that I need to actively take time out to reconnect. I can feel guilty and lazy if I do this too often, and yet, at the same time, I understand that to get my needs met as a woman, I need to be able to surrender to my feminine beingness.

Trust

As I grow, and learn to nourish myself, I'm developing more trust that my needs will be met by a bigger force than myself. Recently, I've been finding I'm naturally affirming and opening to this higher divine power. I'm trusting that my femininity will be respected by life, and by those who are in my life.

Affirmations

I allow my feminine energy
to open and flower.
I allow myself to be supported
in all areas of mothering and womanhood.
I choose to be nourished
on every level of my being.
I allow myself to attract masculine energy which protects and cares
for my feminine energy.
I choose to be surrounded by
supportive, responsible adults,
where there's mutual nourishment.
I choose to be nourished by life in ways that are in alignment with
my highest truth.
I allow myself to be blessed by life.

Living with The Continuum Concept
by Veronika Sophia Robinson

Six months before I met my husband, I was doing a Wellness course, and The Continuum Concept was recommended reading. I'd heard a bit about the theories of the 'in-arms' experience, and was keen to learn more, but hadn't had any luck in sourcing the book.

My husband and I moved in together the day after deciding we wanted to journey through life as a couple. As I helped to clear out his home, he handed me a book and said "You'll like this". It was The Continuum Concept. I was so thrilled! The words rang true to every part of my being. Although it would be another 11 months before I could put the ideas into practice with my own child, I read and re-read what felt to be the ultimate and 'right' way to parent. After I became a mother, I owned three copies of the book, and always had them out on loan to friends. Just the other day I was in my local bookshop, browsing, and saw it sitting on the shelf, like an old friend. I smiled. The Continuum Concept and Joseph Chilton Pearce's Magical Child have defined our style of parenting. It's so hard to imagine having raised our children any other way ~ so counter-intuitive to our biological needs as human beings.

Jean Liedloff, the book's author, had travelled to South America, and lived with the Yequanna, a Stone Age Indian tribe. Here she saw, first-hand, how children were raised. It was in stark contrast to the way most people in Western culture raise their children. She also pointed out how differently the Yequanna children behaved compared to our Western children. I was intrigued. I was hooked.

When my daughter was born, she barely left my arms. If she wasn't in my arms, she was in her father's. We bathed/showered together, slept together, and I kept her in the front pack (a sling attached to the front of the mother's body) inside my seatbelt in the back seat of the car if we had to drive anywhere. Highly illegal I realised some time later, but my instinct for body contact overrode my desire to stay on the right side of the law.

I was determined that my precious baby would have all her biological needs met, to the point I would do ridiculous things like try and get dressed with her in my arms. It's not actually that easy pulling up your knickers when your hands are holding a baby!

By the time number two baby came along, when baby number

one was just a tender, young 22 months old, there was a little problem to deal with regarding the in-arms phase. What would happen to baby number two while I was dealing with baby number one? Toddlers have BIG needs! There was no way baby number two could be carried 24/7 in the way her sister had, simply because there weren't enough arms. I still bathed with both of them, slept with them both, tandem nursed, and yet, it wasn't enough. I discovered I wasn't superhuman, and I certainly wasn't capable of providing all their needs on my own, or as a couple. Nature didn't plan it that way either.

Before long, baby number two would have to be content propped on a pillow beside the shower while I washed my hair and got dressed. Baby number two, along with baby number one, HAD to be in car seats. This in itself was quite traumatic as neither of them were good travellers. They both already expressed a high NEED to be in-arms. Modern life was proving to be a terribly inconvenient adjunct to our natural way of living.

The Continuum Concept has so much to teach us. It's an invaluable guide to parenting and implementing ways to raise our children gently and with respect. Where it goes 'wrong', if I dare suggest it in those terms, isn't so much the book, but our interpretation of its message. Modern, Western mums in nuclear families simply don't have the back-up the Yequanna do, and yet they're trying to do the same style of parenting. You simply can't do it without losing your sanity. It's a very hard thing to hear when you're passionate about an ideal. For some of us, compromise just doesn't seem an option. However, the higher our ideals, the harder we fall when we don't attain them. Our modern lifestyle simply isn't geared up for Yequanna-style parenting. End of story. Or is it?

There are other aspects which make following The Continuum Concept to the letter inadvisable for our culture. Jean Liedloff commented on the happy Yequanna babies and how they never get colic, or have problems socialising. To read such high praise, and then witness our baby screaming its heart out, or our two year old beating up a peer, we wonder what on Earth went wrong, as we'd done 'everything right'.

What makes the theories of The Continuum Concept work for the Yequanna isn't just the practice, it's the environment in which they live. Think about this: while most Westerners with busy lives probably have dreams of being late for work or school, the Yequanna have dreams reflective of their lifestyles. If the day is based around gathering fruit and nuts, or socialising, they simply won't have the same type of stresses that most of us do. They won't be watching the clock to make sure dinner is ready when husband comes home. They won't be racing off to get junior from nursery or the older kids from after-school activities, while frantically filling in a tax return and scheduling an emergency dental appointment.

That colic is so prevalent in our society is because it's a mirror of our culture! Our babies are reflecting to us the complete disharmony of our fast-paced way of life. They're telling us in the very best way that they can that they don't like what's on offer! We need to let our babies off the hook here; the problem isn't with them, it's with us and the culture we live in. If a mother wants to ease her baby's colic, or avoid it altogether, then complete removal of stress is required on the part of the mother ~ assuming and hoping she's the main caregiver at such a tender age.

A young baby is so in-tune with how the mother is feeling, that even if she is carrying him in-arms, breastfeeding on cue, etc., if she's looking at the clock, feeling on edge or needing to get things 'done', rather than just 'being' with her baby, then the baby will build up a nervous energy which needs releasing. Colic cry (scream) is the baby saying "BE STILL" with me.

We take our toddler to play group and he starts biting other children. In our horror we can't help but question why he isn't being sociable when he's had such a good upbringing. Again, the problem isn't that the concept failed, but that we failed the concept, if it can be put in such crude terms. It's no cause for regret for any parent, it's simply a fact. Certainly there's no reason to feel guilty.

However, there are ways to make the most of the wonderful life-affirming messages in The Continuum Concept and raise happy, healthy kids, and nurture yourself as a parent. The key is balance, and a realistic attitude to what it means to raise kids naturally in an unnatural world.

In a nutshell, The Continuum Concept's key philosophy is that of trust. We get so caught up in the words 'in-arms' that we lose sight of what it actually means to be in a mother's arms, and why we're doing it in the first place. Our babies need to be able to trust us. In an ideal world, the main two ways are through constant skin-to-skin contact, and breastfeeding on cue. Unlike me, you can put your baby on the bed while you get dressed, and talk to her, sing to her, even bend over and touch her while making eye contact. She won't feel deprived in the way a baby left abandoned in another room will feel, as she can still hear and see you. When you're dressed, then pick her up. Sometimes we simply have to do jobs around the house that are infinitely easier without a baby in our arms. It's OK to sometimes put baby on the floor (on a pillow), beside you, while you load the washing machine or do the dishes. The key is to make sure she spends the majority of her time in-arms.

When we seek out this way of living, we intuitively seek out our own Yequanna tribe, but for most of us, the only tribe we have is inside the walls of our own home.

We search for support. Yet to examine the culture we're brought up in magnifies exactly why we don't tend to have the village. We were raised in isolation, not taught to be 100% emotionally willing to help and support others. Our cultural message is 'nothing for nothing'. We carry this deep within our being, so much so that most of us don't even recognise it as a driving force in our lives. Most of us are devoid of trust. Often, though, when we point the finger and say "I don't trust you," we're actually affirming that we don't trust ourselves.

We know in our hearts, of course, that this isn't the way forward for humanity, yet to undo our own conditioning in order to create what is our birthright, takes some doing. Raising our children Continuum style allows us the space in which to heal our own childhood of mistrust, of being let down by our parents, as well as breaking the pattern in place.

Our search for a village leads us to support groups, and while they're invaluable and often provide friendships, they're but snippets of time in the course of a week. They don't bring support in the home on a permanent basis. They don't, as a rule, give the extra arms to hold the baby while you dress, or someone to make dinner or sweep the floor.

In an ideal world, mothers would create conscious communities around them before pregnancy. We don't live in an ideal world. However, does that mean we can't at least attempt to bring more love, harmony, acceptance and joy into our own lives, and that of other people? Surely, if ever there was a time for change it is now, in the 2000s.

Society is against us and our baby from the moment we discover we're pregnant. The drive to separate mother and child begins with pregnancy tests, by not allowing a mother to believe what her body is already telling her: she has tender breasts, wees a lot, her period is late, she's feeling emotional…And STILL she can't believe it. Why would a plastic pregnancy kit be more honest than your own body's messages? More importantly, why don't we trust the obvious signs of pregnancy: the signs our foremothers have used since we started cycling to the Moon?

During pregnancy, separation occurs again, when she's not allowed to trust that her baby is growing as Nature planned. A scan steps in between mother and child. A radiographer has to give you the all clear, to let you know if it's OK to continue with your pregnancy. And so it goes on. Separation at birth with the unnecessary weighing of babe on scales, eyes wiped with swabs, vitamin K injection rudely jabbed into baby's tender flesh. And then he's delivered into a crib/cot. Separation continues with a bottle, a dummy, a pram/buggy, a nursery/day care, babysitters, and finally, school. These acts of separation are so much a part of our culture, that very few people stop and question the effect they have on the parent child relationship.

Turning our back on any and all of the devices and intentions which apparently make parenting easier, is almost a societal taboo.

So, if this is the grand cultural message: that 'mother is disposable' ~ is it any wonder that for parents who wish to reclaim humanity's biological need for closeness and trust, they find themselves in a never-never land where trusting the needs of our children is an alien concept?

Gentle alternatives to yelling and hitting
by Veronika Sophia Robinson

If you find that you can't control yourself, and are constantly hitting or shouting at your children, please seek help. The following suggestions should be pasted up somewhere you'll see them regularly, such as a kitchen cupboard.

[] Look for the funny side in a situation. As constant caretakers, we often get overwhelmed, and, consequently, literally cry over spilled milk. Try and get some perspective, and realise that there's nothing your little child/ren can do 'wrong' that will tip the Earth off its axis.

[] Create a calm area ~ this is for when your children aren't coping with situations very well. In this place they can read, lie on a cushion on the floor, do colouring in, listen to a CD, or model something with play clay. Avoid having a TV or computer in this area. You could play some classical music.

[] Remind yourself that you're the adult in the situation. On your side is an ability to 'step outside of the situation', and to bring calm and peace through mindful awareness. Your behaviour is a model for the next generation of parents.

[] Say the alphabet backwards before screaming.

[] Promise yourself that you'll do conscious, connected breathing for five minutes before reacting. When you've done this, ask yourself if you have some needs that haven't been met, such as food, company or sleep.

[] Imagine being your child for a few moments. How does it feel to have the big, red, angry face of a parent yelling at you or shaking your tiny body?

[] Find a seat, sit down, have a cup of calming tea, like chamomile, or a few drops of Rescue Remedy; and tell your children that you'll be with them in a few minutes. If necessary, have them sit in another room (assuming they're safe) while you gather yourself. YOU CAN DO THIS!

Stretch Marks   321

[] Phone a friend or family member (one who doesn't use violence) to ask for emotional support, and to remind you that hands are not for hitting.

[] Hug each other! Children often play up as a way of getting attention. "It's better to be wanted by the police, than not wanted at all."

[] Affirm: "I am calm, loving and able to parent gently."

[] APOLOGISE. No human is ever too big or small to not benefit from apologising or forgiving. In one African culture, when someone in the village has done something 'bad', everyone stops what they're doing, and together they surround the person in question. Each person, in turn, tells him of all the wonderful qualities he has; all the good and marvellous deeds he's done during his life. This ceremony sometimes goes on for days. This is true forgiveness.

Sexuality

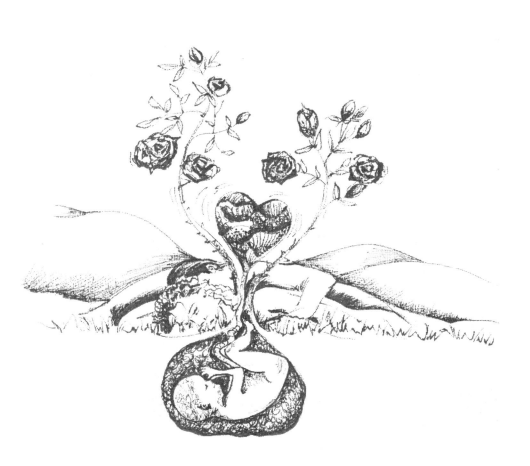

Yin and yang, by Andri Thwaites

My Menstrual Journey
by Sophie Style

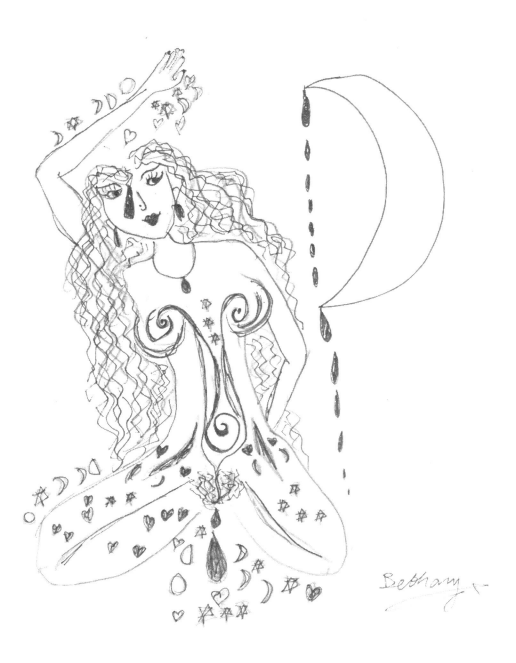

I'll never forget the day during my school holidays, aged twelve, when I found a small brown patch in my underwear. My heart began to race, and I rushed to find my mother, who was in the kitchen. As soon as I saw her, I burst into tears and cried "Mum, I've got the curse!" This was the term my mother used, passed down by my maternal grandmother, and I suppose her mother, grandmother and great-grandmother for many generations before. Mostly I felt scared and unprepared, my body out of my control, suddenly no longer that of a child. Partly I was relieved that I would go back to school and join the clan of over half the 'initiated' girls in my class who already bled each month.

Almost eighteen years later, I sat in a circle with twelve other women during one of our regular gatherings, and we each shared our memories of our First Blood: how we felt; how our parents responded; what we called it. Apart from one of us in the group (whose parents opened a bottle of champagne in celebration!), all of us in our various families and communities were met with a mixture of embarrassment, secrecy, or matter-of-factness ~ the less said about it the better. I sometimes wonder what the following years of my menstrual cycle would have been like had this rite of passage into adolescence and womanhood been recognised and honoured in a meaningful way by my family and community.

Instead, I can only remember my mother telling me that it would be very likely that I would have painful periods as she and my grandmother had both had, but that these would lessen over time. I did indeed have increasingly painful cramps that spread from my womb to my whole pelvic area and down my inner thighs. Every month I spent one or sometimes two days in bed with a hot-water bottle and strong painkillers to relieve the intense aches. When I was nineteen, I decided to go and see my doctor about this, and her only suggestion was to go on the Pill, which I did. During this time, I became more and more disconnected from my body, and convinced that my monthly consumption of tampons and pads was nothing more than a dirty nuisance, waste of money, and yes, a woman's curse. I remember joking to my friends that I couldn't wait until the menopause, when I would be rid of the hassle of periods!

Six years later, a friend of mine gave me a Moon calendar, and suggested that I could keep a record of when I bled each month, and find out which phase of the Moon this coincided with. I thought it was an interesting idea (without feeling any connection at that point between the two things), and as I'd recently stopped taking the Pill, I was curious to see what my cycle would do without the interference of artificial hormones. Initially my cycle was quite long, up to 35 days, and then very irregular, with no obvious bearing on the Moon. I carried on what began as a practical record-taking exercise over the next few years, and gradually began to take note of other details, like how I felt physically and emotionally before and during my period. I began to notice, unsurprisingly, that I'd have more arguments with my partner when I was premenstrual. I also felt bloated, with tender breasts, and craved comfort foods like pizza, pasta and potatoes. As I was still having painful cramps, another friend gave me a list of helpful herbs and aromatherapy oils. I found that hot baths and massaging my womb and inner thighs with clary sage and lavender blends significantly eased the pain. The more I gave time and attention to my cycle, the more I made changes in my diet, and the more I focused on relaxing and breathing with the pain, the less intense my cramps and discomfort became.

Being involved in environmental campaigns, I decided to move from using standard disposable tampons to organic tampons and pads; and then, to my excitement, I found out that I could use a small sea-sponge instead, which would last for at least six months, and meant no more non-biodegradable waste. Most of all, this initiated a new relationship with my own blood, which up until then I had, deep down, viewed as something basically unpleasant and dirty. Rinsing my sponge by hand a few times a day brought me into direct contact with my reddish-brown, fleshy secretions that gradually took on an entirely different quality.

Rather than disdainfully chucking the red water down the sink, whenever I could I started to pour this now magical liquid, full of iron and nutrients, into the Earth, or onto our house-plants, now that we lived in a flat. When I sang the song, "Earth my body, water my blood, air my breath and fire my spirit" as the red water trickled into the soil, it suddenly took on a new meaning to me as a woman: that there really is no separation between me, my body, and the Earth and her cycles.

Little by little, I've taken more and more interest in the different stages of my menstrual cycle, helped especially by exploring a wonderfully insightful series of questions written by a women's health collective, and by filling in, over the past four months, a Moon Dial or Menstrual Mandala. Beginning on the first day I bleed, I write down any notable feelings, dreams, occurrences or changes in my body every day, and choose a colour to represent my overall mood. Although there are many fluctuations and irregularities, dependent also on external circumstances, I feel that I'm slowly beginning to see patterns emerging at each stage: from menstruation, to the start of a new cycle, to ovulation, post-ovulation and pre-menstruation, and slowly feeling in my body the connection between these and the various phases of the Moon.

This connection comes especially to life for me when I bleed just as the Moon is entering her darkest phase. Suddenly I can feel the synchronicity between the end of my cycle and the end of the Moon's cycle, my need to go inward and retreat as the Moon disappears, the shedding of the lining of my womb as the Moon symbolically dies once again. I often feel strongly drawn to write in my journal, to reflect on the previous month, and notice what I need to let go of and what I've learnt. Just before I start bleeding, I frequently have a rush of energy to clean our flat, which somehow feels like the so-called "nesting instinct" before birth, as if to create for myself a harmonious space in which to bleed. It feels like a time of clearing out and releasing, a little death each month, before the rebirth of another menstrual cycle, as the crescent new Moon appears in the evening sky. I love the feel of those first few days when I've finished bleeding: a fresh, rising energy that inspires me to start new projects, or approach ongoing ones afresh, becoming more active after a time of introspection. I particularly love this time if my cycle coincides with the waxing Moon ~ our growing, radiant energies in tandem. Very often there's a very tangible increase in my sexual drive and energy, both in daily life and in my dreams. I can tell when I'm becoming most fertile from the increased flow of vaginal discharge, and now I can sometimes feel myself ovulating, on a few occasions in tune with the full Moon, with a rush of creativity and expansive energy!

Soon after ovulation, I feel I move into quite a different energy, gradually becoming more reflective and slowing down, often tired. Then, as I've now realised, up to 10 days before I bleed I begin to notice that I'm getting more sensitive and more irritable. The infamous "PMT" starts to raise her perilous head, and I move into the most challenging time of the whole month. I've noticed how many people say that the more we honour our cycles and look after our bodies, the less we'll experience premenstrual symptoms. I've certainly found this to be true on a physical level, as much as this can be separated: but on an emotional level, over the past year, I've experienced more intense anger and frustration at this time than ever before in my life. Rather than simply reducing these feelings to the particular levels of oestrogen and progesterone in my body, which is the predominant view, it makes so much more sense to me when women like Christiane Northrup write that this is a time to face our unfinished emotional business, an invitation to look even deeper at imbalances or painful areas in our lives, that often remain hidden the rest of the month. My shadow comes up more strongly than ever, most of all in my relationship, which is of course an opportunity to bring these repressed parts of myself into the light of awareness, to give them the compassion and understanding they never had ~ so much easier to say than to do! My dreams are often full of snakes, unresolved conflicts, inner fears.

In my search for other clues about the sometimes uncontrollable fury I feel, I came across a chapter in Eckhart Tolle's book, The Power of Now, where he describes premenstrual tension as the awakening of what he calls the "collective female pain-body": all the accumulated pain that women have suffered under patriarchy over thousands of years. The rage that surges through me when I'm premenstrual does indeed feel like it goes well beyond my personal experience and wounds. Tolle speaks of transmuting this pain-body so that it no longer comes between you and your true self. The snakes that come to me in my dreams remind me that in the same way as they lose their skin, I also lose the lining of my womb each month, and through this process, can also let go of old patterns that no longer serve me, and transmute the poison into consciousness. My touchstone experience of menstruation came last Summer, during a week long camp in Devon: "Celebrating the Body". For the only time that I can remember, I felt none of the usual tension and unease that precedes my period.

I only felt a growing desire to spend time being quiet, on my own, or with other women ~ reading my tarot cards, writing and singing while lying in a hammock over the babbling stream, Holy Brook. When I began to bleed, I found a tree on the other side of the stream, away from the camp, and asked a friend to bring me food and water, and invite any other women who were bleeding to join me ~ both requests were a big step for me to take, although no-one joined me in the end. I laid out red and orange scarves in a circle around me, and for the first time, allowed myself to bleed directly onto the Earth. Then, having never thought of it before, I spontaneously began to paint my body with my blood as I sat naked in the grass. I felt in that moment that I had stepped through a threshold, into a completely new experience of myself as a woman: my body and spirit transformed over the next hours. That evening, when I joined a group of women, I realised that I was indeed in a new place in myself. It's hard to put into words, but I felt so still and deep and psychically aware, as if I could see into the heart of things. I can only begin to imagine what it would be like to bleed every month in the company of other women, sharing this heightened vision and sensitivity, and what a gift this could be for the wider community, as was the case in many native cultures.

I would love to see more young girls experience their rite of passage into womanhood in beautiful and honouring ways. This could be as simple as being cooked a special meal, being given a present or flowers, or taking a long cleansing bath with oils or rose petals. She could clear her room of any toys, books or clothes she feels she has grown out of, invite her friends to a Red party, or create a ceremony with older women who share with her their experiences of womanhood and their menstrual cycle. Instead of being a curse to begrudge each month, or even to completely suppress, as a new form of the Pill offers, girls would know from the start that their Moontime can be a highly creative, truth-telling time. As women, we carry the cycle of life and death within us ~ we pass through the three phases of woman: maiden, as we begin a new menstrual cycle; mother, as we ovulate; and crone, as we are premenstrual and bleed: repeated again and again until the menopause, just as the Moon makes the same cycle. We need this feminine wisdom, perhaps more than ever, as the structures of patriarchy increasingly crumble around us, and we search for new ways to live in this precious world.

Suggested Resources

The Wise Wound: Menstruation and Everywoman, by Penelope Shuttle & Peter Redgrave
New Moon Rising: Reclaiming the Sacred Rites of Menstruation, by Linda Heron Wind
Shakti Woman: Feeling Our Fire, Healing our World, by Vicki Noble
Women's Bodies, Women's Wisdom, by Christiane Northrup
First Moon: Celebrating the Onset of Menstruation, by Anke Mai & Lorye Keats Hooper (available from Sweet FA)
Walking into Beauty, Resource book for honouring the transition into womanhood, edited

by Anke Mai (available from Sweet FA)
*The Red Tent (novel), by Anita Diamant

Websites
Weaving the Red Web -
www.theredweb.org
(educating women and girls about the positive aspects of menstruation)
Wise Woman Web, Moon Lodge
www.suSunweed.com/Moonlodge.htm
First Moon: Passage to Womanhood - www.celebrategirls.com

Violation of the Feminine:
healing abuse within the family
by Roslyne Sophia Breillat

www.wildheartwisdom.com
Sophia lives, writes and paints from the heart...
Her inspiring articles and powerful images honour the sacredness of the feminine spirit and the beauty of the Earth...Her website offers a wealth of loving wisdom that supports woman's cyclic transformations and the subtle rhythm of the female psyche... Her astrological consultations offer deep insight and the opportunity for real transformation...

Whilst many people in our culture are awakening to a deeper consciousness, abuse towards women and children is becoming more prolific. And the statistics of rape are rapidly increasing in countries where females are supposedly liberated. If freedom is to reign upon this Earth, the heart of the family psyche must be healed. And love is the only answer.

In ancient mythology, the female spirit was revered for her abundant creativity and passionate sensuality.

Her womb was worshipped for its life-giving mystery, and her body was honoured as a sacred temple. Woman's natural power has now become so repressed that she no longer knows who she is. Stripped of her sacredness, she struggles in a world that ignores her true nature. The feminine essence is abused in myriad ways. It's violated whenever the media uses a woman's body to sell a car, a house or a magazine. Woman is abused whenever a man is dishonest with her. She's disrespected whenever a man manipulates or controls her. She's psychically raped whenever a man mentally undresses her or indulges in sexual fantasies. She's dishonoured whenever her perceptive female wisdom remains unseen and unheard. All abuse is denigrating and degrading. All abuse is forceful. All abuse is unloving. All abuse is violent. And all sexual wounding of women creates a dark and empty chasm in the female psyche.

Whenever a girl or woman's body is violated, the feminine essence is dishonoured a little more. Whenever one girl or woman cries out in pain when her body is abused, all women suffer. Whenever any female is treated as a sexual object instead of a Goddess of love, all of humanity suffers. Whenever one woman begins to heal, she contributes to the healing of many other women. For all are united as sisters in a mysterious timeless place. Whenever a man enters a woman's body with true tenderness, sensitivity, reverence, humility and passion, love grows upon this Earth.

Within every young girl rests the sacredness of the female essence. The mystique of her girlish femininity emanates through her actions, and shines through her eyes. The tenderness of her love must only be asked for, never demanded. The purity of her love must only be given, never stolen. As an innocent child, she embodies the delicious wellspring of this love. She spontaneously dances, plays and runs freely as the wind. She delights in the sensual elixir of warm sunshine upon her face, gentle raindrops in her hair, and comforting arms enfolding her body. She is yet untouched by the World's hardness. She's in harmony with her natural sensuality and the innate pleasure of being. She enjoys the sweetness of natural intimacy, secure in the knowledge that she's loved. And she enjoys the sensation of loving touch, for this conveys to her a sense of place upon this Earth.

Like a tiny seedling or budding flower, she needs tender nurturing so as to blossom into the fullness of her femaleness. Trusting her caretakers, she thrives upon their warm embraces, their loving words and their protective influence. Trusting in life, she's open-hearted and unafraid. What happens to her naïve trust when one of these adults violates the tenuous impressions still forming within her innocent young psyche?

When parents discover that their young daughter has been sexually violated, their immediate emotional reactions are usually dramatic. Waves of anger, guilt, grief and disbelief can merge with an overwhelming sense of betrayal, shock and despair. There can be an intense desire for retribution, punishment and retaliation. A disturbed father may react by seeking confrontation and revenge. A distressed mother may react by over-protecting her child. Through unwillingness to face the reality of this trauma they can sink into denial and self-blame. And if they're willing, they can receive an extraordinary opportunity for healing the inherited wounds of the family psyche. This opportunity will challenge the child's parents to open more deeply to love. For many relationships disintegrate when sexual abuse annihilates the comfort and familiarity of daily life.

Suppressed frustration and violent rage often cause an adult male to abuse a young girl. And his actions are commonly created by a lack of love and fulfilment in his sexual relationship with his partner. It's of no comfort to the parents of a daughter traumatised by a trusted carer to know that he/she has also probably been abused. It's particularly devastating when the perpetrator is someone of their own kin with whom child and parents already share a loving closeness. It's difficult to accept that the one who provides warm hugs, cosy evenings, delicious ice creams and adventurous outings is the same one who has violated their daughter and their trust. Statistics reveal that in 95% of cases she already knows the offender, and that girls are most likely to be sexually assaulted by fathers, stepfathers or other male carers. Through fear, denial or shame, relatives, friends and employees often protect the perpetrator rather than the abused child. It's an established fact that children rarely lie about or imagine abuse.

Parents may need counselling for post-traumatic shock disorder, depression or other psychological disturbances triggered by their daughter's traumatic experience. Meditation is beneficial, as this creates calmness, and quietens the mind. Further in their healing they may reap the blessings of forgiveness, surrender and acceptance. True forgiveness is not of the mind. True forgiveness cannot be practised as a structure, or forced before its time. True forgiveness arises naturally, spontaneously and compassionately from the vulnerability of a healing heart and from the infinite wellspring of the spirit within.

Every young girl inherently knows the difference between loving and unloving touch, tenderness and harshness, gentleness and roughness. Sexual violation causes her to feel fragmented, disassociated, broken. She has witnessed graphic dysfunction of the human condition. And she has experienced a loveless act that is raw and primal in its complexity. Life's wisdom and integrity know that the emotional residue of sexual abuse needs to be integrated and healed sensitively and slowly.

The impact of a young girl's sexual trauma hits hard upon the concept of conscious parenting. It shatters cherished beliefs of love. It opens a Pandora's box of opinions about karma, spirituality and healing. It activates pious judgements about right and wrong, good and bad, punishment and shame. It weakens illusory ideals of male and female roles. And most of all, it challenges the structures of a society that denies the difference between abusive sex and intimate sexual loving. The impact of abuse crosses boundaries of morality and faith, innocence and trust. It exposes issues of decency, honesty and integrity. It denies all that is sacred, natural, good and wholesome upon this Earth. Sexual trauma contains the capacity to draw a family together or tear it apart. Its shock waves reverberate through the heart of the home, echoing a disturbance that can last for many generations.

Parents become flooded with much turbulent inner questioning. "Why has this happened to our daughter?" "Will she ever heal?" "Will we ever heal?" "What kind of God has allowed this?" "Why has this happened to us?" "What have we done wrong?" "Why weren't we more careful, diligent, aware, alert?" "Why did we trust our daughter with him/her?" Sometimes it's appropriate to confront the perpetrator and sometimes it's not. There are many sensitive and delicate issues to be faced with straightness, integrity and love. For the shattering discovery of sexual abuse within the family begs for real answers, real healing, honesty and truth.

There is power, purpose and divine intelligence within everything upon this Earth. "There is a purpose to everything under Heaven". There is a purpose within all tragedy, suffering and abuse. For from within the centre of trauma we're called to love more, open more, give more. Profound purpose is revealed within the wound when it's consciously faced. For each wound contains the heart of truth, and the capacity to lead the wounded on a powerful spiritual journey.

Within the complexity of the human condition everyone contains the essence of both perpetrator and victim. The perpetrator is the victim of a society where love is not the ruling power. The victim becomes perpetrator when acting abusively as a reaction to being abused. And those who seek revenge are reacting from the same place of suffering as the perpetrator. For in truth there is no victim and no perpetrator. There is only what is.

Abuse is created by a lack of love. Abuse does not simply appear as an isolated incident within the apparent security of a familial situation. Wherever and whenever it occurs it reflects a repetitive pattern of many generations. Such patterns are deeply hidden. Such patterns run deep, and are difficult to break. Such patterns are cunningly embedded within an insidious façade of prestige, morality, decency and respectability. Such patterns are multidimensional and multifaceted, weaving an intricate web of secrecy and deceit that cries out for exposure and annihilation. And such patterns call for clarity, courage, insight, compassion and transformation. Exposing the ruthless aftermath of abuse breaks the silence of historical past, and crumbles the cement of solid family foundations. The truth is no longer withheld, and a powerful healing can begin.

"The sins of the fathers shall be passed onto the sons." Whenever a girl is sexually traumatised, the fabric binding the dynamics of the family constellation ~ the family psyche ~ is torn asunder. The threads of normality and continuity are broken, and the rich tapestry of family heritage, values and integrity suddenly becomes worn and faded. When a young girl is abused, the veil of illusion parts. And the glow of truth shining through this gap can take her on a potent pilgrimage of spiritual healing.

When a young girl is abused, she experiences a violation of her natural femininity. The female spirit is innately passive and openly receptive. This passivity is not weak or fragile, but a profound emanation of Yin presence. The subtle fluidity of the female psyche is sensitive, sensual and intuitive. The female body opens, surrenders, absorbs, takes in, nurtures, receives.

Whenever a girl's body is sexually violated, this feminine capacity to receive becomes corrupted, clouding her innate discernment of love. Emotional reactions to trauma dim the luminescence of her being, preventing the flowering of her creative potential by damming her feminine flow. She separates from her natural desire to give and receive love. Perceiving her environment as unsafe, she then grows up feeling afraid of others, afraid of the world and afraid of life.

A young girl who has been sexually molested is often so traumatised that she's unable to speak of her experience. Her body and her psyche have been painfully penetrated. She's been spiritually, psychically and physically wounded. Silence becomes her protector and her friend. Terror or shock may silence her. Threats and bribery from her perpetrator may silence her. Denial within her family may silence her. Support of her perpetrator, by other adults, may silence her.

Her natural demeanour changes when she's overwhelmed by the devastating impact of sexual trauma. She may experience depression, bed-wetting, nausea, vomiting, allergies, violent outbursts or suicidal tendencies. She may experience emotional numbness, flashbacks, nightmares, or irrational phobias and anxiety. Secrecy, self-hatred, low self-esteem, panic attacks, post-traumatic stress disorder or self-destructive behaviour may disturb her equilibrium. Terror may arise whenever a particular colour, sound, texture, place or fragrance awakens the incessant memories that haunt her. If she was abused in her bed, she might become afraid of the dark, or have difficulty sleeping.

She may become extremely hyperactive or silently imploded. She might feel lonely, isolated or lacking in motivation. Her innocent faith in the nurturing security of her environment diminishes as she loses her natural ability to trust. She may become fussy about food, and display disordered eating patterns. Anorexia and bulimia frequently manifest as graphic symptoms of sexual abuse.

It's important that she knows she's loved and cherished. She needs to feel safe, and she needs to feel secure. Although sensitive touch will comfort her, this may also trigger memories of abuse. Any force will unnecessarily remind her of her recent trauma. Help her to find her inherent goodness, to feel the well-being in her body, to see the good things in her life. Speak the truth to her, and listen to her perceptions. For within her is the same wisdom and intelligence that is within you.

Art therapy can be healing. Encourage her to use her natural gifts and talents, as creative expression is joyful, fun and therapeutic. A traumatised child will often communicate more easily through painting, drawing, writing, acting, dancing or sand play than through verbal communication. Reiki, massage, re-connective healing, and cranial sacral balancing help create spiritual, physical, emotional and psychological balance. If any of these, or other gentle techniques, feel appropriate, choose your therapist wisely. The true healer is gifted with natural counselling skills, deep insight and sensitive perception. The true healer has been where she is now. Through having penetrated the depths of their own healing they can communicate to her with clarity, detachment, intuition and compassion.

The girl who has experienced abuse walks a different path, and travels a different journey. She sings a different tune, and she dances to a different drum. She sees through the apparent normality and sanity of a society where secrecy and deception mask the truth. She speaks a different language, and she has an entirely different perception of life. She has experienced an intense disintegration of distorted reality at a very young age. She contains the seeds of the true shaman, the true wounded healer. And she often embraces a ruthless desire to penetrate life's mysteries.

The abused girl's pain can act as a powerful catalyst for profound healing. For she easily sees through the lies, the falsity, the sticky glue of illusion holding family conditioning, human conditioning and societal conditioning together.

Within all trauma, tragedy, suffering, abuse, rests a potential gift. And this gift is the blessed gift of true spiritual healing. Throughout her life she'll be given many opportunities to receive this gift. And miraculous blessings may sometimes appear in the guise of challenging circumstances that awaken, stir and deepen in many transforming ways. When her dawning sexuality arises during puberty, she may experience emotional disturbances and menstrual difficulties. She might become obsessive about schoolwork, cleanliness, exercise or extreme diets. She may incessantly strive for perfection on the sports field or in the classroom. She may become addicted to drugs or alcohol. She might become promiscuous as a desperate way of acting out suppressed memories of sexual trauma. Or she may reject all opportunities for nurturing friendships and intimate sexual relating. She may give her love secretly, indiscriminately, or not at all.

She may compulsively attract further abuse from others. Beneath this apparent dysfunction, the wisdom, integrity and intelligence of life bestow an opportunity to resolve unhealed wounding from the original act of sexual trauma. Sadly, many of the adults in her immediate environment never notice her distressed symptoms or her silent cries for help.

If you're a woman healing from sexual abuse, your journey will bless you with gentle faith and infinite courage. You're learning, through the wisdom and strength of spiritual compassion, to surrender to a higher power of love and healing. The depth and beauty of this power is within you right now. No matter how far you've strayed from the wellspring of your inner source, it awaits patiently within, ever calling you home. Beyond your suffering you are the truth of life and the truth of love. You are the muse. You are the shaman. You are the medicine woman. You are the healer.

Your sexual healing is a call to a deeper place beyond all wounding, all trauma, all abuse. This is a place of stillness, forgiveness, compassion. Are you willing to go there? Are you willing to enter this place of grace and freedom? Are you willing to go there, no matter what life takes from you, no matter how it strips the layers of fear and protection from your heart, no matter how painful it is to open to this deeper place? And are you willing to welcome this place, where you'll be stripped naked, raw, bare, before the presence of love?

Those who experience the beauty and liberation of true sexual healing have dared to embrace these wild places, these raw and vulnerable and tumultuous places. For in these places of strength and courage, the spirit never gives up until all is accepted, surrendered, healed. The power of true healing is relentless in its invocation of truth and its desire to birth love.

In our so-called "sexually liberated" society, silence, secrecy, stigma and suppression still surround issues of child sexual abuse.

And yet the graphic distortion of natural sexuality is continually accepted as "normal" in movies, magazines, videos and advertising. The grossness of sex has become the ruling force of the world, instead of the beauty of love being the ruling power.

To the woman who is healing from sexual trauma ~ your healing journey contains potential seeds of gratitude for all of your life experiences, no matter how traumatic or painful. Throughout your healing process you're being freed of negative family structures and inherited patterns of emotional conditioning. Your life-essence is being replenished, creating more joy and vitality for living upon this beautiful Earth.

Although you appear to be a victim of your life circumstances, deep within, beneath the layers of pain and suffering, you are blessed life itself. Profound healing creates spiritual grace. It bestows precious gifts of humility, compassion, openness, surrender, acceptance, peace. These tenderly merge with the innocence and wisdom of your heart's purity. Your perpetrator needs as much love and healing as you. There is only one love upon the Earth. There is only one love that heals.

Whenever a man
enters a woman's body
with true tenderness, sensitivity,
reverence, humility and passion,
love grows
upon this Earth.

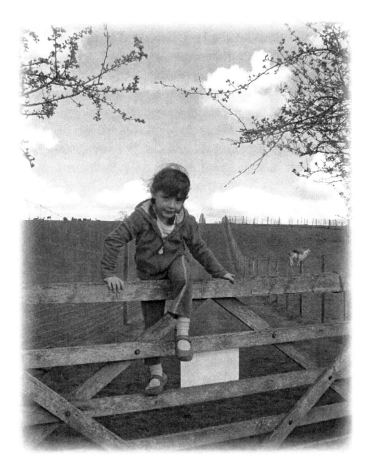

Sophia climbing the gate.

Deep and sensitive lovemaking with a devoted partner slowly and intimately restores a woman's trust. Through being truly loved, acknowledged, and cherished, the beauty of the female essence passionately and sensuously awakens. Such lovemaking opens deep recesses in the psyche, where painful memories hide. The flowing waters of life's integrity will wash these away. For the sweet nectar of this blessed healing balm forgives and transforms.

Dancing allows the spontaneous joy of natural movement to arise. Yoga gifts physical balance, emotional equilibrium and inner peace. Painting, drawing and singing allow your creative wellspring to pour forth. Massage, in a safe situation with someone you trust, opens your body to the sensual pleasure of loving touch. Being with the abundance of Mother Earth reflects your inner beauty. The power of her nurturing presence knows your love, your pain and your desire to heal. Lie upon her soft grass and her solid rocks. Allow her infinite love to hold and support you. Reach out to others. Open your heart to life. Delight in the softness, strength and deliciousness of your femaleness. Know that you are only here for love. Trust in the transforming healing power within, and the Divine integrity of your inner spirit.

Remain open and available, but don't allow anyone to touch you without gentleness, integrity, honesty and love. You are the wise guardian of your vast mystery, and the Divine custodian of your sacred sanctuary. Your body is a beautiful temple. You're worthy of tenderness and respect. Anyone who tries to harm you is not worthy of your love.

There's an exquisite presence within you, beyond all thoughts, doubts, negativity and fear. This is the shining glow of spirit, of truth, of love. Here, you're purity, innocence, silence, power, space, strength. Here, you're the sweetest tenderness, profound stillness and infinite depth of your being. Here, in this blessed place, violation or abuse has never touched you. Here, you're undamaged and unharmed. Here, you're beloved of God. Here, you're free. This same place is also inside your perpetrator, who has perhaps also experienced abuse. The force of suppressed trauma is frequently the cause of abusive actions towards another. You may eventually find forgiveness and compassion for your perpetrator. And as your healing journey deepens, you'll find profound and loving compassion for yourself. You'll eventually embrace life with the sacred purity of an open heart.

Such is the impersonal joy of true healing, and the passionate fire of true transformation. Such is the power of truth. Such is the integrity of life.

Resentment, self-pity and blame will melt into peace, compassion and joy. You'll experience deepening gratitude for the many blessings you receive. You'll become more open to life and love, and less ruled by insecurity and fear. You'll embrace the present moment, and relinquish the past. You'll know the wisdom of the sage and the innocence of the child.

I wish you well on your healing journey as the wise Goddess of love, power, gentleness, strength, wholeness and truth.

You are
the wise guardian
of your vast mystery,
and the Divine custodian
of your sacred sanctuary.

Your body
is a
beautiful temple.

Circumcision:
where sex and violence first meet
by Jeannine Parvati Baker

*From 2002 to 2005, Jeannine Parvati Baker was a loved and valued
columnist for The Mother magazine.*

Jeannine Parvati Baker June 1, 1949 to December 1, 2005
Lay Midwife, Ashtanga Yogini, Astrologer, Founder of Hygieia
College, Herbal Medicine-Woman, Mother of six, Author of
Prenatal Yoga & Natural Childbirth,
Hygieia: A Woman's Herbal , and co-author of Conscious
Conception

**If mothers protected their boys
from the unconscious initiation
into the military cult,
we would create a sustainable future.**

Flowers in the rain. Cold, wet, and tired from the long morning
rally, my eight year-old asks again why we're here. We're standing
with about fifty media people, organisers, and just your ordinary
eccentrics, grandmothers and fathers, university professors,
musicians, nurses and midwives, lawyers, artists, writers, men's
rights activists and children, gathered in the industrial section
of Seattle in November. We're all here for one purpose: to report
about, and demonstrate against, the manufacturers of the plastic
Y-shaped cradle boards used to hold infants immobile during

circumcision. The members of NOHARMM (National Organization to Halt the Abuse and Routine Mutilation of Males) and NOCIRC (National Organization of Circumcision Information Resource Centers, especially the local chapter in Seattle) called the action. We gathered to get here on Veterans' Day to hold a peaceful demonstration at the only place the boards are manufactured in the USA. It was aired on three TV news stations several times the same evening, showing us filling a circumstraint board with flowers.

Previously, there had been talk of doing a guerrilla theatre to get the media and manufacturer's attention. The fantasy scripts ranged from building an adult circumstraint, and staging a mock circumcision of a man, to strapping a dog on the board and circumcising the animal in public. The reasoning behind the dog circumcision was that there would surely be an outcry among animal-rights activists if that were done, which would highlight, in some minds, the insanity of our doing this, unabashedly, to humans as a matter of routine. These gruesome fantasies eventually yielded to the idea of placing cut flowers in a circumstraint in front of the manufacturing offices.

I felt compelled by conscience to attend the demonstration, yet, up until this decision, was uneasy about to what degree, if any, I could participate in an expression of violence. That we chose to prayerfully and respectfully place flowers was an action that I, as a mother and midwife, could wholeheartedly embrace. Taking the idea one step further, as a midwife, it was my practice to advise postpartum visitors to bring potted plants, rather than cut flowers. Flowers, separated from their matrix, the Earth, fade and die ~ while a live plant, like a newborn, is still growing. Being surrounded by growing plants reminds the mother that the baby grows best in her arms, close to the heart. A mother is a baby's Earth. This is why we need more mothers working with the political organisations to end genital mutilation ~ to bring the bigger picture, the connection with our Source, to give a voice to the Earth.

My sacred obligation

For over a generation, I've been devotedly writing and speaking against circumcision. My awakening came in the 1960s, when I was training to be a primal therapist. During one session, I assisted an adult to relive his own circumcision as an infant. Since then, though my mother's religion commands circumcision, I felt I had to honour my sacred obligation and protect my babies from harm. My sons are all intact, and so will be my grandchildren. I used to say that, by nature, I wasn't very political. Of course not, for I was raised female, and became a mother in a patristic culture. We weren't encouraged to be effective in the political arena. When I looked up the definition of politics in Webster's, I was surprised to discover that the second definition is practical wisdom. Who else, but mothers, have been practising wisdom, day and night, by caring for the children? If a country is to politically thrive, it must include the voices of the mothers and grandmothers: those who have an obvious, vested interest (call it cellular or genetic) in sustaining the life that we have brought forth, in ensuring that the Earth is also intact to support that life.

To answer my youngest daughter's question, "Why are we here?", my response was: "How could we not be?" When I learned that only in dominator societies, in warring cultures, does genital mutilation of the young occur, I saw a way I could be a peacemaker, by fulfilling my central responsibility as a mother. By raising peaceful sons, mothers could stop the destruction of our Earth. If mothers protected their boys from the unconscious initiation into the military cult, we would create a sustainable future.

As the Cheyenne Indians say, a nation can fall only when the hearts of the mothers are on the ground. The big problem with circumcision is mothers intuitively know it's wrong, yet they deny this natural impulse to protect their babies. This denial creates a lack of trust in a mother's own capacity to protect him from the knife (sword). She will distrust her own ability to raise her son, enrolling the 'expert' or 'authority', even to the extent of literally cutting off parts of his body so that he'll fit on the Procrustean bed of the mythical normal man, a warrior.

When we abdicate this power to protect our babies in the early postpartum, no wonder there's rampant postpartum depression, i.e., the mother's heart is on the ground.

Just say "no" to circumcision

To raise up the jubilant heart of mothering, we must do everything we can to end circumcision. My daughter and I travelled from our cosy, book-lined home to rainy Seattle to be counted among those who invite the perpetrators of violence against babies via circumcision, to conscience. This was in my mind with each flower I laid on the circumstraint board on Veteran's Day. It has been a long war "the tradition of the fathers" has waged to do violence to children, to do violence to their mothers, and the men these circumcised boys become. It's time to say the war is over, by empowering mothers to just say "no" to circumcision.

After a generation's work to stop circumcision, it's heartening to witness the involvement of the men's rights community; men are giving voice to their experience of the damage done to them without their consent. For several years, at the International Symposia on Circumcision, I've presented a Healing Ceremony for those involved in ending genital mutilation. Seated in a circle, circumcisers, as well as their victims, share their stories. This word-medicine is a deep healing balm on every soul. As men recognise what has been done to them, and the mask of denial slips down, a potent force for healing and protecting the sons of the future emerges. Unmasked, the real men are now present, and can effectively awaken their brothers to the horror of infant-male genital mutilation.

At the strategy meeting in Seattle, attention was given to the words we use in this movement. The term mutilation came up as a red flag which is too startling and offensive. However, again the dictionary tells it like it is: a mutilation is to cut off or damage a body part, or remove an essential part. This is precisely what circumcision does, as the foreskin is the most highly innervated tissue, with specialised secretions which are irreplaceable.

Mutilating the gods of the interior

The etymology of the word penis includes an early meaning from Roman times: the penates are Gods of the Interior, the Inner Household Gods. By mutilating the Gods of the Interior, we're disabling our sons from being in touch with their innermost feelings. A baby who's been circumcised shuts down his capacity to feel, as life, obviously, is just too painfully mutilating. All the immense reservoirs of psychic energy used to repress trauma could, rather, be channelled for sensitive, creative works.

Often I wonder about destiny, and how, on that particular day in the psychology lab almost thirty years ago, I realised that circumcision is devastating to the soul. If I hadn't ever seen a grown man reduced to the infantile rage and pain (to an unfathomable degree), would I have considered circumcising my boys? Having experienced first-hand, in primal therapy, that the traumatic pain of circumcision is imprinted and can be consciously recovered, I knew that I would not inflict such pain upon my own flesh and blood. Flesh and blood is not mere hyperbole: the baby and mother are still one in the early postpartum. What hurts one, harms the other.

This is true for all mothers as well. What we do to one, we do to another. I asked each mother I attended as midwife about circumcision. If the parents insisted on it, then they would have to find another midwife. I couldn't let myself bond to their baby at birth and not be able to protect the new one. This declaration saved many a foreskin.

The benefit of saving foreskins is the creation of a more peaceful society. There are male pheromones which signal to other males their relation. Without the foreskin, which produces these scent molecular messengers, men are more anxious, and quicker to assert dominance upon one another. Keeping our sons intact brings a greater likelihood for co-operative, rather than competitive, behaviours with their fathers, brothers, and all men.

Where sex and violence first meet

There is another psychological benefit to keeping our sons intact. Psychiatrist Rima Laibow finds that men carry an unconscious rage against their mothers for betrayal, abandonment, and the assault of circumcision. In other words, the unconscious mind of the son blames his mother for his circumcision, not the tradition, the circumciser, or the father who wanted his son to look like himself ~ only the mother. It's just like some bad Jewish-mother joke.

Indeed, for a newborn, his world is mother. If she cannot protect him from violation at the beginning, a baby loses trust. And isn't lack of trust an issue in relationships between the genders nowadays? Can circumcision be a symptom of profound resentment between the genders? Can sexuality be healed on a very deep, unconscious level during the perinatal period?

A connection exists between crimes of sexual violence, rape and circumcision. The first heterosexual encounter is when a female nurse prepares the infant penis with antiseptic, often creating an erection, followed by painful cutting! This, and the betrayal by the mother, is revenged in sexual assaults against women. As Marilyn Milos, founder and director of NOCIRC says, "Circumcision is where sex and violence meet for the first time." May our Earth become the garden I know of many courageous parents, who, once informed, not only changed their minds about circumcision, but also became active in helping babies stay whole. Sometimes this means going against tradition. And a family's attachment to tradition can be tenacious. However, we must choose only those rituals from our rich traditions which are best for life. We're free to co-create a new way to show the world what our love looks like, by bringing forth whole children.

By our participation, our marching through Seattle to make a point, my daughter and I were demonstrating more than our desperation that circumcision is still happening. (Believe me, it is a sign of desperation that I'd be motivated to travel from my warm home in the harvest season.) We were also demonstrating that we have trust: trust in people to remember how to be kind to one another, especially to babies.

With every flower I placed on the circumstraint, I thought to myself (then sent through my eyes to one of the workers gathered at the big front office windows), "May you remember to be kind to babies; may you stop circumcision."

In closing, my prayer is for the circumstraint board to go the way of the cradle board. We've been taught that "the hand that rocks the cradle rules the world". But, if we truly want to cease "ruling", i.e., dominating one another, we must keep our babies safe in mothers' arms.

Let the circumstraints become archaic tools, post-industrial museum pieces, depicting torture in a less enlightened time. Or, better yet, let them become planters.

May our Earth become the garden again!

...the
foreskin
is the
most highly innervated tissue,
with specialised secretions
which are irreplaceable.

The spiritual purpose of menopause
by Roslyne Sophia Breillat

Each of the cyclic transformations in a woman's life unfolds through an initial letting go process. And as the past dissolves, the vital spark of the new can ignite. Throughout each of these transformations, a woman enters the mystery of her inner cocoon. Here she prepares for the forthcoming phase that will manifest another facet of her femaleness.

During menarche, the young pubescent woman is asked to let go of her childish ways so as to embrace her maturing years as a menstruating woman. During pregnancy and childbirth the new mother is asked to let go of anything that prevents her giving tenderly, selflessly and open-heartedly to her newborn babe.

During menopause, the mature woman is asked to let go of everything that diminishes her power, ignores her depth, and prevents her wisdom from flourishing.

Throughout the early stages of her menopausal journey, a woman will often experience a period of grief that is seemingly never-ending. The intensity of such grief can be mentally disturbing and emotionally overwhelming. This grief is an important facet of a powerful psychological death/rebirth process. Being present with this process will eventually guide her into a life that supports the power of change. And why does a woman grieve during this phase of her life? She grieves because she has accumulated a complex web of thoughts, emotions and beliefs that don't reflect who she truly is. She grieves because she hasn't wholeheartedly lived her life in alignment with her free spirit. Her self grieves for the familiar comfort of her outer persona. And as many intricate aspects of this self inwardly die, she grieves because she's releasing the pain of the world from her womb. This pain has gathered for many years, releasing shreds of its multiple layers whenever she menstruates. And it releases from a deeper place when she reaches her menopausal years. If she consciously relinquishes her identification with fertility, with being mother, lover, wife, secretary, artist, receptionist, menstruating woman, she's drawn ever deeper into the timeless mystery of her inner realm. And she'll eventually discover, in humility, awe and wonder, that she's the vast and mysterious nothingness of the great void that creates all life. This revelation can be very disturbing if her personality thrives on being recognised as "somebody", rather than sweetly being who she is. The world we live in doesn't recognise the Divine simplicity, truth and purpose contained within the letting go process. We are encouraged to collect, to buy, to shop, to have, to own. We're not encouraged to relinquish, to surrender, to let go, to release, to set free. We're not encouraged to empty our lives of everything that no longer creates nurturing, well-being or fulfillment. The world we live in favours the forceful demands of the outer life. It doesn't honour the mystery and beauty of the inner life. And during menopause, the inner life of the feminine psyche becomes richly potent and vitally important. For its incessant calling is for transition, for transformation, for change.

Woman is a fathomless ocean of love. She's an infinite wellspring of devotion to the immortal source of the Goddess within. In her heart of hearts she naturally desires to live from this place of devoted love. Too often she's forced to leave her infinite sanctuary of lunar feminine darkness. Too often she chases the glaring solar light of the outer masculine worldly dream. Her reality lies within the inner receptivity of an essence that is essentially yin. Her reality is not of existence, clocks, time or linear structures. Her reality is innately cyclic, ovular, circular, spiral. She can easily become attached to the outer world's false opinions and unreal fears of menopause. This prevents her from fully experiencing the simple joy and delicious freedom awaiting her through deeply entering her body and her psyche at this time. Her menopausal journey doesn't signify an ending of her beauty, her femaleness, her femininity. It heralds a potential deepening and empowering of her feminine spirit. Many aspects of her former life will end as they dissolve and disintegrate within the passionate fire of her inner transformation. And many aspects of her personality will die during this powerful phase of inner rebirth. Immersed in the depths of her grieving process, she does not yet see that her menopausal pilgrimage will eventually bestow the expansive freedom of new beginnings. If she believes modern society's ideas that menopause is the end of her life as a real woman, she'll suffer as these ideas are broken down. But if she courageously listens to the wise ways of her muse within, she'll integrate deeper aspects of her femaleness as this powerful transition unfolds. If she consciously embraces the awesome pilgrimage of this profound healing process, life will graciously gift her with the ability to live in the world, but not of it. She will truly know the meaning of being as wise as a serpent, and as gentle as a dove. But first she must grieve.

And so, she grieves. She grieves because the modern world does not honour her gentle, mysterious power. And she grieves because she knows, deep within her heart, there's more to being a woman beyond the superficiality of contemporary society. She grieves because the power of her female wisdom has been suppressed for hundreds of years. And she grieves because she longs to fully experience the beauty and freedom of her deepest female truth.

Her grief arises from the same fathomless place as the grief of an abortion, the grief of a miscarriage, the grief of broken dreams, the grief of a broken heart. It arises from a sacred place deep within the wellspring of the feminine psyche. This place is a sanctuary of release and healing. It brings a woman to her knees, raw, vulnerable and naked before the infinite spirit of her wise inner crone. The sense of loss she may feel throughout this grieving process is the loss of her family structures, her childhood conditioning, her mental ideas, her emotional beliefs. It's not the loss of her true nature, her true being. In fact, her true being will shine forth in all its glory the more she is able to let go.

During her menopausal transition, she's pulled softly, gently, deeply and often tumultuously into her inner Universe of darkness. In ancient mythology, woman was the seductive siren of the sea. She sang sweetly to shipwrecked sailors, enticing them into the dark underworld caverns of her oceanic depths. The menopausal journey is rich with the ancient myths of life. It's a psycho-spiritual disintegration and a holy pilgrimage. It deserves to be honoured for its powerful capacity to clear out the old life, and bestow the new. For many women, it brings the dark night of the soul, and the traversing of the desert, in preparation for a more fulfilling life. As in a traditional shamanic journey, this grieving phase can bring a deep sense of "soul loss" before a woman is ready and willing to discover her true purpose upon this Earth.

Our current civilisation ignores the emerging power of the wise menopausal woman. It cannot reach or acknowledge her depth, for it thrives in the shallow ground of unreality. When the pain of unfulfilled love enters a woman's womb, she suppresses the subtle fragrance of her essence and the passionate fire of her power, to cope in the outer world. This requires a harsh force that is alien to her cyclic female rhythm. And this creates an armoured shell that masks her inherent vulnerability and gentle strength. During her menopausal journey, much repressed pain is released so that her female truth can shine brightly throughout this empowering phase. The wise and loving consciousness within her womb seeks release and freedom during this unique purification.

She'll often experience tears of grief and sorrow as she mourns the loss of all that can never be again. Since her first menstruation, her deeply intimate relationship with her body has innately ebbed and flowed within the cyclic rhythm of tidal, seasonal and lunar phases. Like her beloved Mother Earth, she eternally experiences an endless cycle of birth, death and renewal. Each month she is nourished and replenished by the inherent dance of her menstrual cycle. And each month she potentially moves deeper into the mystery of her being. As menopause draws near, she is nourished by her blossoming gift of power. This gift is not to be used or misused as power over others. It is for serving the truth of life, the truth of her inner source.

Tears of love, regret and remorse may emanate from a profound sorrow that has veiled the female spirit for centuries. If she's a mother who has poured all her love into her children, she may now be faced with the reality of an empty nest. Her heart and her home may feel painfully empty as her babies suddenly grow up, spread their wings, and fly away. Her treasure awaits within her emptiness. Her power awaits within her silence and stillness. Her joy and her radiant light await within her outpouring grief. And why does she grieve? She grieves because this inexplicable loss seems almost unbearable. She does not yet know that her forthcoming blessings will be richly bountiful. For first she must experience emptiness. Her womb and her heart must be emptied of all that no longer serves her deepening truth. Her psyche must be emptied of myriad unreal impressions and distorted perceptions. She must be emptied of all that no longer nurtures her. She must be emptied of all that once filled her with glorious aliveness but now fills her with flatness, deadness and stagnation.

She grieves because she has not been seen, understood, acknowledged, honoured, loved. And she grieves because she needs to be seen, not as the distortion of the world sees her, but as the purity of love sees her. And when this beautiful cup, this holy chalice of her womb, has been emptied of its grief, she's ready for a life of gentled wisdom and grace-filled peace. She now begins to fill her cup with the bounteous fulfillment of new blessings. The experience of this important emptying process is profoundly rewarding for every woman who dares to fully embrace her powerful menopausal transformation. If she's a woman who has never given birth from her womb's ripeness, never felt sweet milk flowing from her breasts, never held her babies gently to her heart and nurtured them into maturity, she may now grieve with the painful finality that she'll never become a mother. Nothing can stop this grief, for now is its time to pour forth. And it must pour forth until it dissolves all that inhibits the birthing of her wise truth and her ripening maturity. She doesn't yet know that although she's not a physical mother, she's beloved within the Divine essence of the Universal Earth Mother.

Why, dear woman, do you grieve so? In truth, you've lost nothing, for you have nothing to lose. And yet, you must grieve now, because it's a necessary part of your birthing of wisdom. You grieve because you're letting go of everything that is unreal within you. You grieve because you're letting go of all attachments to your outer roles and your many accomplishments. You grieve because you no longer know who you are. You grieve for all your dear sisters whose loving power has been repressed and unacknowledged for aeons. You grieve because you're a woman who lives in a male-dominated world. You grieve because you long to be tenderly and passionately reached in the depths of your womb. You grieve because the masculine world is too busy thinking, working, doing and journeying to other planets to stop for one precious moment and tenderly love you and your beloved Mother Earth.

Woman's grieving process during menopause is a purification that washes the past from her body, mind and spirit. The cleansing waters of her tears gift her with an exquisite sense of joy, strength and freedom. Her new life will not fully appear until she consciously and relentlessly lets go of everything she cannot carry on this journey through unknown territory. Her grief is a letting go of all that is no longer real within her psyche, within her heart, within her life. Her grief is the doorway to her wisdom, her power, her freedom.

Fatherhood

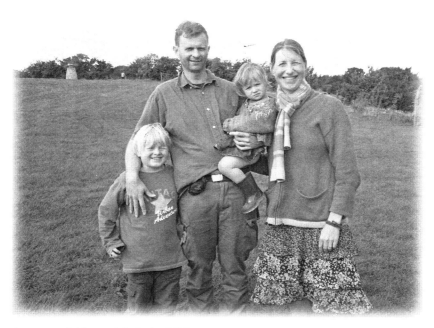

Anton and Alex, with their children Naomi and Hugo, at The Mother magazine family camp, 2009.

Fatherhood at its Best
by Belden Johnson, Fatherhood Vision Circle

Fatherhood Vision Circle was a spontaneous gathering of a very few people at the APPPAH conference: a subgrouping of folks interested in fatherhood. This came out of the images.

A man loving himself and his future children enough to heal himself of his past wounds before he chooses a woman to conceive another soul.

A man nourishing himself by choosing a good woman, and committing to a consciously loving relationship into which to warmly welcome wished-for children.

A man nourishing his woman by speaking total truth, by taking 100% responsibility for his reality, by supporting her highest good as well as his own, by co-creating equally with her the safe nest of home and family.

A man who tells his eight month pregnant wife how beautiful she is.

A man who creates lullabies to sing to his baby in the womb.

A man who wants a homebirth, and is completely present during labour and delivery.

A man who protects children, male and female, from genital mutilation and sexual abuse.

A man who chooses to work half-time so he can parent half-time.

A man who changes all the diapers.

A man who loves skin-to-skin contact with his babies.

A man who welcomes a family bed.

A man who carries his baby in a Heart to Heart Sling.

A man who plays the piano with one hand while holding his baby with the other.

A man who kills the television, and reads his children stories.

A man who wrestles with his children and always lets them win.

A man who coaches co-ed sports teams for his children, and when they ask who won, tells them it was whoever had the most fun.

A man who will gladly teach and gladly learn.

A man who listens.

A man who says it's okay to cry, or be afraid, or angry, or excited.

A man who can cry, be afraid, and be angry without violence or blaming.

A man who celebrates his children's differences from him, and encourages them to become whoever and whatever they wish to become.

A man who, when the time comes, can let the birds fly the nest, and bless them on their way out into the global family.

These images are real and true.
Such fathers are now among us.
Bless them and their fatherhood.

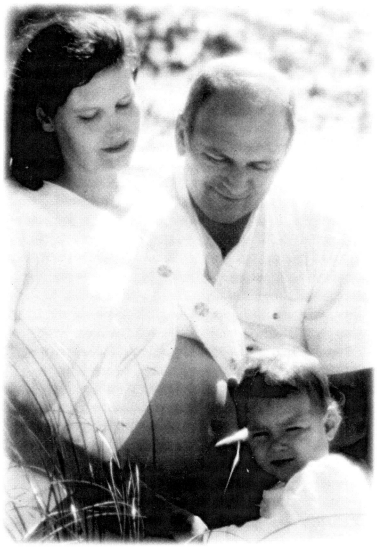

Veronika, Paul and Bethany saying 'hello' to Eliza.

A father's guide to creativity in pregnancy
by Binnie A. Dansby

The process of conception, pregnancy and birth is our most available physical metaphor for the human creative process. When we have an idea, we have conceived. If we add energy and time and attention to the idea, we are pregnant with the possibility. Continued persistence will bring forth a result, a birth. In the light of this understanding, I always encourage pregnant fathers to be aware of the creative energy that is available when their partner is pregnant. At no other time are we more creative than in the co-creative process of 'becoming'. I consider the human body to be the most sophisticated and beautiful of artworks. The energy that was necessary to paint the Sistine Chapel doesn't come close to the energy that is necessary to create a human body. Each father-to-be is in direct contact with that energy when sleeping, when making love and when simply being in daily life. Awareness is the key to the access and use of this valuable resource.

Many years ago, I taught a class called the Conscious Birthing Program, in Santa Monica, California. Fathers were always welcome, and typically comprised one third of those present. The intention of the class was to do process work to facilitate the release of any fears regarding birth. We explored each partner's birth experience as the source of his or her thoughts about birth. Sometimes these thoughts are held just below the level of conscious awareness. I used gentle breathwork, visualisation, and affirmation to help people to remember, release and heal. We also gave attention to societal thinking about birth, and what the people in their lives were telling them about birth. This supported them to acknowledge the influence of the environment on their thoughts and behaviour.

During this time, I had a private client in my counselling and breathwork practice who was a screenwriter with "writer's block". In one of our sessions I suddenly suggested that he come to the Wednesday morning Conscious Birthing class. He was, understandably, in doubt about my sanity, and I admit, I had my doubts, as well. Given some thought, I knew the reason for my invitation was to expose him to all the creative energy generated by 10 to 15 pregnant women. With encouragement, he came, and continued to join us every Wednesday for several months. In a very short time, a quarter of the participants in the program were creative artists of some form. Everyone was pregnant, some with ideas and some with human beings and new lives.

It's been a privilege to work with couples who chose to use the energy of pregnancy to start up new businesses, build new homes, and take art classes together. One couple decided to do The Artist's Way, by Julia Cameron, as they were co-creating a baby. Another went to French class as a couple. Other couples took tango and salsa lessons. They all expressed how easy and enjoyable creative pursuits were for them during pregnancy. An added advantage to learning and creating during pregnancy is that the baby will have an affinity with the language or the activity when they're of an appropriate age. A German woman whom I met spoke English with a British accent. I asked if she had lived in England. She told me that she hadn't. With further inquiry it was revealed that her parents lived in London during her mother's pregnancy with her. They were learning English and speaking it for most of the nine months. They returned to Germany only a week or so before the birth. She reported that one of her easiest classes in school was her English class.

An essential aspect of creativity is curiosity. What do you really want for yourself and your partner and your children? What gives you pleasure? What is something you've been longing to learn about? What is something you've wanted to do with your partner, just the two of you? You have a new life adventure ahead. Be curious about what's happening with your partner. Be curious about the possibilities of giving birth, the world over. Be curious about how to best nourish your pregnant partner and your baby. Be curious about 'fathering' and parenting practices in other cultures. Have fun during pregnancy. Explore the creative possibilities in all parts of your life. Expand and grow during this intense and precious time, and the future will reflect your efforts and commitment.

The Genetic Legacy of Love
by Jeannine Parvati Baker

SIAN WRITES: *I would really appreciate an article on parenting through separation and divorce. My youngest, now four, has been particularly difficult since we left the family home six months ago. Obviously we have all found this very stressful, and I know that the children will be affected, but I'd like to know how best to help them and perhaps avoid some of the trauma. All I ever wanted was to have children with someone I loved, and live in a happy family, so I realise now that everything will always be second best. I want to do what I can for the children's emotional well-being. At the moment, it seems easier for my ten year old, as he can express his emotions and articulate his concerns. We talk about everything (at his level), and he remembers how miserable I was and that his dad just wanted a 'bachelor' lifestyle.*

Dear Sian ~ Your letter showed me a tender spirit, one who is asking the right questions at a most vulnerable time. Next to the death of a spouse, parent, or child, divorce is the most stressful of life's experiences. I feel for you as I've been there myself. Your query letter took me on a trip down mammary lane.

There was one statement in your letter that puzzled me. You wrote, "Everything will always be second best." Forgive my bold question, but how do you know this to be true? "Always" is a very long time, and what does "second best" mean anyway? There's no competition with the God-Us, no contest in life for which a first, second, or third place prize is given when living in the present moment.

With that said, I can empathise with the task at hand. Let me refer to a meeting with a remarkable woman who was my mentor (unbeknownst to her). 20th century author Anais Nin, who I met only once, when I was a young aspiring writer and she a radiant crone, remarked, "When parents fight, it's the equivalent of war to the child." This declaration resonated in my soul then, and still continues to reveal deeper meaning as I watch my children now make me a grandmother.

I may be paraphrasing her statement for it was heard many, many years ago, before I experienced my first divorce. At that time, I had three young children under the age of five years. The farthest thing from my mind when I heard the wise elder speak was that it was my destiny to co-create the psychic equivalence of war for my own children. Divorce is what other people do. Surely I was having some challenges with three youngsters and their father, who at times seemed like the fourth child in the family, and yet I was loyal, determined, and psychologically skilled enough to remain married for almost 10 years, probably forever. Or so I thought.

Yet as our marriage unraveled, so did my pride, and I talked with veterans of divorce and read many a book on how to separate in such a way as to minimise the collateral damage. This is what I now share with you, for it was almost 30 years ago that I began the co-parenting journey. I learned too much the hard way.

What I learned was that each of my children has both parents within every cell of their bodies. This is the genetic legacy of love. Though the prevailing biological story is that mothers provide more genetic material than fathers do (mothers give our mitochondria, the food factory of cell metabolism to our offspring), we're almost in equal proportion composed of both of our parents' DNA.

Knowing this, when I speak about my children's father, I'm being heard on a cellular level. There are ears within the ten billion cells of my children that take the stories in deeply. Not only in my children dwell the DNA of their father, but in my brainstem and bloodstream as well. Did you know that when a woman conceives a baby, the father's genetic material migrates into her? If she gives birth, there's a massive transmigration of the father's DNA into her body. Each child adds more of his genetics into the mother.

This brings me to the second most powerful statement from my inspiration, Anais Nin: "We don't see the world as it is, we see the world as we are."

There's a natural tendency to tell children my side of the story. Yet what seems to be the truth of what happened to the original lovers is merely a story, and my side of it at that. Yet "my side" is not so clearly delineated, especially in light of the current research in cellular biology.

In the tour down the mammary lane of my first divorce, I encounter my regrets. How I wish that I'd been more consistent in telling the story of our dissolution with respect and honour for the man whom I once invited into the softest tissues of my self, shared my bed, and my very soul. Yet I shocked myself to hear the words that fell out of my mouth in reaction to the several custody battles we engaged in for yet another decade. Indeed, it came to me that with the continual fighting, we had to some degree wasted our divorce.

Stretch Marks   361

One of the major battles was centered on the (verbal) agreement we had at the time of divorce, and my ex-husband's eventual change of mind regarding how our children would be raised. I eventually brought him to court to secure a judgment that he cease to vaccinate our children on their weekend and summer visits to his home. That is an entire article in itself, to be shared at another time, for one of the consequences of those hidden vaccinations was the introduction of the live viral Sabin polio into my new healthy baby when I remarried. It was the only time he was seriously ill as child.

Now I know more about forensic psychology and natural health than I ever consciously wanted to, and continue to this day to consult with many separating families to assist them in learning from my mistakes. The good news was that I was successful in protecting my children from not only vaccination, but from also being "disciplined" by my ex-husband's second wife, who nowadays would be considered a child abuser. But this was back in the 1980s, when I had to trailblaze my radical ideas through the court system, paying top dollar to educate my attorneys, who were clueless about the hazards of vaccination.

As I reflect upon the harsh judgments I held about my ex-husband, I see the results of those stories in my grown children. They were hardly able to speak with their father for many years; and only after I had done the work to understand him, could they begin.

More recently, one is closer to her father, yet the other two are still quite estranged. This is sad for me, as I feel accountable. Now we work to become good grandparents, for it benefits all our relations when we do.

My children have had a hard time forgiving their father, and what I've learned is that they're not supposed to. They just need to understand, and then forgiveness is like grace ~ it will flow as a gratuitous psychic event. To accomplish this, focus on what you love(d) about your children's father. When your children ask you questions, respond as if their father was present ~ for he is, in every fibre of your children's being ~ not to mention in your own reptilian brain. Be generous with praise for your ex-husband's fine qualities, the ones you were attracted to, and the ones he still has. Allow your children to learn who he is now, and will become, directly from their own experience.

Be aware that the tendency to judge his desire to be a bachelor (as a violation of the sacred marriage contract) is superseded by what is presently happening. You have the rest of your life to share your values with your children, and if they are optimal for them, they will know it.

What allowed me to heal from the devastation of divorce was gratitude ~ gratitude for my marriage ~ for our love made it possible for me to be a mother. Each time I saw my children's faces, I could see the original love for their father that called them to me in the first place ~ or not. The choice was mine ~ as it is yours. Be patient with yourself, for this is the supreme challenge ~ to stay in the present and allow your jubilant heart to come out to greet your children each day. If you can be grateful for what is, you'll have found a shortcut to enlightenment.

So I'll leave you with this: divorce and single parenting are for the courageous. Be consoled, for this journey is akin to giving birth: if there's too much pain to handle, the mother will simply become unconscious. So no worries, gentle mother, this is your destiny as it was mine. However, it's worth the pain to stay conscious and learn the workings of soul; for when we do, we'll be guided in how to sustain our sacred agreement as possible mothers. For the sake of not only our own children and grandchildren, but for all our relations, we will come out the other side wiser, kinder, and more fully ecstatic. We may indeed realise that life, without the fathers of our children, is the best it can be: maybe even better.

The Enneagram of Personality Types:
how it's helped my parenting
by Paul Robinson

The Enneagram Of Personality Types ~ well that sounds pretty boring, dry and technical: but it's not. The Enneagram has given me a deep understanding of myself. It's a tool for life ~ in that it can accurately and succinctly highlight the potentials and pitfalls for every one of us. It can also be very useful in the understanding of other people, and the development of empathy. Beyond personal growth and understanding, it's usefully employed in any relationship ~ family, in the classroom or in the workplace. It's capable of taking us to the doors of spirituality.

If this system were more widely known and understood, the world would be a more peaceful place. The Enneagram is dynamic, and all-encompassing; it defines personalities, without stereotyping. It doesn't put people into personality pigeon holes, it's fluid. In this system there are nine basic personality types, each of which is influenced to a greater or lesser degree by the adjacent types ~ or wings, as they're known. So, in fact, you could say that there are really 27 types, because, for example, personality Type One is observably different to a Type One with a strong Nine wing, and different to a Type One with a strong Two wing. All three have Type One as the core of their personalities, but the "colouring" is different. In fact, the personality of everyone, falls somewhere on the circumference of the diagram opposite. The chances of it falling directly on one of the types are slim; almost certainly it will be between two of the basic types.

In addition, each type has several healthy, average and unhealthy levels. A personality in the average levels is going to function quite differently to the same personality type in its healthy and unhealthy levels. There's a further refinement. Each personality type has a direction of integration and of disintegration. For example, personality Type One, when functioning very healthily, tends to assume some of the characteristics of a healthy Type Seven; and an unhealthy Type One tends to be overlaid with some of the unhealthy characteristics of Type Four. To give a personal example, I'm Type One. This explains why I'm the proof-reader of this magazine ~ and you should see how I hang out the washing! Amongst other things, Ones tend to be orderly, and have a fine sense of detail. We also tend not be spontaneous, we suppress anger, and could benefit from lightening up a bit. When we're functioning in a healthy (psychological) way, we go in our direction of integration, which for a Type One is Type Seven. Lo and behold, Type Seven tends to be full of energy, very animated, and the life and soul of the party. And the qualities of a healthy Type Seven (which the healthy Type One gravitates towards), are all those jolly things, without any of the drawbacks of average and unhealthy Sevens.

The diagram shows all of human nature at a glance! Each basic type has been assigned a title, to give a flavour of how it functions. The four adjectives below each title give a broad idea of how that personality sees the world when they're emotionally healthy, average, and unhealthy. For me (Type One), I see myself encapsulated in those four words; they never fail to raise a wry smile. Of course, there's a lot more to me than 'idealistic, orderly, perfectionist, intolerant', but as someone who likes to think he's progressing along a spiritual path, those words are a sober reminder.

The lines in the diagram show how the Types are linked. The arrows show the directions of integration. So, for example, the lively, extroverted Type Seven, when functioning healthily, focuses all the energy and ideas that are associated with Sevens, and behaves in an accomplished manner; on top of that, their behaviour also tends towards the higher features of Type Five: perceptiveness, visionary. The direction of disintegration is in the opposite direction. An unhealthy Type Seven would not only demonstrate excessive and manic behaviour, but also tend to have the intolerant attitude of an unhealthy Type One. Most brief overviews of the Enneagram tend to make the subject seem quite complex, and I suppose this is no exception; but the main thing is to work out what your Type is. If you never went further than that, the insights gained could be life-changing.

The origins of the Enneagram are hazy. Part of the tradition can be traced back into antiquity through the mystical arm of Sufi. Gurdjieff certainly had some knowledge of it, but the Enneagram as we know it today can be fully explained in terms of contemporary psychological thought. Up to a point you could say that there's not much in the Enneagram Of Personality Types that you couldn't find elsewhere. But you couldn't find all of it in one place elsewhere, and it wouldn't be expressed so clearly and succinctly.

I first encountered it in the early 90s. A friend, knowing I was looking for answers to 'Life, The Universe, and Everything' (after the end of my first marriage), pointed me in the direction of an architect who gave consultations as a passionate sideline. We spoke for a while. He explained the ins and outs, and then got me to fill in a questionnaire ~ which he then studied. From this chat, and the questionnaire, it was clear to him that I was a Type One, probably with a Two wing. This meant nothing to me; and he apologised for not having a photocopy of the chapter on Type Ones to send me home with. He said he'd post it out. A week passed, and I'd almost forgotten about the Enneagram, when the chapter arrived. I decided to read it in a café I went to occasionally. I sat down with my coffee and cake, but no expectations. The chapter was about 20 pages long. Over the course of the first four pages, my jaw dropped. I was incredulous. It was as if the writer had been spying on me, and had meticulously noted my traits and foibles. What he'd written in those pages turned out to be the broader brush strokes of my personality. In recognising those, I was softened up for what was to follow. I became open to the more subtle (and not always palatable) aspects of myself which were reflected to me in those pages. I was converted immediately; and like many converts, set about converting the people around me. Looking back now, I can see that those with my personality type would tend to do that. Many people I spoke to thought it was very interesting, and they, too, were astonished at how accurately it described them; but in almost all cases, it ranked alongside a magazine quiz ~ a nice bit of entertainment, but they weren't interested in the potential to change and grow.

One of the most elementary things I learnt was that there are nine completely different ways of looking at the world and its events (there are many shades of grey between these). That simple fact was an eye-opener. So if nine people, each with one of the nine personality types, were to observe an event, they'd have nine quite dissimilar experiences to report. They might describe the broad details similarly, but their perceptions of those details, and what was important, would differ enormously. Nine people all of the same type would tend to give similar reports.

A couple of years later, I met Veronika, who was also on a quest for personal and spiritual growth. I shared the Enneagram with her. She realised its potential immediately. We've used it to understand ourselves, each other, and the people around us. My eldest daughter (then 19) did an Enneagram test with me. Between us, we worked out her type. She was very fond of Veronika, and decided that she wanted to come and live with us. We were thrilled, but the dynamics didn't work. It was just one of those things, where no-one was to blame ~ the mix of personalities not suitable to be under one roof. After a month, she moved out, the relationship between her and Veronika apparently irreparable. Not so! Because of the Enneagram, Veronika understood my daughter fairly well, and herself, very well. There was no discussion between them at the time, but Veronika was able to modify her behaviour and attitude. Relationships are very like equations. If one side changes, the other has to. Because of her insights, the relationship was saved. (One of my greatest joys of recent times was when that daughter came from New Zealand to visit us, last year ~ and to hear her and Veronika, in the next room, laughing their heads off about something.)

When our daughters, Bethany and Eliza, came along, we were able to work out their personality types by observing them. (It's said by some specialists in this field that the personality type displayed by a child is not necessarily the one they'll have as an adult. I take the view of others who assert that a child's personality may be modified by circumstances, but it will stay within the parameters of that basic personality. It's the old nature/nurture issue. There's a longitudinal study which was started in Dunedin [New Zealand] in the 1970s, involving various regular check-ups on all babies born at that hospital. As far as I know, this study is still running. I heard one of the professors being interviewed about some of the conclusions he'd drawn from his observations of the thousands of children and adults who had taken part in that study. One of his comments stood out like a beacon. He said that when he first became involved with the project, he would have asserted that human nature/personality was, say, two thirds nurture, and one third nature. After over twenty years of observation, he stated that he now thought it was the other way round. This is my layman's conclusion, too.) Bethany and Eliza, still, at 12 and 10, exhibit the same traits that we observed when they were tiny. They came out wired that way. By being able to pinpoint their basic type (we'd expect to refine that, and to identify their sub-type when they're older, if they're interested, and want to put the work in), we're able to understand them better ~ both to help us in our day-to-day relationships with them, and to help them, as they mature, to know where their strengths and challenges lie: and have insights into, and empathy with, the behaviour of other people (especially their parents!). It's very easy, as parents, to expect our children to be like us in their attitudes and behaviour; or we might expect them to be like each other. Even now, knowing that their personalities aren't the same as the rest of their family, I have to remind myself that they don't see the world through my lenses. I constantly have to revisit the insights into their perceptions of the world that I've gained through the Enneagram, in order to stop myself from trying to impose my world view on them.

Here are some very brief descriptions of the nine types.

1: Reformers, Judges, Perfectionists

Ones are focused on personal integrity, and can be wise, discerning and inspiring in their quest for the truth. They also tend to dissociate themselves from their flaws or what they believe are flaws (such as negative emotions), and can become hypocritical, and hypercritical of others, seeking the illusion of virtue to hide their own vices. The greatest fear of Ones is to be flawed, and their ultimate goal is perfection.

2: Helpers, Givers, Caretakers, Assistants

Twos, at their best, are compassionate, attentive, generous and caring, but they can also be particularly prone to clinginess, neediness and manipulation. Twos want, above all, to be loved and needed. They fear being unworthy of love.

3: Achievers, Performers, Status Seekers

Threes tend to be especially adaptable and changeable. Some walk the world with confidence and authenticity; others wear a series of public masks, acting in ways they think will bring them approval, but losing track of their true self. Threes are motivated by the need to succeed and to be seen as successful.

4: Romantics, Individualists, Aesthetes, Artists

Fours are driven by the desire to understand themselves, and find a place in the world. They often fear that they have no identity or personal significance. Fours embrace individualism, and are often profoundly creative and intuitive, and at best they are very humane. However, they have a habit of withdrawing to internalise, searching desperately inside themselves for something they never find, and creating a spiral of depression.

5: *Experts, Thinkers, Investigators, Observers*

Fives are motivated by the desire to understand the facts about the world around them. Believing they are only worth what they contribute, Fives have learned to withdraw, to watch with keen eyes, and speak only when they can shake the world with their observations. Sometimes they do just that. However, some Fives are known to withdraw almost completely from the world, becoming reclusive hermits and fending off social contact with abrasive cynicism. Fives fear incompetence or uselessness, and want to be capable and knowledgeable, above all else.

6: *Loyalists, Heroes/Rebels, Defenders, Sceptics, Questioners*

Sixes long for safe stability above all else. They exhibit unwavering loyalty and responsibility, but once betrayed, they're slow to trust again. They're particularly prone to fearful thinking and emotional anxiety, as well as reactionary and paranoid behaviour. Sixes tend to react to their fears either in a phobic manner by avoiding fearful situations, or by confronting them in a counter-phobic manner.

7: *Enthusiasts, Adventurers, Sensationalists*

Sevens are adventurous, constantly busy with many activities, with all the energy and enthusiasm of Peter Pan. At their best they embrace life for its varied joys and wonders, and truly live in the moment; but, at their worst, they dash frantically from one new experience to another, too scared of disappointment to actually enjoy themselves. Sevens fear being unable to provide for themselves or to experience life in all of its richness.

8: *Bosses, Mavericks, Challengers, Asserters*

Eights value their own strength, and desire to be powerful and in control. They concern themselves with self-preservation. They're natural leaders, who can be either friendly and charitable, or dictatorially manipulative, ruthless and willing to destroy anything in their way. Eights seek control over their own lives and destinies, and fear being harmed or controlled by others.

9: *Mediators, Peacemakers, Preservationists, Peace Seekers*

Nines are ruled by their empathy. At their best they're receptive, gentle, calming and at peace with the world. They also, however, tend to dissociate from conflicts and to indifferently go along with other people's wishes. They may also simply withdraw, and try to shut down emotionally and mentally. They fear the conflict caused by their ability to simultaneously understand opposing points of view, and seek peace of mind above all else. Nines are especially prone to dissociation and passive-aggressive behaviour.

One of the lessons I'm at last learning about personal/spiritual growth is that it's all very well to read interesting books, full of great ideas of how to do this and that; but it's very easy to keep on reading more books ~ it's a great distraction, which means I can put off the hard work of actually knuckling down and starting to implement the changes necessary to live a fulfilling, happy and balanced life. We have a deep-seated fear of becoming unbalanced by fundamental changes ~ better the devil you know. So, with regards the Enneagram, it's possible to gain insights into the depths of ourselves; but unless we take the next step, and put those insights to work, then we'll be off again, reading the next book, going to the next seminar. And the same applies to our relationships. The challenge is to put oneself into the other person's shoes, to try, using the knowledge gained from the Enneagram, to feel what life is like for that other person. Without that step being taken, only lip-service has been paid, and we'll continue to see that person through our prejudices; if we won't see them as they really are, they'll appear to continue to behave as we think they shouldn't.

There are many writers on the subject of the Enneagram, and there are many interpretations of its wisdom. The books I've found most useful, are Personality Types, by Don Richard Riso and Russ Hudson (Houghton Mifflin), The Wisdom of the Enneagram, also by Riso and Hudson (Bantam Books) and The Enneagram Of Parenting, by Elizabeth Wagele (HarperSanFransisco).

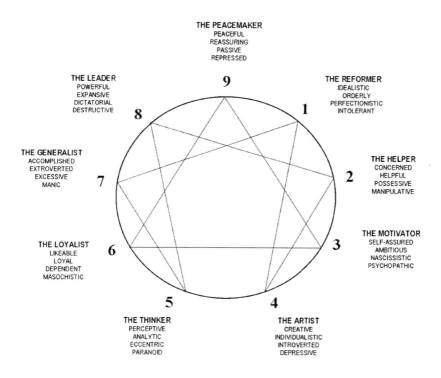

THE PEACEMAKER
PEACEFUL
REASSURING
PASSIVE
REPRESSED

THE LEADER
POWERFUL
EXPANSIVE
DICTATORIAL
DESTRUCTIVE

THE REFORMER
IDEALISTIC
ORDERLY
PERFECTIONISTIC
INTOLERANT

THE GENERALIST
ACCOMPLISHED
EXTROVERTED
EXCESSIVE
MANIC

THE HELPER
CONCERNED
HELPFUL
POSSESSIVE
MANIPULATIVE

THE LOYALIST
LIKEABLE
LOYAL
DEPENDENT
MASOCHISTIC

THE MOTIVATOR
SELF-ASSURED
AMBITIOUS
NASCISSISTIC
PSYCHOPATHIC

THE THINKER
PERCEPTIVE
ANALYTIC
ECCENTRIC
PARANOID

THE ARTIST
CREATIVE
INDIVIDUALISTIC
INTROVERTED
DEPRESSIVE

Stretch Marks

Education and Learning

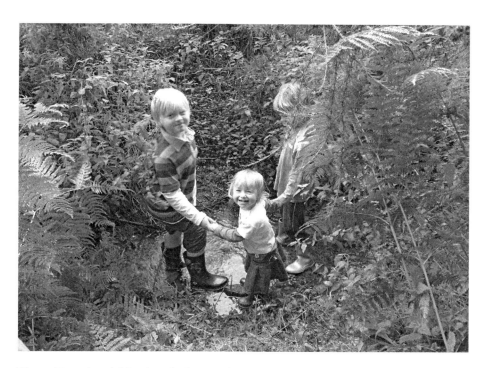

Hugo, Naomi and friend exploring at The Mother magazine family camp, 2009

The gifts of learning at home
by Siobhán Kramer

Siobhán Kramer lives with her partner and two small children in rural Ireland. They home educate, grow vegetables, and live off the grid. To read more or get in touch, please visit:
http://bloginthebog.wordpress.com

What leads a family to decide not to send their children to school? Parents of many different educational backgrounds may come to this decision. A tendency to challenge the received wisdom of the day might be one precipitating factor: possibly a certain amount of stubbornness. In other cases, parents don't start out by questioning the education system much, but the system doesn't suit their child in some way, which forces them to think critically about something which most people take utterly for granted. My own parents had very different individual experiences of school. My mother was academically gifted and successful, but saw that the education system didn't suit everyone. Individual learning styles weren't catered for, and practical, artistic and other non-academic skills weren't highly valued. She objected greatly to the apparent premise that the teacher "gives" knowledge to the student, rather than drawing out their innate capabilities. My father, on the other hand, had a very negative experience of school. He and his classmates experienced terrorisation and brutality at the hands of the religious order that ran his school during the 1940s and '50s. He loved horses, working the land and growing things, but such talents and inclinations weren't prized by the education system. He left school early and was successful in many ventures, without qualifications. When they had children of their own, my parents saw that we were learning lots of things quite happily at home. They also found the local school inflexible when they were investigating enrolment, and so they kept my sister and I at home for the time being. I was the first of ten children, all of whom were "unschooled" (though my parents hadn't heard this term at the time!).

It's hard to convey how different the cultural climate in Ireland was toward this path 30 years ago, than it is today. Many people, of course, still dismiss home education, organic gardening, homebirth and other such choices as hippy nonsense, or some other damning label. Nowadays, however, there's a definite movement associated with such lifestyles ~ visible in magazines, such as The Mother, or on the Internet. There was no Home Education group or magazine in Ireland when my parents started their family. They anticipated a trend which was not yet trendy! Their families didn't agree with what they were doing, and weren't shy about telling them so. They were given dire warnings about how they were compromising our futures, and cutting us off from "the real world". My parents spent the majority of their time at home with us. They owned a modest house, and focused on acquiring skills such as organic growing, over university degrees and possessions. They rejected many of the consumerist values of the culture they lived in ~ which seemed to bring up anger and defensiveness in their peers. So, did I live in the real world? Certainly, the older siblings in our family didn't have a huge amount of early contact with popular culture. I didn't know how credit cards worked, or have a mobile phone, until I went to university. I may have been embarrassed by this fact at different times, but I now see it as an advantage rather than a disadvantage. Playing video games and eating processed foods, for example, are aspects of this culture which I prefer my children to come into contact with as slowly and minimally as possible. I believe that minimal early exposure to these things gives them a sporting chance of choosing or rejecting them, rather than doing them addictively and without awareness. If there is a "real world", in my opinion, it is the world of Nature, of which we're a part.

Learning about our interconnectedness to other living things and our planet may be the most important lesson we learn, not just as children, but for our survival as a species. Of course, the intersection between making choices for our children as little ones and giving them the space to freely choose or reject things as they grow is another important issue.

Growing up home educated, in a large, close family, wasn't always idyllic. The vast majority of response by school educated children to my situation was positive, in that they considered me lucky. My extreme love of reading and writing were not, however, always compatible with a life which required us to be outdoors a lot; helping with younger siblings; gardening; and caring for animals. I found it hard to honour my needs for solitude and quiet in such a chaotic house, where privacy and peace were endangered species. My parents departed a long way from the conformist, authoritarian culture they grew up in, which took great effort and commitment.

Still, this departure was not always enough for me. La Leche League, The Mother magazine and books and forums of equality between parents and children represent my truth more accurately. I find this struggle between how I was raised, my aspirations, and good old reality, to be very difficult at times. My parents support my efforts and listen to what I have to say, despite the challenges my choices present to their values. It's a gift to have this dialogue, rather than the one-sided communication which still goes on between many adult children and their parents. I found out the hard way, by having my children 18 months apart, that short gaps between children, as in my family of origin, were not suited to my own aspirations of peaceful parenting and meeting everyone's needs. In ways, I think that close families are equally blessed and cursed. While there's much one wants to emulate in the style and practices of one's parents, finding out where they end and you begin can be a painful process. Just as our strength is our weakness, however, our weakness is also our strength. When I talk to some friends about the pain of opposition of one's family to one's choices, I count my blessings in that I have a supportive family. For better or for worse, I think that home educating families tend to have an intimacy which is alien to many modern families.

I had fears around starting school at the age of seventeen. I was afraid of not fitting in, or not being able to keep up. I can see clearly now, over ten years down the line, that as the oldest child of one of the older Irish home educating families, I felt a certain amount of pressure to prove that I could perform at school as good as or better than the next person. My four years of University education may have also been partly born of this need to prove myself. I sometimes wish I hadn't been so influenced by the opinions of others and desperate to prove myself, but this is a feature of mine in many areas of my life. To wish it away would be to wish myself other than I am. Separating the decision to home educate from the personality of the parent is not always an easy task. Because home education requires a certain amount of doggedness and persistence, these tend to be a feature of home educating parents. Feeling like a misfit may be another feature of taking such a counter-cultural decision. As a home educating parent, you'll probably spend far more time in the company of your child than most of your peers, which will set you apart. The decision to forgo one parent's income often goes hand in hand with home education, which also goes against the cultural grain. Therefore, in a home educating family, the parents will probably be one of the main influences on the child's life, compared to the not inconsiderable influence of persons outside the family in a school situation. The chances of the parents being determined and persistent in a home educating family are also quite high. These factors all point to an intensity of relationship between the home educating family which is uncommon in most Western nuclear families. Although this can be a mixed blessing, I personally am grateful to my parents for the gift of the inestimable time and energy given to us in their decision to home educate. No parents are perfect, but their refusal to passively swallow received wisdom has greatly helped to inform my questioning nature. Having grown up at some distance from many aspects of our culture has helped me to make informed choices which have brought me much fulfilment, empowerment and joy. Having been home educated is very much a part of who I am, and I wouldn't change it for the world.

*I think that
home educating families
tend to have
an intimacy
which is alien
to many modern families.*

The Central Place of Play
in Early Learning and Development
by Dr. Richard House

The prominent early years academic, Professor Tina Bruce, has said that 'Play cannot be pinned down, and turned into a product of measurable learning. This is because play is a process [which] enables a holistic kind of learning, rather than fragmented learning' (in Ward, 1998: 22, 24; see House, 1999).

It's often said that play is, paradoxically, a very serious business indeed. One reason why this might be so is strikingly described by David Elkind: '[Play] is young children's only defence against the many real or imagined attacks and slights they encounter... [It] is always a transformation of reality in the service of the self' (quoted in Oldfield, 2001: 96).

It follows from this that we interfere with and impinge upon the 'genius' of children's free play at our ~ and their ~ peril...

'Play' has certainly been in the news a lot in recent years ~ both through the educational authorities in their move towards an organised so-called 'curriculum' for the early years (as typified by the Curriculum Guidance for the Foundation Stage document ~ hereafter referred to as 'CGFS' ~ DfEE and QCA, 2000), and also in the works of a number of commentators bemoaning the degradation of authentic play in modern culture (e.g. Elkind, 1990; Jenkinson, 2000).

The key debate that has recently dominated early years practice has been over the very nature of play itself ~ with Waldorf and other 'holistic' approaches arguing forcefully that, to be authentic, play must be an unintruded-upon, self-directed activity and experience for the young child; whereas the current fashion within mainstream early years thinking embraces so-called 'structured (or extended) play', in which adults actively and consciously intervene into the play of young children, guiding and manipulating it towards pre-determined 'learning goals' and experiences that the adult thinks the young child should have for its own good. There's hardly a better example of the incommensurable world views demonstrated by current mainstream approaches to early learning, on the one hand, and that of Steiner Waldorf philosophy on the other.

From a holistic and Steiner Waldorf perspective, self-directed imaginative play is therefore crucial for children's healthy physical, emotional and social development: as Rawson and Rose (2002: 71) put it,

'The way we allow… children to play is of spiritual concern. The health of the body; the life processes [including healthy breathing ~ RH]; mental, emotional, social, and moral competence; and conscience and the innermost sense of self ~ all are developed through play'.

It will be useful to highlight the attitude to play demonstrated in the British Government's CGFS document, as it enables us to make a highly revealing comparison with the Waldorf approach to play. As already mentioned, 'free play' is central to the Waldorf early years learning environment. CGFS, however, displays a very different view.

Early on in CGFS, we are told that 'The role of the practitioner includes… supporting and extending children's play…' (p. i); then on page 7, 'Well-planned play is a key way in which children learn…'; 'The role of the practitioner is crucial in… supporting children's learning through planned play activity, extending and supporting children's spontaneous play…' (p. 25).

This latter is a quite extraordinary statement ~ an unintended oxymoron that reveals quite conclusively that, despite the manifold representations made to the Government on play (not least from the Steiner Waldorf movement), there's an almost wilful misunderstanding (or deliberate ignoring?…) of the nature of authentic play. The very idea, for example, that it's the adult's place to 'extend spontaneous play' for children!

In my view, the likely long-term impoverishing effects on the healthy development of the unfortunate children subjected to this fundamentally misguided regime can scarcely be dreamt of.

Later in CGFS, we are told that 'practitioners need to take part in children's play… and encourage children to sort, group and sequence in their play ~ use words such as "last", "first", "next", "before", "after", "all", "most", "each", "every"' (p. 53).

Not only is this a quite grotesque case of control-freakery gone mad (perhaps the practitioner will have a checklist to tick off each word when she has 'taught' it to the child?), but it again represents a quite fundamental misunderstanding of the nature of authentic play. And later still: 'practitioners need to… play alongside children, using words and actions to represent objects, for example say, "Mmmm, I'd like some more cake", while pretending to cut a slice and pass it…; (and to) prompt children's thinking and discussion through involvement in their play' (p. 57); and practitioners should make 'good use of opportunities to talk "mathematically" as children play' (p. 72)!

Adult intrusion into child's play is, then, seen as being perfectly acceptable: thus we read that practitioners encourage 'children's mathematical development by intervening in their play'…: 'Intervening in children's play includes asking appropriate questions such as, "How many people have you drawn?", "Are any of those shapes the same?" and "Have all the trucks got the same number of wheels?"' (ibid.).

Later, we read that practitioners need to 'participate in children's play to encourage use of number language' (p. 75). Later still, the following 'Stepping stone' is set out: 'Introduce a story line or narrative into their play' (p. 124), and the injunction, 'Be interested [i.e. feign it? ~ RH] and participate in children's play' (p. 125).

In contrast, there's a host of literature ~ non-Waldorf as well as Waldorf ~ which explains at length just why free play is so crucial. First, creativity and freedom are inextricably linked, and the roots of creativity lie in the capacity to play in what the celebrated psychoanalyst and paediatrician Donald Winnicott called the 'transitional space' (e.g. Winnicott, 1971).

In Waldorf terminology, authentic play can only occur within a 'dream' or 'mythological' consciousness (sometimes also called 'participative consciousness'), from which the child should not be prematurely 'awakened' through inappropriate, adult-centric intrusions.

The distinguished child psychologist Susan Isaacs wrote eloquently and with perennial wisdom about the true nature of play and its central role in healthy child development: for Isaacs, the child's imaginative play 'is a starting point [or foundation ~ RH] not only for cognitive development but also for the adaptive and creative intention which when fully developed marks out the artist, the novelist, the poet' (1930: 104).

The psychic process involved in play is seen by Isaacs as both crucial and highly complex: thus, in play the child is 're-creating selectively those elements in past situations which can embody his emotional or intellectual need of the present, [as] he adapts the details moment by moment to the present situation' (ibid., original emphasis).

Several years later, Isaacs was to write that the lessening of inner tension and anxiety resulting from free dramatic play 'makes it easier for the child to control his real behaviour [i.e. he learns self-regulation ~ RH]..., helps to free the child from his personal schemas, and to enhance his readiness to understand the objective physical world for its own sake' (Isaacs, 1933: 210).

On pages 425-7 of her Social Development in Young Children, Isaacs sets out a truly magnificent and inspiring statement on the crucial importance of free play in healthy child development and learning, which should be required reading for each and every early years worker and policy-maker (see House, 2000: 12). Thus, there are also quite crucial self-healing and emotional-developmental aspects to authentic play, as Jenkinson points out in Chapter 3 of The Genius of Play, which she fittingly titles 'Teaching the heart'.

For as Rawson and Rose write, 'The activities and games that express the heart are also the games that develop the heart, together with the whole of our rhythmical system' (2002: 77). Both prominent psychoanalytic theorists (typified in this case by Isaacs; but see also Winnicott's important work, 1971) and Rudolf Steiner viewed fantasy as a crucial indissoluble accompaniment to authentic play.

Thus we see Steiner saying that 'Our willing depends on sympathy..., [and] out of sympathy there arises fantasy' (quoted in Konig, 1998: 65).

For Karl Konig, such sympathy takes the form of a 'continuous joy of existence..., uniting ever anew with the world around' (ibid.), as is the origin of all fantasy. The child takes her fantasy from her 'ceaseless need for lively activity... fantasy is born out of [her] limb system' (ibid.: 65, 66).

Further, 'Each... form of movement is embedded in a story that... begins without ending, and ends without having begun' (p. 65). Indeed, in all play, 'there is no beginning and no ending, and yet all is happening' (ibid). According to Rawson and Rose (2002: 75), fantasy begins to arise as the child approaches her fourth year, and they define it as 'the child's ability to project her increasingly conscious inner life onto the world around her' (ibid.).

Fantasy has a special place in infancy: it 'takes hold of any kind of material, movements as well as ideas, for activating itself;...

[and] fantasy without play and play without fantasy are almost unthinkable…play enlivens fantasy…, [and] fantasy kindles and diversifies play' (Konig, 1998: 64).

Moreover, 'Real experiences have their sources only in the child's fantasy… [T]he child can grasp his environment only as interpretation of his fantasy, and existence gains its true meaning and becomes experience in this way alone' (64). As Konig graphically puts it, 'Without [fantasy] all ideas stagnate… Concepts remain rigid and dead, sensations raw and sensuous' (Konig, 1998: 66).

And here is one of the last century's greatest minds, Albert Einstein:

'I have come to the
conclusion that the
gift of fantasy has
meant more to me than any talent for abstract,
positive thinking'
(quoted in Rawson and Rose, 2002: 21).

What seems quite unarguable is that as soon as an external (adult-centric) agent intrudes upon those crucial self-regulative and intrinsically healing processes triggered in and through authentically free play (as occurs in 'structured' play), then these processes will at the very least be significantly distorted ~ and at worst their value to the young child will be largely destroyed.

In this spirit, I agree wholeheartedly with Frommer when, writing of the child's 'time of magic and omnipotence' between three and six, she writes, 'The clumsy adult must be careful not to destroy this web of magic by stupid and tactless intervention… It's a world we adults have lost, and we can only regain understanding of it… by sympathetic intuitive insight and faithful non interference' (Frommer, 1994: 24).

The form taken by play also changes and evolves through the early years. Fantasy play around ages four to five is spontaneous, often based on imitation and the inspiration gleaned from stories and the archetypal fairy tales. The five year old is normally content to adapt to reality as he finds it, whereas there's a discernible shift in the six year old, when his play becomes more inward and idea-based, with fewer props needed, and with the child becoming more interested in creating a reality through play.

So what are the implications of these views for the way in which the Waldorf Kindergarten environment is organised? First, the provision of space and unhurried opportunity is crucial.

In most if not all Waldorf Kindergartens, there's an extended period of free play near or at the start of the Kindergarten session, in which as far as is possible, and within sensible boundaries of safety and sociality, adults don't intrude into the children's play unless they're specifically asked for assistance by the children; and then the tacit guiding principle is that the adult intrudes only to the absolutely minimal extent that is required by the specific situation, and should continually reflect inwardly on their own behaviour and its appropriateness.

The mature self-awareness and self-development of the teacher is crucial here; for teachers and assistants need to know their own 'inner child' and her/his needs very well, in order that they do not unconsciously 'act out' their own issues with the children.

I believe that this is in fact what is often happening when adults do over-intrude (and when policy-makers advocate it!) into the worlds of the young children in their charge. Rudolf Steiner himself recognised this danger early in the last century: [the teacher] yearns to have something in its own nature as vital as the wisdom of the child. (It goes without saying that he will never admit this.) In his subconscious life…, longings for the wise life forces of the children play a great part, though he may not know it… He begins to prey upon the young souls as a vampire… Anyone who looks into the life of the classroom freely and without bias will be driven to… corroborate this statement…[T]hey will see how the teachers rob the children of force, instead of giving it. ~ Rudolf Steiner, 1931: 37.

It's important that there's an adequate and appropriate range of play resources available for the range of ages (three to six) which is typically present in the mixed-age Waldorf Kindergarten.

In the Waldorf Kindergarten, children are also provided with simple and unelaborated, natural play materials and 'props' ~ ones which encourage the children freely to engage their developing and fertile imaginations and fantasy lives, and which avoid, if at all possible, 'dead' human-made materials like plastic, nylon material, and so on. Dolls are a case in point. What the child needs in its play is something which can reflect her own condition and her own unfolding developmental potentials, and she'll find this in a doll made of soft natural material, with no more than the slightest hint of a face, which can then be made to represent whatever expression the child needs it to have at any given time (Rawson and Rose, 2002: 74).

Steiner also had prescient remarks to make about the kinds of toys that children should ideally be provided with: 'Our materialistic age produces few good toys... [The] work of the imagination moulds and builds the forms of the brain. The brain unfolds as the muscles of the brain unfold... Give the child the so-called "pretty" doll, and the brain has nothing to do' (quoted in Grunelius, 1991: 45).

A recent German research project gave compelling corroboration of the Steinerian approach to toys and play. In this so-called 'nursery without toys', children were left with spartan resources (blankets, tables, chairs...), and before long it was found that their imaginations thrived, their interactive social skills developed dramatically, and their sense of purpose and capacity to concentrate improved greatly (Roberts, 1999: 6; see also Mowafi, 2001; Clark, 2002).

What is so interesting is how the findings of modern empirical research are progressively confirming so many of the principles of Waldorf educational philosophy and practice ~ especially in the early years; and what is so galling is how little public recognition still seems to be received by an educational approach which in many ways seems to have 'had it right' all along.

In sum, and quoting Rawson and Rose, 'Children who are allowed to play freely will demonstrate a genius for lateral thinking and problem solving of which we adults should be envious. All too often..., well-intentioned adults are too quick to intervene..., and on both sides important possibilities remain unrealised' (2002: 78).

This, in turn, highlights just how important are the sensitive attunement and subtle, sometimes intuitive nuances entailed in healthy adult-child relating ~ or what Steiner evocatively called 'the intangibles of education', which demand of the parent, adult and teacher qualities of openness; self-awareness; the capacity to listen and not unconsciously project; of empathy; and, above all, of unconditional non-possessive love (Carl Rogers).

Letting Divinity out to play
by Tish Clifford

We have become a world obsessed with education, and I've recently had some stark reminders of this.

I DON'T EDUCATE ~ or I should say, I don't in the traditional Western, left-hemisphere way. In fact, I can't stand it, and the minimal reading, writing, and maths that I do with my eldest child often leaves us both feeling a bit 'off colour'.

You see, I don't draw my sense of self from academia and education, and I certainly don't draw my children's sense of self from academia and education.

If you study ancient spiritual scriptures, you'll notice parallels in the stories. We are divine beings of 'God' (Source/Spirit ~ use whatever word fits), and it's our labelling, educated (programmable) mind that takes us away from who we really are. No spiritual techniques say "now go and label this and go and label that, and learn it inside out so that you can be intelligent and academic and know yourself!" No, they say the opposite. They say forget the rational mind, forget the labels ~ become the experience. Breathe life. Live.

If we get our sense of self through our ego, then we'll value education highly, because we don't have another reference point for that which we truly are. We'll 'think' we're our thoughts, our concepts, and our delusions.

Education is generally brought about through the fear that if we're not educated we'll not be able to get on in this world and provide for ourselves. To some degree, this is true, but only because the world has become dominated by a system that highly values what education you have, and then pays in accordance to this.

But this system is flawed; it's flawed because the Earth doesn't care how educated you are, or how much money you earn. A time is coming, soon, when what will be valued will be highly different to what is currently valued. Those who have an understanding of natural biological laws, who know which wild foods one can eat; who know how to connect with spirit; who know which herbs will heal; and how to build natural shelter, etc., are the people who'll be valued. This system will crash, is crashing, has to crash; there's no choice in the matter.

Giving our children a real education means 'teaching' them about Nature, and how to feed and provide for themselves from her system. It means allowing our children space to connect with their true inherent natural self. A self that can't be educated in there, as it is in there from conception. Life is about allowing this inherent self time to be: free.

On the flip side, and for anyone who still feels they really want their little Johnny to be 'good' at something, let's take a look at autistic savants[*1]. Savants are basically autistic individuals who display incredible genius abilities. These abilities can be musical, artistic, mathematical, language-based, memory-based, or scientific; there's also evidence that some appear to have extra-sensory abilities. But they all have one thing in common: they didn't have to learn a thing. These skills appeared naturally, and they weren't given 'art lessons' at three to be able to draw like Leonardo, or given 'visual text-book' music lessons to play Mozart, or 'rational maths lessons' to 'do' complex mathematical sums better than a calculator, or taught languages to be able to learn Icelandic in two weeks. And here is the interesting bit for all of us 'normal folk': some world authorities, in investigating this phenomenon, have come to a startling conclusion: that these skills are present within every one of us, and they're present in the right hemisphere of our brain.

You see, it would appear that the left hemisphere filters out these skills by being dominant, (and, some would say, deluded, dysfunctional, and exceptionally limited!). Savants seem to have partial release from the tyranny of this hemisphere, and so they manifest these inherent and extraordinary skills effortlessly. Others can discover these skills, too. It's labelled 'acquired savants', and interestingly and tellingly it happens when there's been some kind of damage to the left hemisphere through an accident or stroke, so the right side has to then compensate. These skills appear completely spontaneously.

Alan Synder, from the Centre of the Mind in Australia[*2], has for some years been trying to access these savant traits in 'normal' individuals. His research has sent shock waves around the scientific community. He basically 'shuts down' areas of the left hemisphere for periods of time using magnetic stimulation, and, lo and behold, these genius traits appear as if by magic!

It has to be said here, that savant autistics also experience great social difficulties, and I'm not in any way trying to say it would be beneficial to create savants out of us all! But we do live in a world that rewards the left brain, and the current way that we teach children is taking them directly away from the place where they may discover these inherent skills naturally, for themselves. Recently, I expanded my daughter's drawing ability dramatically within one hour by teaching her a few of the lessons out of Drawing From The Right Side Of The Brain. I did this more out of curiosity than because I want her to be able to draw accurately. It also means our children, if we choose to educate them in a traditional left-hemisphere, Western way, will experience more stress than they need to, especially when we consider the ease at which the right hemisphere can do the very things we're trying to teach.

To get free and natural access to this phenomenal hemisphere can be quite tricky. It would appear that for some reason, (and scientists normally try to explain this away within the generally accepted adaptive selection model$_{(*3)}$, the left hemisphere in all individuals around the world is dominant. In babies and small children, it's less so, but as they grow, it naturally takes charge, as it's the hemisphere that speaks. And speech is obviously the pinnacle of our evolutionary right, or so we're conditioned to believe by the very hemisphere that speaks, and wants to stay in control!

Ancient and modern mystics, however, don't share that same belief; and silencing the talking mind (meditation) is a technique that's been used through the ages to get access to our more profound nature.

I believe, as parents, we need to consider and ponder this all very carefully if we want to create happy, spiritually-connected children who have a deep access to a profound level of functioning very rarely seen. The Indigo Children seems to be a concept that alternative folk are interested in. I propose these are children who have more heightened right hemisphere access, for whatever reason.

Activities which help to allow this hemisphere time out of the 'shackles' of the dominant left are: being in Nature…silently; meditation; singing and playing music; picking wild food; dancing; massage and sensual touch or any body 'work'; relaxation; visualisation; chanting; gardening; being creative, etc. By bringing these activities into our daily lives, and the lives of our children, we nurture them in a way which will bring more peace and happiness to our families.

As for education: pah! I say let divinity out to play…

I trust that as our modern world collapses before our very eyes (isn't it already?), it will be these divine 'children' and spiritually-minded, Earthly parents who lead humanity forward…to paradise on Earth, where we value each other and all that truly sustains us…

*1 For more info on savants visit this amazing web site - http://www.wisconsinmedicalsociety.org/savant/faq.cfm
And of particular interest for this article visit:
http://www.wisconsinmedicalsociety.org/savant/eachus.cfm
*2 For more info on Synder's research: http://www.centreforthemind.com/
*3 For an alternative to this standard model, please visit: www.kaleidos.org.uk

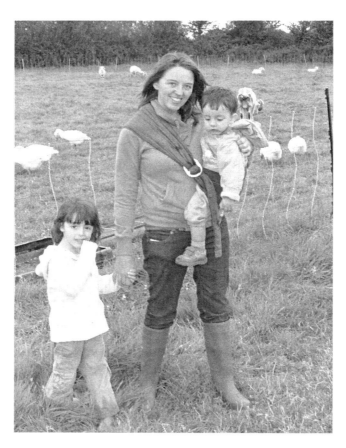

Amelia and her children, Sophia and Nicholas

Touch the Future:
basic trust, learning and the intelligence of play
by Michael Mendizza

Michael Mendizza is an educational and documentary filmmaker, writer, photographer and founder of Touch the Future.
www.nurturing.us   www.ttfuture.org

Touch the Future was founded to explore the question: how has childhood changed since World War II? Recent studies in learning and brain development demonstrate that when the environment changes, we adapt. The greater the change, the greater the pressure to adapt. With this in mind, we can look at changes in the outer environment, and explore how they affect learning, sense of place, relationships, feelings of empathy, and values: factors implicit in the formation of one's all-important self-image.

How have changes in the environment we call 'childhood' affected the self-image of young people today? What is the environment of childhood? What do we mean when we say 'childhood'?

Consider that it's adult culture ~ beliefs, behaviours and assumptions ~ that creates the box we call childhood. If a child's intelligence and capacity to learn is infinite, we should look at the box, rather than the child, when we attempt to define childhood. Childhood is more a set of limitations than a period of life suited to expansive, adaptive learning. If our focus were on learning, rather than limiting, our systems of education, athletic programs, and just about everything we call childhood, would change dramatically.

We live in a culture based on comparison and contrast: contest. Life is a contest. We get grades. We line up in class. Who is tallest? Fastest? Most attractive? We measure everything. This is part of the box we call childhood. Whenever one is in a contest ~ being measured, tested, and compared ~ there exists the possibility of fear, failure, judgment, and the need to be defensive. This need to defend is woven into the environment. The greater the risk, the greater the need to invest energy in the defence structure we call our ego ~ which comes with a corresponding loss of learning ability and performance.

Clearly, the level of contest has increased, demanding that more and more attention be devoted to self-defence. If contest implicitly strengthens the self-centred ego, as a defence reflex, then the question arises: is it possible to raise or educate a child in a way that prevents this ego-defence reflex from developing? In child's play, or the zone ~ the flow state of peak performance ~ the ego disappears as the whole body and mind focus on the task or challenge. We might consider that what we think of as the ego only pops up along with the need to defend or justify. The less security there is, the louder it screams, and the more dominance it asserts in order to protect its image ~ which seems quite natural for a defence structure.

Is it possible to raise a child in such a way that this defensive self-image isn't needed? With this question, we begin to look at childhood in terms of basic trust, safety and threat. Remember, however, that in a contest-culture, threat is ever-present. It's always there. There is a right way, and if you don't do it that way, you're wrong.

When the child first tries to do anything, most often they don't succeed. Failure is built into the system. The parent feels it's really important to tell the child the right way to do things. I did so yesterday when my son washed the car. He didn't do it my right way, and I had to tell him. I couldn't help myself. The concept of right and wrong is built into the structure. School and grades, judgments, reinforce the need for this psychological defence mechanism.

Five years ago, we began a project called The Intelligence of Play. A colleague happened to be an athletic performance specialist. His proven methods involve helping top golfers get out of their own way, and free their innate intelligence to perform as it was designed to. With this placed under the microscope, it became obvious that the ego gets in the way of learning and performance. It wastes attention and energy, usually on psychological fears, which are only as real as we make them. What are they going to think of me?

This is the big question we ask when someone is looking, a question which brings us back to basic trust and safety, and the defence reflex called the ego. All of us have had moments when that defence structure is not there, and we enter the zone (or flow; there are many names for it.)

I think the best and most basic name for this egoless state is play. Real child's play, and what athletes call the zone, are the same thing. The child at play is completely entrained. Their body, their emotions, their intellect are all coherently focused on what's going to happen next? There's a sense of deep relationship and mystery, a burning curiosity to discover what's next. I've been interviewing professional golfers, asking what it was about the way they were raised that allowed them to reach an extraordinary level of performance.

Two things came up in every interview with professional athletes. The first was love of the game, love of the pure experience. They got involved because mum and dad just loved to play golf. This was the space in which they saw dad at home and at peace, and they simply wanted to become a part of that. The second aspect was no fear of censor. In other words, it didn't matter what their score was. It didn't matter how well they did. What mattered was that they were participating in the experience, enjoying and learning from every shot.

When they came back from a tournament, their parents didn't ask them, "What did you shoot, what's your score?" There was no equation of score to self-worth. The score didn't matter. They were unconditionally accepted as human beings. Competition came much later, and enabled them to pull and test themselves further. Competition is not about beating another person ~ the root of the word competition means to strive together. The competitor is your friend, providing the resistance necessary to draw out hidden potential. It's hard to fully realise potential when playing alone. Three aspects of great learning and performance became very clear ~ love of the game, of the experience itself, no fear of censor, and a complete sense of entrainment: flow.

Have you ever looked at the mountain, and just seen the mountain, without the witness sitting there, saying, 'gee, it's a nice day, isn't it?' without that split taking place? That is what we mean by complete attention, entrainment. The play state, the flow state is that direct, complete engagement in relationship without fear of censor or measurement.

Another colleague, Joseph Chilton Pearce, author of many books (including a national best-seller, The Magical Child), was quick to point out that in our contest culture we've replaced learning with conditioning ~ conditioning being a predetermined, "correct" way to do something. It's common knowledge that we use a fraction of our potential; some say only five percent of our mental potential at any one time.

Part of the reason that we use so little is that we're often repeating what we know. Most of the time we're conditioning ourselves, and our children, rather than really learning. Culture censors and prevents most of us from stepping outside of this conditioning. People are censored, rather than encouraged to learn and develop.

Childhood is plagued by our insistence that children accept the limitations we long ago adopted for ourselves. And we beat it into them.

Joseph Chilton Pearce also offered that the essence of real learning is real play. So we have conditioning, which is what our schools and athletic programs are based on. And we have adaptive learning, which occurs in the state of play. And play can only take place in complete safety. Play as a state requires, first and foremost, that you be safe. You can't be safe if somebody's there measuring and censoring, judging, evaluating.

When we replaced self-organising child's play, sandlot games, for example, and organised them into Little Leagues, we replaced real learning with conditioning, judgment and fear, which implicitly strengthens the defensive reflex we call 'me', the ego ~ and real learning slowed. The world is growing more complex. Levels of fear and threat are increasing. Parents don't feel safe letting children out into the front yard simply to mess around; they need to know exactly where their kids are, and what they're doing, at all times. So they place their children in adult-organised programmes, which can be as damaging ~ in terms of public fear and humiliation ~ as they are beneficial.

Fred Donaldson has spent the last twenty five years playing with special needs kids, and wild animals ~ bears, elk, seals, dolphins, foxes, and wolves. The reason he seeks out these children ~ autistic, with cerebral palsy, and so on, is that he has to step out of his cultural model to relate to, and really play with, them. The cultural self-image of "Fred" has to disappear in order to play with a wild animal or a special child. Krishnamurti said, "Love exists when I disappear." Fred says, "I can't play until Fred disappears." And, "I can't play with you, because you think you're who you are and I think I'm who I am, and we're locked into these identities, which limits our relationship." So Fred seeks out wild animals as playmates, because they too demand that he be fully present, which means that he can't be Fred. He's done this for many years, all over the globe.

Knowing some of these things, is it possible to create learning environments that don't cause this ego defence-reflex to kick in? Currently, it's built into the system, along with its implicit aggression and violence. We're all stuck in a structure, which demands that the defence reflex be ever-present. Most can't even conceive of an alternative. The level of threat determines how much energy and attention has to be diverted into defence. It takes a minimal amount of attention and energy to swing a bat. If you're asking the big question "what are they going to think of me?", that attention and energy is fragmented. Part is going into defence; performance diminishes. The question is, "how do we create increasingly challenging environments without strengthening this fear reflex?"

I think a greater understanding of The Intelligence of Play is a way of doing that. We need to begin with the prenatal relationship between mother and her unborn child. Is it one of fear and anxiety and worry and concern, or is it one of joy and play? If play is the foundation, rather than worry and contest ~ tension is removed.

In play there's no possibility of failure. It doesn't matter what you're doing. The purpose of play is to learn, not to achieve a predetermined result. You can't do learning wrong. There's no possibility of error in real play, or real learning. The ego isn't there, only complete attention.

We are asking top athletes, not how they hit the ball, but how they were raised. What kind of environment were they raised in that allowed them to love the game, and not waste attention and energy on self-defence? There are several hundred million parents and kids involved with the "organised anxiety programs" we collectively call athletics. They're brutal. Talk about contest, and fear reaction. It's rampant. It's gotten so bad that athletes are saying we shouldn't have these kinds of organised sports until kids are perhaps eleven or twelve years old. Today we're enrolling kids at four and five.

Childhood has become more censored, more restricted, more limited: less playful in every way, with a corresponding increase in fear, self-defence, ego, me-first, aggression and violence. Fred is very clear his intention, when he takes his work to gangs or corporations, is to help people be safer. Fear and lack of basic trust are core issues. We separate babies from mothers at birth; this induces insecurity right from the start. The defence system kicks right in. Then there is abandonment to daycare, and abandonment to television. How do we reframe what we think of as childhood in terms of basic trust? To a parent or educator this means, how do you create a relationship in which there is no fear? Without fear, play as learning can expand, infinitely. Otherwise, we're just conditioning.

Authentic play, original play, is a complete flip on how we view ourselves as individuals, how we think of learning, how we look at development. It forms the basis of a relationship, which is more authentic than the cultural limitations we accept about ourselves and impose on our children. The intelligence of play means learning without limits, every day, with the entire world as a playmate. Now that's a good idea...

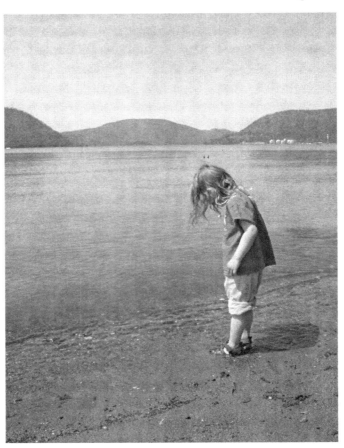

Rocco exploring the Hudson River, New York.

About Starflower Press

Starflower Press is dedicated to publishing material which lifts the heart, and helps to raise human consciousness to a new level of awareness.

Starflower Press draws its name and inspiration from the olden day herb, Borage (Borago Officinalis), commonly known as Star-flower. It's still found in many places, though it's often thought of as a wild flower, rather than a herb.

Starflower is recognisable by its beautiful star-like flowers, which are formed by five petals of intense blue (sometimes it's pink). The unusual blue colour was used in Renaissance paintings. The Biblical meaning of this blue is *heavenly grace*.

Borage, from the Celtic borrach, means courage. Throughout history, Starflower has been associated with courage. It's used as a food, tea, tincture and flower essence to bring joy to the heart, and gladden the mind.

Visit www.starflowerpress.com for books, Starflower tea and Starflower Essence.

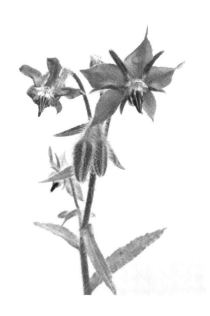

About The Mother magazine

Each issue of The Mother is gestated and birthed within the walls of our home. Articles are edited, photos and illustrations chosen, and pages are laid out, all against the backdrop of our family life: the simmering of leek and potato soup in the kitchen, great conversations, riotous laughter on the family bed. Throughout the early years, while I edited, my girls would play with cloth dolls by the fireside, a cat would be tucked up on my lap as I typed; a child's fingers made music on a violin or piano; great works of art were painted beside me on the dining room table; and for the first few years, there was lots of breastfeeding!

The essence of this grass roots approach to a professional publication brings heart and soul to the families around the world who read The Mother.

The purpose of The Mother is not to prescribe a way of parenting, but to help women and men access their deep, intuitive knowing, and find a way to parent optimally. We cover many topics and aspects of natural family living ~ beginning with fertility awareness, conscious conception, peaceful pregnancy and ecstatic birthing. The natural consequences of these are: full-term breastfeeding; the family bed; and bonded family life. We encourage natural immunity and vaccine awareness.

The Mother magazine recognises that modern technology is here to stay, and aims to inform readers about how these can impact on child development.

We encourage deliberately conscious and aware consumerism, including the use of natural products (toys, cleaning and body care). We value and recognise that children learn best in informal, child-led situations. Our articles reflect the value of small schools, forest schools and home education. At times, most of us compromise the optimal, both in terms of parenting, and life in general. We encourage taking responsibility for the outcomes of our choices, actions and inaction.

If you've enjoyed reading *Stretch Marks*, then we invite you to join The Mother magazine's family. www.themothermagazine.co.uk

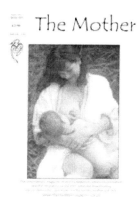 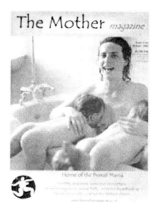 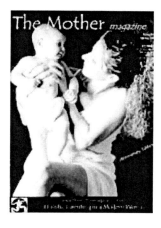

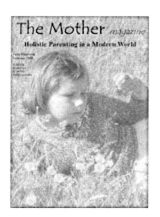 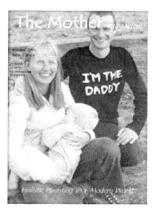 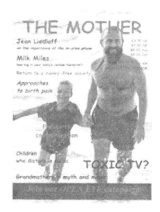

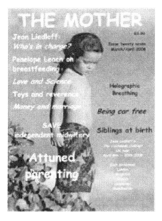 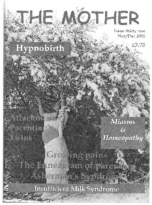 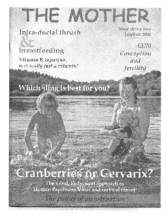

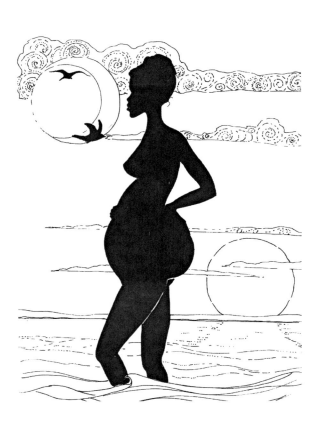

Lightning Source UK Ltd.
Milton Keynes UK
03 June 2010

155064UK00001BB/57/P